WHEELER'S

DENTAL ANATOMY, PHYSIOLOGY AND OCCLUSION

WHEELER'S

DENTAL ANATOMY, PHYSIOLOGY AND OCCLUSION

SEVENTH EDITION

MAJOR M. ASH, Jr., DDS, MS, Dr.h.c.

Marcus L. Ward Professor of Dentistry
and Research Scientist, EMI
School of Dentistry
University of Michigan

W.B. SAUNDERS COMPANY

A Division of Harcourt Brace & Company

Philadelphia   London   Toronto   Montreal   Sydney   Tokyo

W.B. SAUNDERS COMPANY
A Division of
Harcourt Brace & Company

The Curtis Center
Independence Square West
Philadelphia, PA 19106

Library of Congress Cataloging-in-Publication Data

Ash, Major M.

Wheeler's dental anatomy, physiology and occlusion / Major M.
  Ash, Jr.—7th ed.
      p. cm.
    Includes bibliographical references and index.

ISBN 0-7216-4374-4
1. Teeth.   2. Occlusion (Dentistry).   I. Title.   II. Title: Dental
anatomy, physiology, and occlusion.
    [DNLM: 1. Dental Occlusion.   2. Tooth—anatomy & histology.
3. Tooth—physiology.   WU 101 A819w]
RK280.A74   1993

611'.314—dc20

DNLM/DLC   92-19497

WHEELER'S DENTAL ANATOMY,   ISBN   0-7216-4374-4
PHYSIOLOGY AND OCCLUSION

Printed in the United States of America

Last digit is the print number: 9   8   7   6   5   4   3

Dedicated To
Fayola

≡ *Special Acknowledgments*

It is a pleasure to make special acknowledgment of the following individuals who have suggested valuable information from their own special field of knowledge. Discussions about the need for changes or addition of material to my manuscript were most helpful and I wish to specify these individuals and their particular field of interest.

George M. Ash, B.S., D.D.S., M.S., A.B.O. (Orthodontics)
Jeffrey L. Ash, B.S., D.D.S., M.S. (Endodontics)
Carolyn M. Ash, B.S., D.D.S., M.S. (Prosthodontics)
Sally Holden, R.D.H., R.D.A., M.S. (Dental Hygiene)
Hans Graf, Dr. Med. Dent., P.D. (Periodontics)
Jose dos Santos, D.D.S., M.S.C., P.D. (Restorative)
Stanley J. Nelson, D.D.S., M.S. (Occlusion)

≡ *Preface*

One of the challenges of a new edition is to make changes that reflect current thinking in the field, and to delete material that is no longer pertinent to what is being taught. Much of the guidance for change comes directly from teachers of dental anatomy, some comes from the section on dental anatomy and occlusion of the American Association of Dental Schools, and still more comes from an assessment of current literature.

A recurring problem in teaching dental anatomy is the inability of the student, and often the clinician, to relate variations in the natural dentition to the restorations for various patients, especially anterior teeth. Incisors look like incisors, but because of variations in size, color, wear, position, and shape, they may appear quite different in various individuals. Such differences have continued to be recognized in this edition.

One of the major goals of previous editions has been to provide details about the morphology of human teeth that are relevant to the practice of dentistry. The importance of specific anatomical features of a particular tooth to the diagnosis and treatment of oral diseases has received very little attention in dental research and hypotheses regarding such associations go untested and remain to be verified by appropriate research. Past assumptions about the relationship between contours and periodontal health continue to be reflected clinically in restored contours that have very little relationship to function or aesthetics. Additional coverage of this subject has been provided in this edition.

Relationships between developmental grooves, occlusal relations, pulp chamber and root canal morphology, and the development of cracked teeth and pain (cracked tooth syndrome) remain virtually unresearched. How then does the clinician prevent cusp fracture or approach the restoration of a tooth (e.g., the distolingual cusp of the mandibular first molar) with silver (amalgam)? Part of the answer must relate to the anatomy of developmental grooves, occlusal relations, facets of wear, and bruxism. Potential lines of fracture in developmental grooves have been included in this edition.

Of particular interest in this edition are the recent approaches to data concerning standards of human tooth formation and dental age assessment. These kinds of data have relevance to some clinical problems, as well as to other fields. Although the dentition may be the single best indicator of chronological age in juveniles, there are important gaps in available sources of tooth formation chronologies. For a comprehensive review of methodologies by which critical choices among the chronologies can be made, the reader is directed to the references cited in Chapter 2, especially those of B. Holly Smith (1991) and Lunt and Law (1974).

The eruption of a tooth is a continuous process that involves the movement of a tooth in the bud stage to its emergence through the gingiva and finally into occlusal contact. However, as a parameter of dental maturity, data on eruption generally refers to the clinical appearance of the emergence of the tooth in the oral cavity. Although the term *eruption* is used erroneously to denote clinical emergence, there appears to be no confusion as to what the term *eruption* means in tables of the chronology of the human dentition. No attempt will be made in this edition to change the term *eruption* to *emergence* in the tables and illustrations.

References that appear at the end of the chapters relate to specific citations in the body of the text, as well as general support for the material presented. Some of the older citations relating to descriptive studies have been replaced where appropriate literature was available.

Special thanks are given to the teachers of dental anatomy who have made suggestions for correction or change in this edition, including Drs. E. M. Wilkins and Stanley Nelson. Also acknowledged is the preparation of illustrations by Professor William Brudon who, as always, has turned rough sketches into works of art. Thanks is given to Per Kjeldsen and Keary Campbell for photographic services and Joanne Kazlauskas for her assistance in typing the revisions for the present edition.

Major M. Ash, Jr.

Contents

1 ≡ *Introduction*

The first step in understanding dental anatomy is to learn the nomenclature, or the system of names, used to describe or classify the material included in the subject. When a term is used for the first time, it is emphasized in italics. Additional terms will be discussed as needed in subsequent chapters. The term *mandibular* refers to the lower jaw, or *mandible;* the term *maxillary* refers to the upper jaw, or *maxilla*.

Nomenclature

The Primary (Deciduous) Teeth

The formation of the teeth, development of dentition, and growth of the craniofacial complex are closely related in the prenatal as well as the postnatal development period. At birth there are usually no teeth visible in the mouth, but many teeth in various stages of development are found in the jaws. The postnatal period of development of the primary dentition spans about 2½ years. This primary dentition remains intact until a child is about 6 years of age, when the transition to the permanent dentition begins. The number of primary teeth present in the child is usually 20 if none are congenitally missing or lost as a result of disease.

The denomination and number of teeth for all Mammalia are expressed by formulae. The denomination of each tooth is represented by its initial letter, I for *incisor,* C for *canine,* P for *premolar,* M for *molar;* each letter is followed by a horizontal line and the number of each type of tooth is placed above the line for the maxilla (upper jaw) and below the line for the mandible (lower jaw). The formula includes one side only.

The dental formula for the primary teeth in humans is:

$$I \frac{2}{2} C \frac{1}{1} M \frac{2}{2} = 10$$

This formula should be read thus: Incisors, two maxillary and two mandibular; canines, one maxillary and one mandibular; molars, two maxillary and two mandibular—or ten altogether on one side, right or left (Fig. 1–1, *A*).

In clinical practice, the primary teeth in the maxillary arch, beginning with the right second molar, are designated by letters A through J. Beginning with the left mandibular second molar, the teeth are designated by letters K through T. The "Universal" system notation for the entire primary dentition is

1

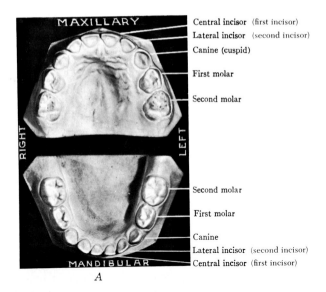

MAXILLARY

Central incisor (first incisor)
Lateral incisor (second incisor)
Canine (cuspid)

First molar

Second molar

RIGHT   LEFT

Second molar

First molar

Canine
Lateral incisor (second incisor)
Central incisor (first incisor)

MANDIBULAR

A

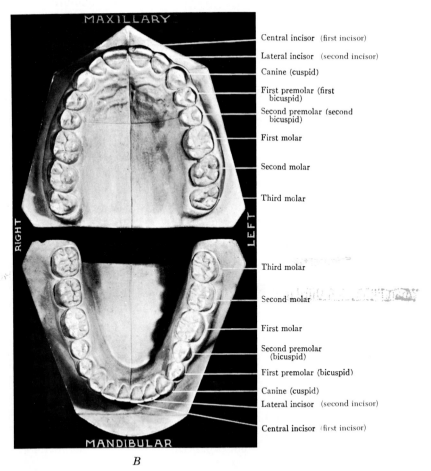

MAXILLARY

Central incisor (first incisor)

Lateral incisor   (second incisor)

Canine (cuspid)

First premolar (first bicuspid)

Second premolar (second bicuspid)

First molar

Second molar

Third molar

RIGHT   LEFT

Third molar

Second molar

First molar

Second premolar (bicuspid)

First premolar (bicuspid)

Canine (cuspid)
Lateral incisor (second incisor)

Central incisor (first incisor)

MANDIBULAR

B

Figure 1–1. *A*, Casts of deciduous, or primary, dentition. *B*, Casts of permanent dentition.

A	B	C	D	E	F	G	H	I	J
T	S	R	Q	P	O	N	M	L	K

Another notation system divides the arches into quadrants with the entire dentition notated as

E	D	C	B	A	A	B	C	D	E
E	D	C	B	A	A	B	C	D	E

Thus, for a single tooth, such as the left maxillary central incisor the designation is ⌊A . For the mandibular right second molar, the notation is given as E⌉ .

The Permanent Teeth

The transition to permanent dentition begins with the eruption and emergence of the first permanent molars, shedding of the deciduous incisors, and emergence and eruption of the permanent incisors. After the shedding of the deciduous canines and molars, emergence and eruption of the permanent canines and premolars, and emergence and eruption of the second permanent molars, the permanent dentition is completed except for the third molars. This process requires about 20 years to complete. The permanent, or *suc-cedaneous*, teeth replace the exfoliated deciduous teeth in a sequence of eruption that exhibits great variety. The number of teeth in adults, including third molars when present, is 32.

The *permanent dental formula* in humans is:

$$I \frac{2}{2} C \frac{1}{1} P \frac{2}{2} M \frac{3}{3} = 16$$

Premolars have now been added to the formula, two maxillary and two mandibular, and a third molar has been added, one maxillary and one mandibular (Fig. 1–1, *B*).

In the Universal notation system for the permanent dentition, the maxillary teeth are numbered from 1 through 16, beginning with the right third molar. Beginning with the mandibular left third molar, the teeth are numbered 17 through 32. Thus, the right maxillary first molar is designated as 3, the maxillary left central incisor as 9, and the mandibular right first molar as 30. The entire dentition is designated by the notation

1	2	3	4	5	6	7	8	9	10	11	12	13	14	15	16
32	31	30	29	28	27	26	25	24	23	22	21	20	19	18	17

Another notation system uses the quadrant system, in which, beginning with the central incisors, the teeth are numbered 1 through 8 (or more). For example, the maxillary right first molar is designated 6⌋ and the maxillary right central incisor as 1⌋ . The Palmer notation for the entire permanent dentition is:

8	7	6	5	4	3	2	1	1	2	3	4	5	6	7	8
8	7	6	5	4	3	2	1	1	2	3	4	5	6	7	8

The Universal system is acceptable to computer language, whereas the Palmer notation is generally incompatible with computers and wordprocessing systems. Each tooth in the Universal system is designated with a unique number, leading to much less confusion than with the Palmer notation. A two-digit system proposed by Federation Dentaire Internationale (FDI) for both the primary and permanent dentitions has been adopted by the World Health Organization and accepted by other organizations such as the International Association for Dental Research. The FDI system of tooth notation is:

Primary Teeth

Upper Right   *Upper Left*

55	54	53	52	51	61	62	63	64	65
85	84	83	82	81	71	72	73	74	75

Lower Right   *Lower Left*

Permanent Teeth

Upper Right   *Upper Left*

18	17	16	15	14	13	12	11	21	22	23	24	25	26	27	28
48	47	46	45	44	43	42	41	31	32	33	34	35	36	37	38

Lower Right   *Lower Left*

In the two-digit FDI system the first digit indicates the quadrant (1 to 4) for the permanent dentition and for the primary dentition (5 to 8). The second digit indicates the tooth within a quadrant: 1 to 8 for the permanent teeth and 1 to 5 for the primary teeth. Thus, the permanent upper right central incisor is 11 (pronounced "one-one," not "eleven").

The Crown and Root

Each tooth has a *crown* and *root* portion. The crown is covered with *enamel,* and the root portion is covered with *cementum*. The crown and root join at the *cementoenamel* junction. This junction, also called the *cervical line* (Fig. 1–2), is plainly visible on a specimen tooth. The main bulk of the tooth is composed of *dentin,* which is clear in a cross section of the tooth. This cross section displays a *pulp chamber* and a *pulp canal,* which normally contain the *pulp tissue*. The pulp chamber is in the crown portion mainly, and the pulp canal is in the root (Fig. 1–3). The spaces are continuous with each other and are spoken of collectively as the *pulp cavity*.

The four tooth tissues are *enamel, cementum, dentin,* and *pulp*. The first three are known as *hard tissues,* the last as *soft tissue*. The pulp tissue furnishes the blood and nerve supply to the tooth. The tissues of the teeth must be considered in relation to the other tissues of the orofacial structures (Figs. 1–4, 1–5) if the physiology of the teeth is to be understood.

The *crown* of an incisor tooth may have an incisal *ridge* or *edge,* as in the *central* and *lateral incisors;* a single *cusp,* as in the canines; or two or more cusps, as on premolars and molars. Incisal ridges and cusps form the cutting surfaces on tooth crowns.

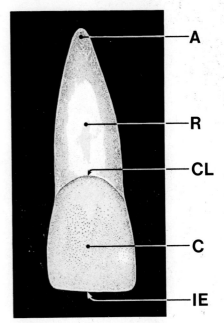

Figure 1–2. Maxillary central incisor (facial aspect). *A*, Apex of root; *R*, root; *CL*, cervical line; *C*, crown; *IE*, incisal edge.

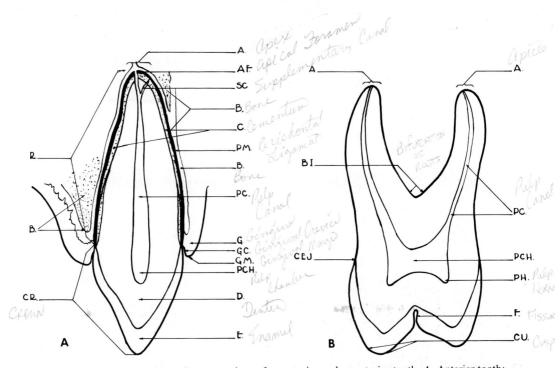

Figure 1–3. Schematic drawings of cross sections of an anterior and a posterior tooth. *A*, Anterior tooth; *A*, Apex; *AF*, apical foramen; *SC*, supplementary canal; *C*, cementum; *PM*, periodontal ligament; *B*, bone; *PC*, pulp canal; *G*, gingiva; *GC*, gingival crevice; *GM*, gingival margin; *PCH*, pulp chamber; *D*, dentin; *E*, enamel; *CR*, crown; *R*, root. *B*, Posterior tooth; *A*, Apices; *PC*, pulp canal; *PCH*, pulp chamber; *PH*, pulp horn; *F*, fissure; *CU*, cusp; *CEJ*, cementoenamel junction; *BI*, bifurcation of roots.

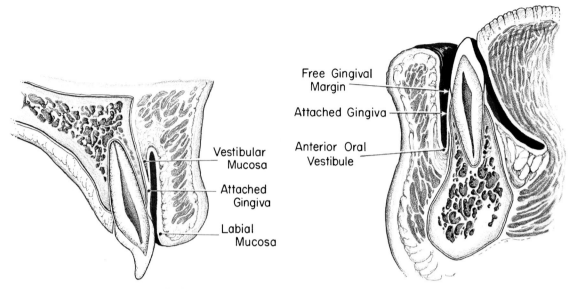

Figure 1–4. Sagittal sections through the maxillary and mandibular central incisors.

The *root* portion of the tooth may be *single,* with one *apex* or terminal end, as usually found in *anterior* teeth and some of the premolars; or *multiple,* with a *bifurcation* or *trifurcation* dividing the root portion into two or more extensions or roots with their *apices* or terminal ends, as found on all molars and in some premolars.

The root portion of the tooth is firmly fixed in the bony process of the jaw, so that each tooth is held in its position relative to the others in the *dental arch.* That portion of the jaw which serves as a support for the tooth is called the *alveolar process.* The bone of the tooth socket is called the *alveolus* (plural, *alveoli*) (Fig. 1–6).

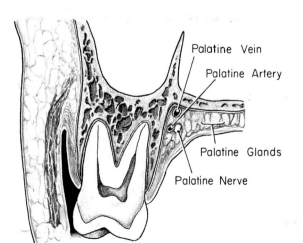

Figure 1–5. Section through the second maxillary molar and adjacent tissues.

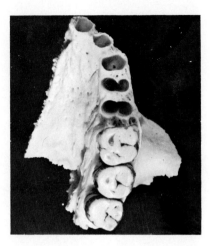

Figure 1–6. Left maxillary bone showing the alveolar process with three molars in place and the alveoli of the central incisor, lateral incisor, canine, and first and second premolars. Note the opening at the bottom of the canine alveolus, an opening that accommodates the nutrient blood and nerve supply to the tooth in life. Although they do not show up in the photograph, the other alveoli present the same arrangement.

The crown portion is never covered by bone tissue after it is fully erupted, but it is partly covered at the *cervical third* in young adults by soft tissue of the mouth known as the *gingiva* or *gingival tissue,* or *gum tissue.* In older persons, all of the enamel and frequently some cervical cementum may be exposed in the oral cavity.

Surfaces and Ridges

The crowns of the incisors and canines have four surfaces and a ridge, and the crowns of the premolars and molars have five surfaces. The surfaces are named according to their positions and uses (Fig. 1–7). In the incisors and canines, the surfaces toward the lips are called *labial surfaces;* in the premolars and molars, those facing the cheek are the *buccal surfaces.* When labial and buccal surfaces are spoken of collectively, they are called *facial surfaces.* All surfaces facing toward the tongue are called *lingual surfaces.* The surfaces of the premolars and molars which come in contact with those in the opposite jaw during the act of closure (called *occlusion*) are called *occlusal surfaces.* In incisors and canines, those surfaces are called *incisal surfaces.*

The surfaces of the teeth facing toward adjoining teeth in the same dental arch are called *proximal* or *proximate surfaces.* The proximal surfaces may be called either *mesial* or *distal.* These terms have special reference to the position of the surface relative to the *median line* of the face. This line is drawn vertically through the center of the face, passing between the central incisors at their point of contact with each other in both the maxilla and the mandible. Those proximal surfaces which, following the curve of the arch, are faced toward the median line, are called *mesial surfaces,* and those most distant from the median line are called *distal surfaces.*

Four teeth have mesial surfaces that contact each other: the maxillary and mandibular central incisors. In all other instances, the mesial surface of one tooth contacts the distal surface of its neighbor, except for the distal surfaces of third molars of permanent teeth and distal surfaces of second molars in deciduous teeth, which have no teeth distal to them. The area of the mesial or distal surface of a tooth which touches its neighbor in the arch is called the *contact area.*

Central and lateral incisors and canines as a group are called *anterior teeth;* premolars and molars as a group, *posterior teeth.*

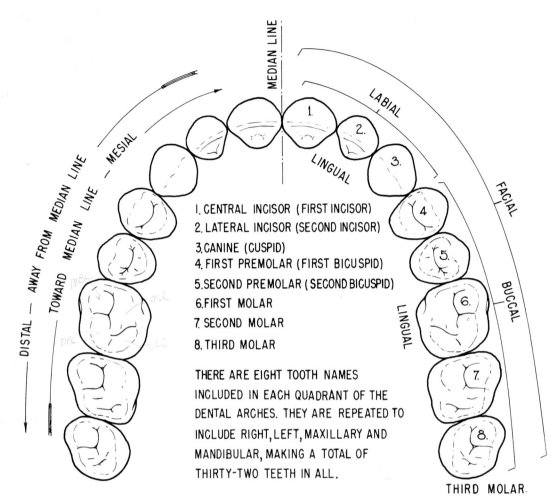

MEDIAN LINE

LABIAL

LINGUAL

FACIAL

BUCCAL

LINGUAL

MESIAL — TOWARD MEDIAN LINE

DISTAL — AWAY FROM MEDIAN LINE

1. CENTRAL INCISOR (FIRST INCISOR)
2. LATERAL INCISOR (SECOND INCISOR)
3. CANINE (CUSPID)
4. FIRST PREMOLAR (FIRST BICUSPID)
5. SECOND PREMOLAR (SECOND BICUSPID)
6. FIRST MOLAR
7. SECOND MOLAR
8. THIRD MOLAR

THERE ARE EIGHT TOOTH NAMES
INCLUDED IN EACH QUADRANT OF THE
DENTAL ARCHES. THEY ARE REPEATED TO
INCLUDE RIGHT, LEFT, MAXILLARY AND
MANDIBULAR, MAKING A TOTAL OF
THIRTY-TWO TEETH IN ALL.

THIRD MOLAR

Figure 1–7. Application of nomenclature. Tooth numbers ⌐1 to ⌐8 indicating left maxillary teeth. Tooth surfaces related to the tongue (lingual), cheek (buccal), lips (labial), and face (facial) apply to four quadrants as well as to the upper left quadrant. The teeth or their parts or surfaces may be described as being away from the midline (distal) or toward the midline (mesial).

Other Landmarks

In order to study an individual tooth intelligently, we must be able to recognize all landmarks of importance by name. Therefore, at this point it will be necessary to become familiar with additional terms, such as:

cusp	triangular ridge	developmental groove
tubercle	transverse ridge	supplemental groove
cingulum	oblique ridge	pit
ridge	fossa	lobe
marginal ridge	sulcus	

A *cusp* is an elevation or mound on the crown portion of a tooth making up a divisional part of the occlusal surface (Figs. 1–3 and 1–8).

Figure 1–8. Some landmarks on the maxillary first molar. *BG*, Buccal groove; *MBC*, mesiobuccal cusp; *SG*, supplemental groove; *TF*, triangular fossa; *MLC*, mesiolingual cusp; *DG*, developmental groove; *DLC*, distolingual cusp; *OR*, oblique ridge; *DMR*, distal marginal ridge; *DBC*, distobuccal cusp; *CF*, central fossa; *BCR*, buccocervical ridge.

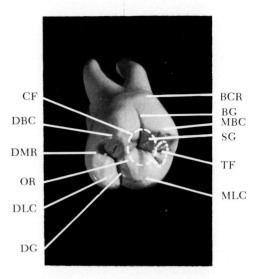

A *tubercle* is a smaller elevation on some portion of the crown produced by an extra formation of enamel (see Fig. 4–21, *A*). These are deviations from the typical form.

A *cingulum* (Latin word for *girdle*) is the lingual lobe of an anterior tooth. It makes up the bulk of the cervical third of the lingual surface. Its convexity mesiodistally resembles a girdle encircling the lingual surface at the cervical third (see Figs. 1–9 and 4–20, *A*).

A *ridge* is any linear elevation on the surface of a tooth and is named according to its location (e.g., *buccal* ridge, *incisal* ridge, *marginal* ridge).

Marginal ridges are those rounded borders of the enamel that form the mesial and distal margins of the occlusal surfaces of premolars and molars and the mesial and distal margins of the lingual surfaces of the incisors and canines (Figs. 1–9, *A*, and 1–10).

Triangular ridges descend from the tips of the cusps of molars and premolars toward the central part of the occlusal surfaces. They are so named because the slopes of each side

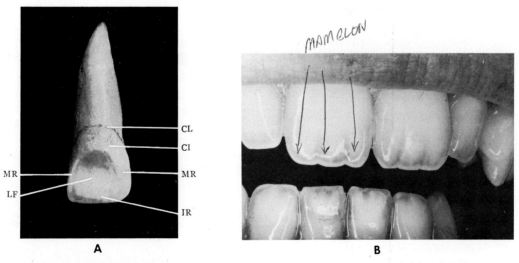

A   **B**

Figure 1–9. Maxillary right central incisor (lingual aspect). *CL*, Cervical line; *CI*, cingulum (also called the linguocervical ridge); *MR*, marginal ridge; *IR*, incisal ridge; *LF*, lingual fossa. *B*, Mamelons on erupting, noncontacting central incisors.

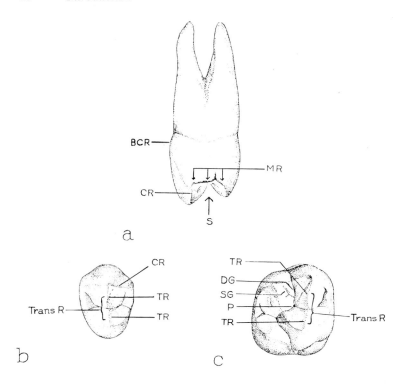

Figure 1–10. *a,* Mesial view of a maxillary right first premolar. *S,* Sulcus traversing occlusal surface; *MR,* marginal ridge; *CR,* cusp ridge; *BCR,* buccocervical ridge. *b,* Occlusal view of maxillary right first premolar; *CR,* cusp ridge; *TR,* triangular ridges; *Trans R,* transverse ridge, formed by two triangular ridges crossing the tooth transversely. *c,* Occlusal view of a maxillary right first molar. *TR,* triangular ridge; *DG,* developmental groove; *SG,* supplemental groove; *P,* pit formed by junction of developmental grooves; *TR,* triangular ridge; *Trans R,* transverse ridge.

of the ridge are inclined to resemble two sides of a triangle (Figs. 1–10, *B* and *C,* and 1–11). They are named after the cusps to which they belong, e.g., the triangular ridge of the buccal cusp of the maxillary first premolar.

When a buccal and a lingual triangular ridge join, they form a *transverse* ridge. A transverse ridge is the union of two triangular ridges crossing transversely the surface of a posterior tooth (Fig. 1–10, *B* and *C*).

The *oblique ridge* is a ridge crossing obliquely the occlusal surfaces of maxillary molars. It is formed by the union of the triangular ridge of the distobuccal cusp and the distal cusp ridge of the mesiolingual cusp (Fig. 1–8).

A *fossa* is an irregular depression or concavity. *Lingual* fossae are on the lingual surface of incisors (Fig. 1–9). *Central* fossae are on the occlusal surface of molars. They are formed by the converging of ridges terminating at a central point in the bottom of the depression, where there is a junction of grooves (Fig. 1–11). *Triangular* fossae are found on molars and premolars on the occlusal surfaces mesial or distal to marginal ridges (Fig. 1–8). They are sometimes found on the lingual surfaces of maxillary incisors at the edge of the lingual fossae where the marginal ridges and the cingulum meet (see Fig. 4–21, *A*).

A *sulcus* is a long depression or valley in the surface of a tooth between ridges and cusps, the inclines of which meet at an angle. A sulcus has a developmental groove at the junction of its inclines. (The term *sulcus* must not be confused with the term *groove.*)

A *developmental groove* is a shallow groove or line between the primary parts of the crown or root. A *supplemental groove,* less distinct, is also a shallow linear depression on the surface of a tooth, but it is supplemental to a developmental groove and does not mark the junction of primary parts. *Buccal* and *lingual grooves* are developmental grooves found on the buccal and lingual surfaces of posterior teeth (Figs. 1–8 and 1–11).

Pits are small pinpoint depressions located at the junction of developmental grooves or

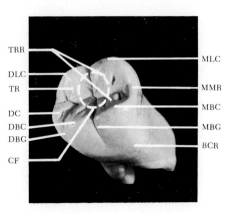

Figure 1–11. Mandibular right first molar. *MLC,* Mesio-lingual cusp; *MMR,* mesial marginal ridge; *MBC,* mesiobuccal cusp; *MBG,* mesiobuccal groove; *CF,* central fossa; *DBG,* distobuccal groove; *DBC,* distobuccal cusp; *DC,* distal cusp; *TR,* triangular ridge; *DLC,* distolingual cusp; *TRR,* transverse ridge; *BCR,* buccocervical ridge.

at terminals of those grooves. For instance, *central pit* is a term used to describe a landmark in the central fossa of molars where developmental grooves join (Fig. 1–9, *C*).

A *lobe* is one of the primary sections of formation in the development of the crown. Cusps and mamelons are representative of lobes. A *mamelon* is any one of the three rounded protuberances found on the incisal ridges of newly erupted incisor teeth (Fig. 1–9, *B*). (For further description of lobes, see Figures 4–19 through 4–21).

The *roots* of the teeth may be single or multiple. Both maxillary and mandibular anterior teeth have only one root each. Mandibular first and second premolars and the maxillary second premolar are single-rooted, but the maxillary first premolar has two roots in most cases, one buccal and one lingual. Maxillary molars have three roots, one mesiobuccal, one distobuccal, and one lingual. Mandibular molars have two roots, one mesial and one distal. It must be understood that description in anatomy can never follow a hard-and-fast rule. Variations frequently occur. This is especially true regarding tooth roots, e.g., facial and lingual roots of mandibular canine.

Division into Thirds, Line Angles, and Point Angles

For purposes of description, the crowns and roots of teeth have been divided into thirds and junctions of the crown surfaces are described as *line angles* and *point angles.* Actually, there are no angles or points or plane surfaces on the teeth anywhere except those that appear from wear (*abrasion*) or from accidental fracture. *Line angle* and *point angle* are used only as descriptive terms to indicate a location.

When the surfaces of the crown and root portions are divided into *thirds,* these thirds are named according to their location. Looking at the tooth from the *labial* or *buccal* aspect, we see that the crown and root may be divided into thirds from the incisal or occlusal surface of the crown to the apex of the root (Fig. 1–12). The *crown* is divided into an incisal or occlusal third, a middle third, and a cervical third. The *root* is divided into a cervical third, a middle third, and an apical third.

The crown may be divided into thirds in three directions: inciso- or occlusocervically, mesiodistally, or labio- or buccolingually. Mesiodistally, it is divided into the mesial, middle, and distal thirds. Labio- or buccolingually it is divided into labial or buccal, middle, and lingual thirds. Each of the five surfaces of a crown may be so divided. There will be one middle third and two other thirds, which are named according to their location, e.g., cervical, occlusal, mesial, lingual.

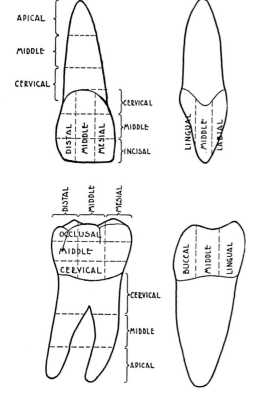

Figure 1–12. Division into thirds.

A *line angle* is formed by the junction of two surfaces and derives its name from the combination of the two surfaces that join. For instance, on an anterior tooth, the junction of the mesial and labial surfaces is called the *mesiolabial line angle* (Fig. 1–13, *A*).

The *line angles* of the *anterior teeth* are:

mesiolabial	distolingual
distolabial	labioincisal
mesiolingual	linguoincisal

Because the mesial and distal incisal angles of anterior teeth are rounded, *mesioincisal line angles* and *distoincisal line angles* are usually considered nonexistent. They are spoken of as *mesial* and *distal incisal* angles only.

The *line angles* of the *posterior teeth* are:

mesiobuccal	distolingual	bucco-occlusal
distobuccal	mesio-occlusal	linguo-occlusal
mesiolingual	disto-occlusal	

A *point angle* is formed by the junction of three surfaces. The point angle also derives its name from the combination of the names of the surfaces forming it. For example, the junction of the mesial, buccal, and occlusal surfaces of a molar is called the *mesiobucco-occlusal point angle* (Fig. 1–14, *B*).

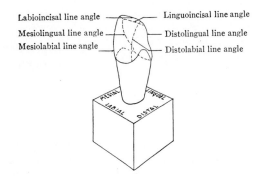

Labioincisal line angle — — Linguoincisal line angle

Mesiolingual line angle — — Distolingual line angle

Mesiolabial line angle — — Distolabial line angle

Figure 1–13. Line angles.

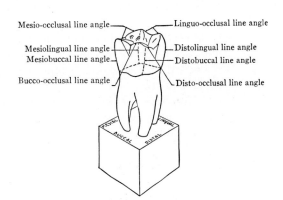

Mesio-occlusal line angle — — Linguo-occlusal line angle

Mesiolingual line angle — — Distolingual line angle

Mesiobuccal line angle — — Distobuccal line angle

Bucco-occlusal line angle — — Disto-occlusal line angle

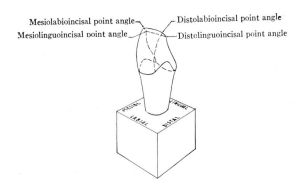

Mesiolabioincisal point angle — — Distolabioincisal point angle

Mesiolinguoincisal point angle — — Distolinguoincisal point angle

Figure 1–14. Point angles.

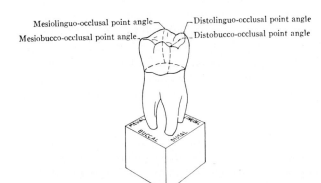

Mesiolinguo-occlusal point angle — — Distolinguo-occlusal point angle

Mesiobucco-occlusal point angle — — Distobucco-occlusal point angle

The *point angles* of the *anterior teeth* are:

        mesiolabioincisal   mesiolinguoincisal
        distolabioincisal   distolinguoincisal

The *point angles* of the *posterior teeth* are:

        mesiobucco-occlusal   mesiolinguo-occlusal
        distobucco-occlusal   distolinguo-occlusal

The subject of tooth drawing and carving is being introduced at this point because it has been found through experience that a laboratory course in tooth morphology (dissection, drawing, and carving) should be carried on simultaneously with lectures and reference work on the subject of dental anatomy. Illustrations and instruction in tooth form drawing and carving, however, will not be included in this volume. A manual covering the subject is published in a separate binding (*An Atlas of Tooth Form,* W. B. Saunders Company, Philadelphia).

The basis for the specifications to be used for carving individual teeth is the table of average measurements for permanent teeth given by Dr. G. V. Black. However, teeth carved or drawn to these average dimensions cannot be set into place for an ideal occlusion. Therefore, for purposes of producing a complete set of articulated teeth carved from ivorine, minor changes have been made in Dr. Black's table. Also, carving teeth to natural size, calibrated to tenths of a millimeter, is not practical. The adjusted measurements are shown in Table 1–1. The only fractions listed in the model table are 0.5 mm and 0.3 mm in a few instances. Fractions are avoided whenever possible to facilitate familiarity with the table and to avoid confusion. Teeth that were carved to adjusted measurements and set up in arch form in an articulator are shown in Figures 1–15 through 1–17.

A table of measurements must be arbitrarily agreed upon so that a reasonable comparison can be made when appraising the dimensions of any one aspect of one tooth in the mouth with that of another. It has been found that the projected table functions well in that way. For instance, if the mesiodistal measurement of the maxillary central incisor is 8.5 mm, the canine will be approximately 1 mm narrower in that measurement; if by chance the central incisor is wider or narrower than 8.5 mm, the canine measurement will correspond proportionately.

Photographs of the five aspects of each tooth (mesial, distal, labial or buccal, lingual, and incisal or occlusal) superimposed on squared millimeter cross-section paper reduces the tooth outlines of each aspect to an accurate graph, so that it is possible to compare and record the contours (Figs. 1–18 and 1–19).

Close observation of the outlines of the squared backgrounds shows the relationship of crown to root, extent of curvatures at various points, inclination of roots, relative widths of occlusal surfaces, height of marginal ridges, contact areas, and so on.

Although there is no such thing as an established invariable norm in nature, in the study of anatomy it is necessary that there be a starting point; therefore, we must begin with an *arbitrary criterion,* accepted after experimentation and due consideration. Since restorative dentistry must approach the scientific as closely as manual dexterity will allow, models, plans, photographs, and natural specimens should be given preference over the written text in this subject.

Every curve and segment of a normal tooth has some functional basis, and it is important to reproduce them. The successful operator in dentistry or, for that matter, any designer of dental restorations should be able to mentally create pictures of the teeth from

Table 1–1. Measurements of the Teeth: Specifications for Drawing and Carving Teeth of Average Size*

	Length of Crown	Length of Root	Mesiodistal Diameter of Crown†	Mesiodistal Diameter of Crown at Cervix	Labio- or Bucco-lingual Diameter	Labio- or Bucco-lingual Diameter at Cervix	Curvature of Cervical Line—Mesial	Curvature of Cervical Line—Distal
Maxillary Teeth								
Central incisor	10.5	13.0	8.5	7.0	7.0	6.0	3.5	2.5
Lateral incisor	9.0	13.0	6.5	5.0	6.0	5.0	3.0	2.0
Canine	10.0	17.0	7.5	5.5	8.0	7.0	2.5	1.5
First premolar	8.5	14.0	7.0	5.0	9.0	8.0	1.0	0.0
Second premolar	8.5	14.0	7.0	5.0	9.0	8.0	1.0	0.0
First molar	7.5	b l / 12 13	10.0	8.0	11.0	10.0	1.0	0.0
Second molar	7.0	b l / 11 12	9.0	7.0	11.0	10.0	1.0	0.0
Third molar	6.5	11.0	8.5	6.5	10.0	9.5	1.0	0.0
Mandibular Teeth								
Central incisor	9.0‡	12.5	5.0	3.5	6.0	5.3	3.0	2.0
Lateral incisor	9.5‡	14.0	5.5	4.0	6.5	5.8	3.0	2.0
Canine	11.0	16.0	7.0	5.5	7.5	7.0	2.5	1.0
First premolar	8.5	14.0	7.0	5.0	7.5	6.5	1.0	0.0
Second premolar	8.0	14.5	7.0	5.0	8.0	7.0	1.0	0.0
First molar	7.5	14.0	11.0	9.0	10.5	9.0	1.0	0.0
Second molar	7.0	13.0	10.5	8.0	10.0	9.0	1.0	0.0
Third molar	7.0	11.0	10.0	7.5	9.5	9.0	1.0	0.0

* In millimeters. This table has been "proved" by carvings shown in Figures 1–15 and 1–16.
† The sum of the mesiodistal diameters, both right and left, which gives the arch length, is: maxillary, 128 mm; mandibular, 126 mm.
‡ Lingual measurement is approximately 0.5 mm longer.

MEASUREMENTS OF THE TEETH: AN EXAMPLE*

	Length of Crown	Length of Root	Mesiodistal Diameter of Crown†	Mesiodistal Diameter of Crown at Cervix	Labio- or Bucco-lingual Diameter of Crown	Labio- or Bucco-lingual Diameter at Cervix	Curvature of Cervical Line—Mesial	Curvature of Cervical Line—Distal
Maxillary Teeth								
Central incisor	10.5	13.0	8.5	7.0	7.0	6.0	3.5	2.5

* In millimeters.

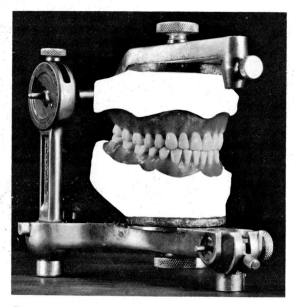

Figure 1–15. Carvings in Ivorine of individual teeth made according to the table of measurements (Table 1–1). Since skulls and extracted teeth show so many variations and anomalies, an arbitrary norm for individual teeth had to be established for comparative study. Hence, the 32 teeth were carved, natural size, in normal alignment and occlusion, and from the model a table of measurements was drafted.

any aspect. Complete pictures can be formed only when one is familiar with all details in tooth form.

It should be possible to draw reasonably well an outline of any aspect of any tooth in the mouth. It should be in good proportion without reference to another drawing or three-dimensional model.

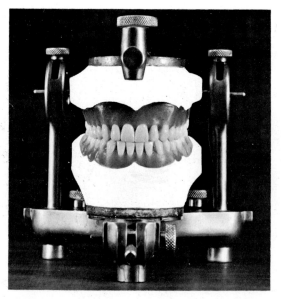

Figure 1–16. Another view of the models shown in Figure 1–15.

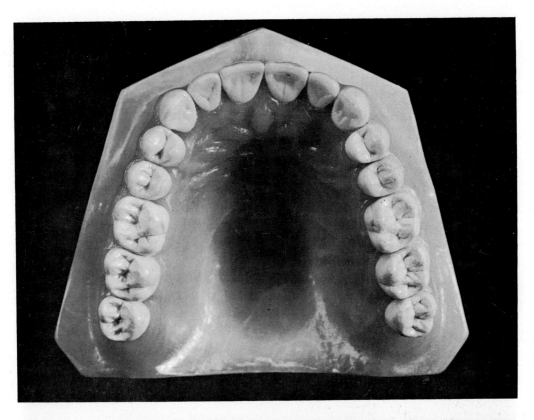

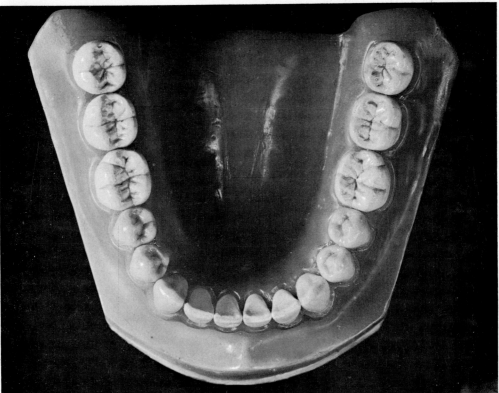

Figure 1–17. Occlusal view of the models shown in Figures 1–15 and 1–16.

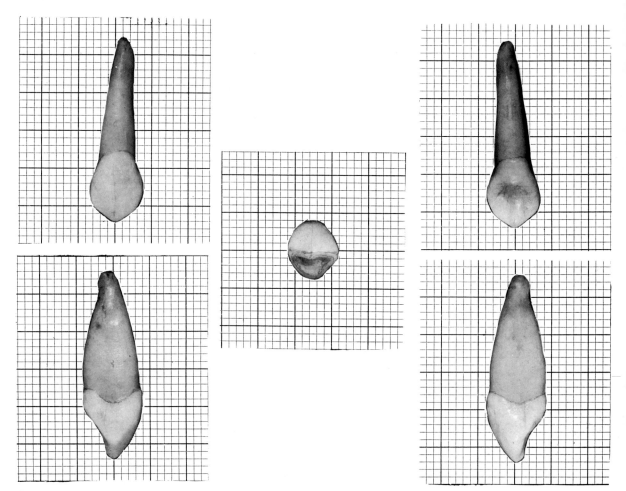

Figure 1-18. Maxillary left canine. When viewing the mesial and distal aspects, note the curvature or bulge on the crown at the cervical third below the cementoenamel junction. This is called the *cervical ridge,* or the *cervicoenamel ridge.*

For the development of skills in observation and in the restoration of lost tooth form, a student must:

1. Become so familiar with the table of measurements that it is possible to make instant comparisons mentally of the proportion of one tooth with another from any aspect.
2. Learn to draw accurate outlines of any aspect of any tooth.
3. Learn to carve with precision any design one can illustrate with line drawings.

Readers who are not familiar with the *Boley gauge* should study its use before reading the following instructions on the use of the table of measurements.

To understand the table, let us demonstrate the calibrations as recorded and the landmarks they encompass. There are *eight calibrations* of each tooth to be remembered. These measurements are shown in the accompanying example for the maxillary central incisor.

The method for measuring an anterior tooth will be shown first (Figs. 1–20 through 1–26), then the posterior method will be shown (Figs. 1–27 through 1–33).

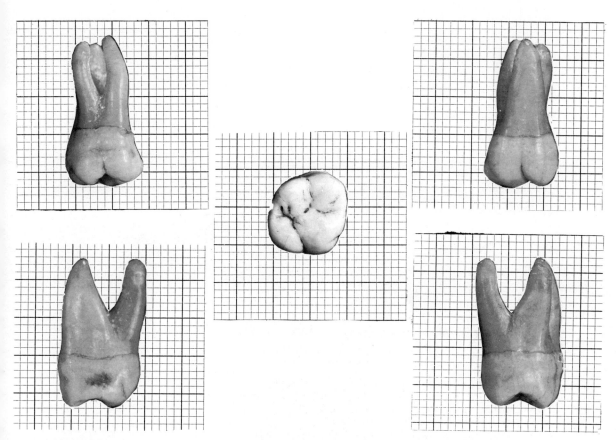

Figure 1–19. Maxillary right first molar. When viewing the mesial and distal aspects, note the curvature or bulge on the crown at the cervical third below the cementoenamel junction.

Method of Measuring an Anterior Tooth

(Keep the long axis of the tooth vertical.)

1. LENGTH OF CROWN (LABIAL)*

Measurement { Crest of curvature at cemento-enamel junction
Incisal edge

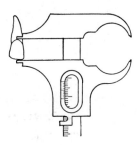

Figure 1–20. Length of crown.

2. LENGTH OF ROOT

Measurement { Apex
Crest of curvature at crown cervix

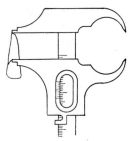

Figure 1–21. Length of root.

* Use the parallel beaks of the Boley gauge for measurements whenever feasible. The contrast of the various curvatures with the straight edges will help to make the close observer more familiar with tooth outlines.

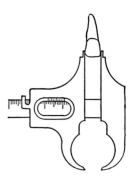

3. MESIODISTAL DIAMETER OF CROWN

Measurement { Crest of curvature on the mesial surface (mesial contact area)
Crest of curvature on the distal surface (distal contact area)

Figure 1–22. Mesiodistal diameter of crown.

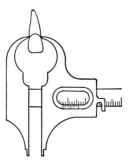

4. MESIODISTAL DIAMETER OF CROWN AT THE CERVIX

Measurement { Junction of crown and root on mesial surface
Junction of crown and root on distal surface (use caliper jaws of Boley gauge in this instance instead of parallel beaks)

Figure 1–23. Mesiodistal diameter of crown at cervix.

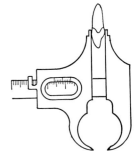

5. LABIOLINGUAL DIAMETER OF CROWN

Measurement { Crest of curvature on the labial surface
Crest of curvature on the lingual surface

Figure 1–24. Labiolingual diameter of crown.

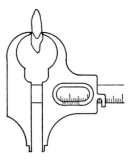

6. LABIOLINGUAL DIAMETER OF CROWN AT THE CERVIX

Measurement { Junction of crown and root on labial surface
Junction of crown and root on lingual surface (use caliper jaws in this instance also)

Figure 1–25. Labiolingual diameter of cervix.

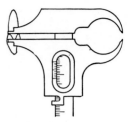

7. CURVATURE OF CEMENTOENAMEL JUNCTION ON MESIAL*

Measurement {
Crest of curvature of cementoenamel junction, labial and lingual
surface
Crest of curvature of cementoenamel junction on the mesial
surface

Figure 1–26. Curvature of cementoenamel junction on mesial.

8. CURVATURE OF CEMENTOENAMEL JUNCTION ON DISTAL

(Turn the tooth around and calibrate as in Fig. 1–26.)

Measurement {
Crest of curvature of cementoenamel junction on the labial and
lingual surfaces
Crest of curvature of cementoenamel junction on the distal surface

Method of Measuring a Posterior Tooth

(Keep the long axis of the tooth vertical.)

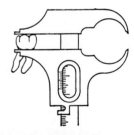

1. LENGTH OF CROWN (BUCCAL)

Measurement {
Crest of buccal cusp or cusps
Crest of curvature at cemento-
enamel junction

Figure 1–27. Length of crown.

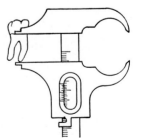

2. LENGTH OF ROOT

Measurement {
Crest of curvature at crown cervix
Apex of root

Figure 1–28. Length of root.

---

* *This measurement is most important because normally it represents the extent of curvature approximately of the periodontal attachment when the tooth is in situ.*

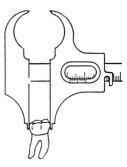

3. MESIODISTAL DIAMETER OF CROWN

Measurement
$\left\{\begin{array}{l}\end{array}\right.$
Crest of curvature on mesial surface
(mesial contact area)
Crest of curvature on distal surface
(distal contact area)

Figure 1–29. Mesiodistal diameter of crown.

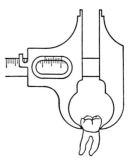

4. MESIODISTAL DIAMETER OF CROWN AT THE CERVIX

Measurement
$\left\{\begin{array}{l}\end{array}\right.$
Junction of crown and root on mesial surface
Junction of crown and root on distal
surface (use caliper jaws of Boley
gauge instead of parallel beaks)

Figure 1–30. Mesiodistal diameter of crown at cervix.

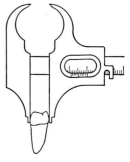

5. BUCCOLINGUAL DIAMETER OF CROWN

Measurement
$\left\{\begin{array}{l}\end{array}\right.$
Crest of curvature on the buccal
surface
Crest of curvature on the lingual
surface

Figure 1–31. Buccolingual diameter of crown.

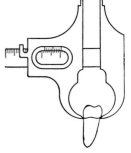

6. BUCCOLINGUAL DIAMETER OF CROWN AT THE CERVIX

Measurement
$\left\{\begin{array}{l}\end{array}\right.$
Junction of crown and root on
buccal surface
Junction of crown and root on
lingual surface (use caliper jaws)

Figure 1–32. Buccolingual diameter of crown at cervix.

7. CURVATURE OF CEMENTOENAMEL JUNCTION ON MESIAL

Measurement $\left\{\begin{array}{l} \text{Crest of curvature of cemento-} \\ \text{enamel junction on the mesial} \\ \text{surface} \\ \text{Crest of curvature of cemento-} \\ \text{enamel junction, buccal and lingual} \\ \text{surfaces} \end{array}\right.$

8. CURVATURE OF CEMENTOENAMEL JUNCTION ON DISTAL

(Turn tooth around and measure as in Fig. 1–33.)

Measurement $\left\{\begin{array}{l} \text{Crest of curvature of cemento-} \\ \text{enamel junction on the distal surface} \\ \text{Crest of curvature of cemento-} \\ \text{enamel junction on the buccal and} \\ \text{lingual surfaces} \end{array}\right.$

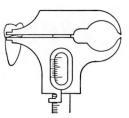

Figure 1–33. Curvature of cementoenamel junction on mesial.

References

American Dental Association, Committee on Dental Education and Hospitals (1968 [1968]). Tooth numbering and radiographic mounting. Am. Dent. Assoc. Trans. 109:25;109:247.

American Dental Association, Committee on Nomenclature (1947). Committee adopts official method for the symbolic designation of teeth. J. Am. Dent. Assoc. 34:647.

Atchison, J. (1950). *Dental Anatomy and Physiology for students,* 2nd ed. London: Staples Press.

Black, G. V. (1897). *Descriptive Anatomy of the Human Teeth,* 4th ed. Philadelphia: S. S. White Dental Manufacturing.

Broomell, I. N., and Fischelis, P. (1923). *Anatomy and Histology of the Mouth and Teeth,* 6th ed. Philadelphia: Blakiston's.

Dewey, M. (1916). Dental Anatomy. St. Louis: Mosby.

Elerton, R. J. (1989). Keeping up-to-date with tooth notation. Brit. Dent. J. 166:55.

Federation Dentaire Internationale two-digit system of designating teeth (1971). Int. Dent. J. 21:104.

Gaddes, T. (1981 [1881]). Extracts from the last century: A course of lectures on dental anatomy and physiology. Br. Dent. J. 151:5; Br. J. Dent. Sci. 24:1.

Goodman, P. (1987). A Universal system for identifying permanent and primary teeth. J. Dent. Child. 34:312.

Harrison, W. P. (1930). Developing dental anatomy into a basic dental subject. J. Am. Dent. Assoc. 17:897.

Palmer's dental notation (1891). Dental Cosmos 33:194.

Schrocer, C. (1959). Practical application of tooth morphology. J. Prosthet. Dent. 9:867.

Schwartz, R. (1935). Practical Dental Anatomy and Tooth Carving. London: Henry Kimpton.

Tims, H. W., and Henry, C. B. (1923). *Tomes' Dental Anatomy.* New York: Macmillan.

Tomes, C. S. (1898). *A Manual of Dental Anatomy, Human and Comparative,* 5th ed. Philadelphia: Blakiston's.

Tonge, C. H. (1981). Oral anatomy: Progress of a discipline. Br. Dent. J. 151:3.

Thorton, D. (1921). Teaching dental anatomy. J. Natl. Dent. Assoc. 8:45.

Wheeler, R. C. (1928). Some fundamentals in tooth formation. Dental Cosmos 70:889.

World Health Organization (1987). Oral health surveys: Basic methods, 3d ed. Geneva: WHO.

2 Development and Eruption of the Teeth

A knowledge of the development of the teeth and their emergence into the oral cavity is applicable to clinical practice, as well as to archaeology, demography, forensics, and paleontology. However, the latter applications will be considered only briefly here. It is assumed that the histology of tooth formation and concepts of tooth eruption have been covered elsewhere. Historically the term *eruption* has been used to denote emergence of the tooth through the gingiva although it denotes more completely continuous tooth movement from the dental bud to occlusal contact (Demirjian, 1986). However, the terms *eruption* and *emergence* will be used here at this time in such a way as to avoid any confusion between historical use of *eruption* and its more recent expanded meaning.

Dental age has been assessed on the basis of the number of teeth at each chronological age (Demirjian, 1986) or on stages of the formation of crowns and roots of the teeth (Smith, 1991). Dental age during the mixed dentition period may be assessed on the basis of which teeth have erupted, the amount of resorption of the roots of primary teeth, and the amount of development of the permanent teeth (Proffit et al., 1986).

Calcification or mineralization (most often visualized radiographically) of the organic matrix of a tooth, root formation, and tooth eruption are important indicators of dental age. Dental age can reflect an assessment of physiologic age comparable to age based on skeletal development, weight, or height (Demirjian et al., 1973). However, when forming, the crowns and roots of the teeth appear to be the tissues least affected by environmental influences (nutrition, endocrinopathies, etc.), and dentition may be considered to be the single best physiological indicator of chronological age in juveniles (Smith, 1991).

Dental development may be based also on the emergence (eruption) of the teeth; however, because caries, tooth loss, and severe malnutrition may influence the emergence of teeth through the gingiva (Ronnerman, 1977; Alvarez and Navia, 1989), chronologies of the eruption of teeth are less satisfactory for dental age assessment than those based on tooth formation. In addition, tooth formation may be divided appropriately into a number of stages that cover continuously the development of teeth (Nolla, 1952; Moorrees et al., 1963a) in contrast to the single episode of tooth eruption.

The importance of the emergence of the teeth to the development of oral motor behavior is frequently overlooked, no doubt partly as a result of the paucity of information available. However, the appearance of the teeth in the mouth at a strategic time in the maturation of the infant's nervous system and its interface with the external environment must have a profound effect on the neurobehavioral mechanisms underlying the infant's development and learning of feeding behavior, particularly the acquisition of masticatory skills.

Tooth Formation Standards

Events in the formation of human dentition are based primarily on data from studies of dissected prenatal anatomic material and from radiographic imaging of the teeth of the same subjects over time (longitudinal data) or of different subjects of different ages seen once (cross-sectional data). From these kinds of studies both descriptive information and chronological data may be obtained. To assemble a complete description or chronology of human tooth formation it would seem necessary to use data based on more than one source and methodology. However, it is not easy to define ideal tooth formation standards from studies based on different variables and many different statistical methods. Subjects surveyed in most studies of dental development are essentially of European derivation, and population differences can only be established by studies that share methodology and information on tooth formation in nonwhite/non-European-derived populations (Smith, 1991).

Chronologies of Human Dentition

The chronology of human dentition (Logan and Kronfeld, slightly modified by McCall and Schour) that appears in Table 2–1 has been revised to reflect more recent data about the chronology of the primary dentition. Table 2–1 and related chronologies (Logan and

Table 2–1. **Chronology of Human Dentition***

Dentition	Tooth	First Evidence of Calcification	Crown Completed	Eruption	Root Completed
		(Weeks in Utero)[c]	(Months)	(Months)[a,d]	(Years)
Primary (upper)	i1		14 (13–16)	1½	10 (8–12)	1½
	i2		16 (14⅔–16½)b	2½	11 (9–13)	2
	C		17 (15–18)b	9	19 (16–22)	3¼
	m1		15½ (14½–17)	6	16 (13–19)♂ (14–18)♀	2½
	m2		19 (16–23½)	11	29 (25–33)	3
Primary (lower)	i1		14 (13–16)	2½	8 (6–10)	1½
	i2		16 (14⅔–)b	3	13 (10–16)	1½
	C		17 (16–)b	9	20 (17–23)	3¼
	m1		15½ (14½–17)	5½	16 (14–18)	2¼
	m2		18 (17–19½)	10	27 (23–31)♂ (24–30)♀	3
Permanent (upper)	I1	3–4 mo.		4–5 yr.	7–8 yr.	10
	I2	10–12 mo.		4–5 yr.	8–9 yr.	11
	C	4–5 mo.		6–7 yr.	11–12 yr.	13–15
	P1	1½–1¾ yr.		5–6 yr.	10–11 yr.	12–13
	P2	2–2¼ yr.		6–7 yr.	10–12 yr.	12–14
	M1	at birth		2½–3 yr.	6–7 yr.	9–10
	M2	2½–3 yr.		7–8 yr.	12–13 yr.	14–16
	M3	7–9 yr.		12–16 yr.	17–21 yr.	18–25
Permanent (lower)	I1	3–4 mo.		4–5 yr.	6–7 yr	9
	I2	3–4 mo.		4–5 yr.	7–8 yr.	10
	C	4–5 mo.		6–7 yr.	9–10 yr.	12–14
	P1	1¾–2 yr.		5–6 yr.	10–12 yr.	12–13
	P2	2¼–2½yr.		6–7 yr.	11–12 yr.	13–14
	M1	at birth		2½–3 yr.	6–7 yr.	9–10
	M2	2½–3 yr.		7–8 yr.	11–13 yr.	14–15
	M3	8–10 yr.		12–16 yr.	17–21 yr.	18–25

*From Logan, W., and Kronfeld, R. J. (1933), slightly modified by McCall and Schour (Orban, 1944) and reflecting other chronologies by Kronfeld, 1935; Kronfeld and Schour, 1939; Schour and Massler, 1940; (a) Lysell et al., 1962; (b) Nomata, 1964; (c) Kraus and Jordan, 1965; and Lunt and law, 1974. (d) = mean age in months ± ISD.

Table 2–2. **Modification of the Table "Chronology of the Human Dentition" (Logan and Kronfeld), slightly modified by McCall and Schour), Suggested by Lunt and Law (1974), for the Calcification and Eruption of the Primary Dentition**

Deciduous Tooth	Hard Tissue Formation Begins* (Fertilization Age in Utero, Weeks)		Amount of Enamel Formed at Birth	Enamel Completed (Mos after Birth)	Eruption (Mean Age† in Months,†1 SD)	Root Completed (Yr)
Maxillary						
Central incisor	14	(13–16)	• Five-sixths	1½	10 (8–12)	1½
Lateral incisor	16	(14⅔–16½)‡	• Two-thirds	2½	11 (9–13)	2
Canine	17	(15–18)‡	• One-third	9	19 (16–22)	3¾
First molar	15½	(14½–17)	• Cusps united; occlusal completely calcified plus a half to three fourths crown height*	6	16 (13–19) boys (14–18) girls	2½
Second molar	19	(16–23½)	• Cusps united; occlusal incompletely calcified; calcified tissue covers a fifth to a fourth crown height*	11	29 (25–33)	3
Mandibular						
Central incisor	14	(13–16)	• Three-fifths	2½	8 (6–10)	1½
Lateral incisor	16	(14⅔–)‡	• Three-fifths	3	13 (10–16)	1½
Canine	17	(16–)‡	• One-third	9	20 (17–23)	3¾
First molar	15½	(14½–17)	• Cusps united; occlusal completely calcified*	5½	16 (14–18)	2¼
Second molar	18	(17–19½)	• Cusps united; occlusal incompletely calcified*	10	27 (23–31) boys (24–30) girls	3

* From Kraus, B. S., and Jordan, R. E. (1965). *The Human Dentition before Birth*. Philadelphia; Lea & Febiger, pp. 107, 109, and 127 (except variation ranges of lateral incisors and canines).

† Adapted from Lysell, L., Magnusson, B., and Thilander, B. (July 1962). Time and order of eruption of the primary teeth. A longitudinal study. *Odontol. Revy* 13:217.

‡ Variation ranges of lateral incisors and canines from Nomata, N. (March 1964). A chronological study on the crown formation of the human deciduous dentition. *Bull Tokyo Med. Dent. Univ.* 11:55. (Fetal length-to-age conversions were made; no values are available for late onset in mandibular lateral incisors and canines since all values from Nomata's data are earlier than the mean values from Kraus and Jordan.) Fetal length-to-age data from Patten, B. M. (1946). *Human Embryology*. Philadelphia: Blakiston's. p. 184.

Table 2–3. **Available Values for Prenatal Formation of Primary Teeth**

| Tooth | Age of Attainment Schedule | | Stage for Age Schedule | |
| | Beginning Calcification (Weeks Postfertilization) Sunderland et al., 1987 | | Amount of Crown Formed at Birth | |
	50th %tile	Range[a]	Kronfeld and Schour, 1939[b]	Kraus and Jordan, 1965
di1	15	13–17	⅗	—
di2	17	14–19	⅗	—
dc	19	17–20	⅓	—
dm1	16	14–17	Cusps united	Occlusal united
dm2	19	18–20	Cusp tips isolated	Cusps united

[a] Earliest age at which mineralization is seen through age at which 100 percent of the sample shows initial mineralization.
[b] These values are based on "tooth ring analysis"; they remain almost the only nonpictorial data available for deciduous incisors. (Smith, 1991)

Kronfeld, 1933; Kronfeld, 1935; Kronfeld and Schour, 1939; Schour and Massler, 1940; McCall and Schour [Orban, 1944]) reflect an interesting history of development and compilation (Garn, 1959; Lunt and Law, 1974). A number of deficiencies in samples and methods used have prevented the acceptance of a chronology that may be considered ideal for standards of normal growth. The suggestions for revision made by Lunt and Law (1974) in their modification of the calcification and eruption schedules of the primary dentition (Table 2–2) have been incorporated into the Logan and Kronfeld chronology shown in Table 2–1. The problems associated with revising a table completely or "plugging in" revised data is apparent when it becomes necessary to make critical choices from among available sources as illustrated in Tables 2–3 and 2–4 by Smith (1991).

Table 2–4. **Ages for Postnatal Development of Mandibular Deciduous Teeth Expressed in Decimal Years**

| Mandibular Tooth | Age Crown Completed (Yr) | | | Age Root Completed (Yr) | | |
| | Moorrees et al., 1963b[a] | | Kronfeld and Schour, 1939[b] | Moorrees et al., 1963b[a] | | Kronfeld and Schour, 1939[b] |
	Mean	−2s.d.-+2s.d.		Mean	−2s.d.-+2s.d.	
di1	—	—	0.1–0.2	—	—	1.5
di2	—	—	0.2	—	—	1.5–2.0
dc	—	—	0.7	—	—	3.25
Males	0.7	0.4–1.0	—	3.1	2.4–3.8	—
Females	0.7	0.4–1.0	—	3.0	2.3–3.8	—
dm1	—	—	0.5	—	—	2.25
Males	0.4	02.–0.7	—	2.0	1.5–2.5	—
Females	0.3	0.1–0.5	—	1.8	1.3–2.3	—
dm2	—	—	0.8–0.9	—	—	3.0
Males	0.7	0.4–1.0	—	3.1	2.4–3.9	—
Females	0.7	0.4–1.0	—	2.8	2.2–3.6	—

[a] These data comprise an age-of-attainment schedule.
[b] The basis of these values may be some combination of "tooth ring analysis" and observation of an infant sample; no other values could be located for deciduous incisors in studies with documented methods (Smith, 1991).

The pictorial charts of the development of the human dentitions (Figs. 2–1 and 2–2) are not intended to be used as ideal standards of normal development, although the illustrations could be redrawn to be more comparable with statistical studies such as those of Moorrees et al. (1963a,b). Present use of the charts is directed more to illustrating to patients general aspects of development than for precise guidance of clinical procedures, age prediction, or maturity assessment.

Radiographic studies of tooth formation (Fig. 2–3) have used at least three stages: beginning calcification, crown completion, and root completion. Nolla (1952) expanded the number of stages to eleven and Gleiser and Hunt (1955) to thirteen, which has served as the basis for several studies, including that of Moorrees et al. (1963a), who developed fourteen stages of permanent tooth formation (Fig. 2–4). The fourteen stages are not numbered but designated by abbreviations: C = cusp; Cr = crown; R = root; Cl = cleft; A = apex; subscripts: i = initiated; co = coalescence; oc = outline complete; and c = complete. Moorrees et al. (1963b) studied the development of mandibular canines and provided normative data.

The age of attainment of a growth stage is not easily determined because in a proportion of the cases that are observed the attainment of the stage has not occurred and in others the stage is over. Several procedures to answer the question as to when a growth stage did occur have been used to construct chronologies of tooth formation, but many of these methods lead to chronologies which are not comparable for various reasons, including the problem of having fundamentally different underlying variables. Thus, the major statistical methods used to construct different statistically based chronologies of tooth formation relate to fundamentally different variables and should be used for different purposes (Smith, 1991).

Age-of-attainment type of chronologies may be produced by cumulative distributive functions or probit analysis (Smith, 1991), as well as by the average of age at first appearance less one-half interval between examinations (Anderson et al., 1976). Cumulative distributive functions, which have been used by a number of investigators, including Garn et al. (1958, 1959), appear to be the best method of determining the age of attainment (Tanner, 1986). An example of this type of chronology is a schedule of tooth emergence as illustrated in Figure 2–5, where the proportion of subjects that have attained a particular stage is plotted against the midpoint of each age group. A chronology of age of attainment of tooth formation for females is shown as an example of this type of chronology (Table 2–5). Age of attainment schedules are useful clinically where it is necessary to avoid damage to developing teeth during treatment.

Chronologies of tooth formation based on the average age of subjects in a stage of development have been suggested by several investigators (Gleiser and Hunt, 1955; Demisch and Wartman, 1956; Haartaja, 1965; Fass, 1969). Although these kinds of chronologies are better suited for *age prediction* than age of attainment, no chronology is ideal for this purpose, and an alternate strategy suggested by Goldstein (1979) has been used by Smith (1991) to calculate age prediction tables for mandibular tooth formation. Values for predicting age in females are presented in Table 2–6. Such a table is useful to answer the question, how old is this individual? In this schedule each tooth is assessed independently and the mean of all available ages is assigned as the dental age. In Table 2–6 the age related to a stage reflects the midpoint between mean age of attainment of the current stage and the next one. Age prediction chronologies are used for assessing unknown ages of patients and for forensic and archaeological applications.

Chronologies of maturity assessment have been based on mean stage for age where stages are averaged rather than subject ages (Nolla, 1952, 1960). However, to avoid problems associated with the calculation of mean age or mean stage, maturity scales have

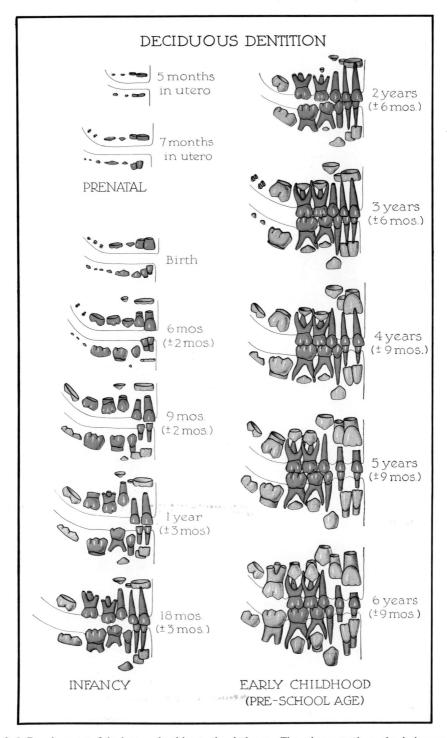

DECIDUOUS DENTITION

5 months
in utero

7 months
in utero

PRENATAL

Birth

6 mos.
(±2 mos.)

9 mos.
(±2 mos.)

1 year
(±3 mos)

18 mos.
(±3 mos.)

INFANCY

2 years
(±6 mos.)

3 years
(±6 mos.)

4 years
(±9 mos.)

5 years
(±9 mos.)

6 years
(±9 mos.)

EARLY CHILDHOOD
(PRE-SCHOOL AGE)

Figure 2–1. Development of the human dentition to the sixth year. The primary teeth are the darker ones in the illustration. (From Schour, I., and Massler, M.: The development of the human dentition. J. Am. Dent. Assoc., 28:1153, 1941.)

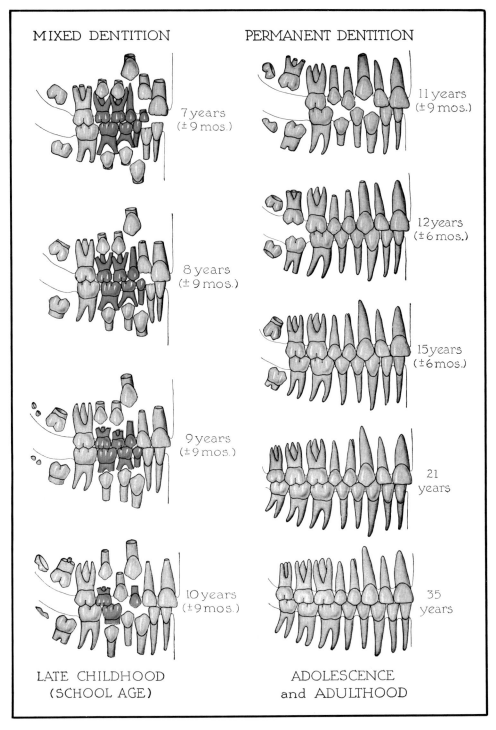

MIXED DENTITION

PERMANENT DENTITION

7 years
(± 9 mos.)

11 years
(± 9 mos.)

8 years
(± 9 mos.)

12 years
(± 6 mos.)

9 years
(± 9 mos.)

15 years
(± 6 mos.)

10 years
(± 9 mos.)

21
years

LATE CHILDHOOD
(SCHOOL AGE)

ADOLESCENCE
and ADULTHOOD

35
years

Figure 2–2. Development of the human dentition from the seventh year to maturity. Note the displacement of primary teeth by succedaneous permanent teeth. (From Schour, I., and Massler, M.: The development of the human dentition. J. Am. Dent. Assoc., 28:1153, 1941.)

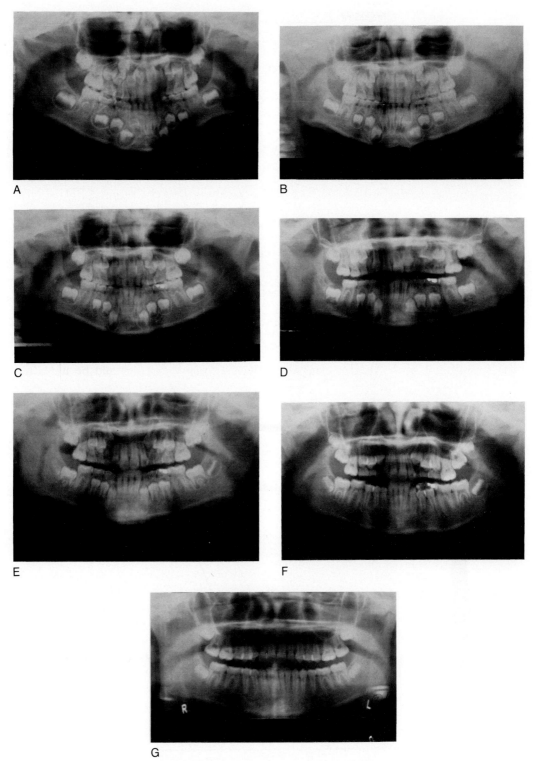

Figure 2–3. Radiographic series of the developing permanent dentition: *A*, 9/78. *B*, 10/79. *C*, 9/80. *D*, 9/81. *E*, 9/82. *F*, 9/83. *G*, 10/85.

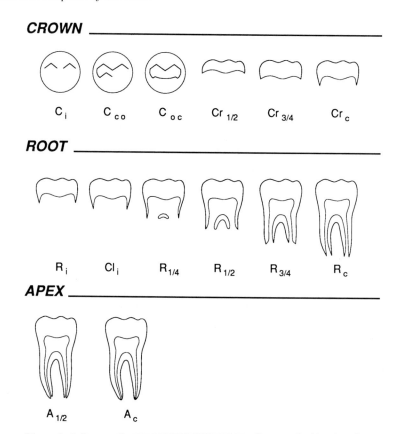

Figure 2–4. Stages of permanent tooth formation. See text for identity of abbreviations (after Moorees et al, 1963a)

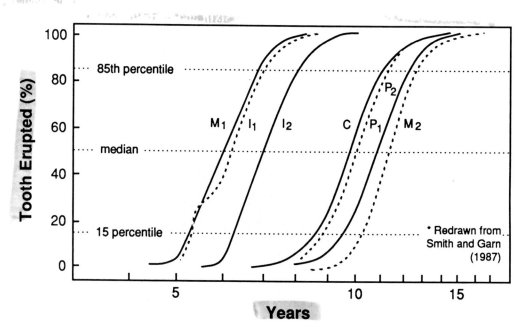

Figure 2–5. Age of attainment of a growth stage using a cumulative distribution function where data represents tooth emergence

Table 2–5. Mean Age of Attainment of Developmental Stages for Females (Permanent Mandibular Teeth)[a]

Developmental Stage	I1	I2	C	P1	P2	M1	M2	M3
Ci	—	—	0.5	1.8	3.0	0.0	3.5	9.6
Cco	—	—	0.8	2.2	3.6	0.3	3.7	10.1
Coc	—	—	1.2	2.9	4.2	0.8	4.2	10.7
Cr½	—	—	2.0	3.6	4.8	1.0	4.8	11.3
Cr¾	—	—	3.0	4.3	5.4	1.5	5.4	11.7
Crc	—	—	4.0	5.1	6.2	2.2	6.2	12.3
Ri	—	—	4.7	5.8	6.8	2.7	7.0	12.9
Rcl	—	—	—	—	—	3.5	7.7	13.5
R¼	4.5	4.7	5.3	6.5	7.5	4.5	9.2	14.8
R½	5.1	5.2	7.1	8.2	8.8	5.1	9.8	15.7
R⅔	5.6	5.9	—	—	—	—	—	—
2¾	6.1	6.4	8.3	9.2	10.0	5.7	10.7	16.6
Rc	6.6	7.6	8.9	9.9	10.6	6.0	11.2	17.2
A½	7.4	8.1	9.9	11.1	12.0	7.0	12.5	18.3
Ac	7.7	8.5	11.3	12.2	13.7	8.7	14.6	20.7

[a] Values interpolated from Moorrees et al. (1963a); all ages in years. (Smith, 1991)

been designed by several investigators, including Wolanski (1966), Demirjian et al. (1973), Healy and Goldstein (1976), and Nystrom et al. (1986). Such scales are useful when maturity is assessed for subjects of known age but are not designed for anthropological or forensic applications (Smith, 1991).

The Primary Dentition

Calcification of the primary teeth begins in utero 13 and 16 weeks (Table 2–1). By 18–20 weeks postfertilization, all the primary teeth have begun to calcify. Emergence of the primary dentition takes place between the sixth and thirtieth months of postnatal life. It takes from 2 to 3 years for the primary dentition to be completed (Fig. 2–6), beginning with

Table 2–6. Values for Predicting Age from Stages of Permanent Mandibular Tooth Formation—Females[a]

Developmental Stage	I1	I2	C	P1	P2	M1	M2	M3
Ci	—	—	0.6	2.0	3.3	0.2	3.6	9.9
Cco	—	—	1.0	2.5	3.9	0.5	4.0	10.4
Coc	—	—	1.6	3.2	4.5	0.9	4.5	11.0
Cr½	—	—	2.5	4.0	5.1	1.3	5.1	11.5
Cr¾	—	—	3.5	4.7	5.8	1.8	5.8	12.0
Crc	—	—	4.3	5.4	6.5	2.4	6.6	12.6
Ri	—	—	5.0	6.1	7.2	3.1	7.3	13.2
Rcl	—	—	—	—	—	4.0	8.4	14.1
R¼	4.8	5.0	6.2	7.4	8.2	4.8	9.5	15.2
R½	5.4	5.6	7.7	8.7	9.4	5.4	10.3	16.2
R⅔	5.9	6.2	—	—	—	—	—	—
2¾	6.4	7.0	8.6	9.6	10.3	5.8	11.0	16.9
Rc	7.0	7.9	9.4	10.5	11.3	6.5	11.8	17.7
A½	7.5	8.3	10.6	11.6	12.8	7.9	13.5	19.5
Ac	—	—	—	—	—	—	—	—

[a] Values interpolated from Moorrees et al. (1963a); all ages in years. (Smith, 1991)

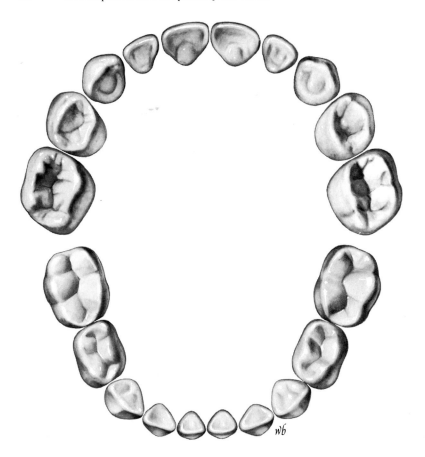

Figure 2–6. Composite artistic rendition of primary dentition taken from skull material. Bilateral differences are not unusual.

the initial calcification of the primary central incisor to the completion of the roots of the primary second molar (Table 2–1). However, each permanent tooth takes 8–14 years to complete if the third molar is considered (Table 2–1). Normally at birth no teeth are visible in the mouth; however, occasionally infants are born with erupted mandibular incisors.

Investigations of the chronology of emergence of the primary teeth in different racial and ethnic groups reflect considerable variation (Demirjian, 1986), and there is very little information available on tooth formation in nonwhite/non-European-derived populations (Smith, 1991). World population differences in tooth standards suggest that there are patterned differences that may not be large (Smith, 1991). Tooth size or tooth morphology, as well as tooth formation, is highly inheritable (Garn et al., 1965). There are few definitive correlations between primary tooth emergence and other physiologic parameters such as skeletal maturation, size, and sex (Falkner, 1957).

The eruption or emergence of primary mandibular central incisors through the gingiva occurs at a mean age of eight months (Table 2–1). In Tables 2–1 and 2–2 values for eruption are presented as the mean age and a range of variation based on plus or minus one standard deviation, after rounding all values to the nearest month. The eruption of these teeth is followed about two months later by the maxillary central incisors at a mean age of 10 months, and then by the mandibular lateral incisors at a mean age of 13 months. In some instances babies may display four mandibular incisors before the maxillary teeth erupt.

At a mean age of 16 months (Table 2–1) the primary first molars erupt with the maxillary molar tending most often to erupt earlier than the mandibular first molar (Lunt and Law, 1974). There is some evidence for a difference by sex for the first primary molars but there appears to be no answer for the question: Why does the first molar have a different pattern of sexual dimorphism? (Demirjian, 1986).

The primary maxillary canine erupts at a mean age of 19 months and the mandibular canines at 20 months (Table 2–1).

The primary second mandibular molar erupts at a mean age of 27 months with evidence that there is difference between boys and girls (Table 2–1). The primary maxillary second molar follows at a mean age of 29 months.

The predominant sequence of eruption of the primary teeth in the individual jaw is central incisor (A), lateral incisor (B), first molar (D), canine (C), and second molar (E), as depicted in Table 2–1. Variations in that order may be due to reversals of central and lateral incisors, first molar and lateral incisor, or eruption of two teeth at the same time (Lysell et al., 1962). Jaw reversals in eruption of canines and first molars have been found to be important in increasing the variety of sequences (Lysell et al., 1962; Sato and Ogiwara, 1971). When differences according to jaws are considered, Lunt and Law (1974) conclude that the lateral incisor, first molar, and canine tend to erupt earlier in the maxilla than in the mandible. Sato and Ogiwara (1971) found a characteristic order in about a third of their sample of children:

AB	D	C	E
A	B	D	CE

However, this arrangement of mean ages of eruption to yield a mean order of eruption was found to occur only in a small percentage of the subjects in the study by Lysell et al. (1962).

The completed primary dentition may show evidence of bruxing wear, especially of the anterior teeth (Fig. 2–7, *A*). Spacing of the teeth may be beneficial for the subsequent eruption of the permanent successors.

The premature loss of primary teeth because of caries may not only reflect an unfortunate lack of knowledge as to the course of the disease but also establishes a negative attitude about preventing dental caries in the adult dentition. Loss of primary teeth may lead to lack of space for the permanent dentition. It is sometimes assumed by lay persons that the loss of primary teeth, which are sometimes referred to as "baby teeth" or "milk teeth," is of little consequence because they are only temporary. However, the primary dentition may be in use from the age of 2 to 2½ years until the age of 7, or about 5 years in all. Some of the teeth are in use from 6 months until 12 years of age, or 11½ years in all. Thus,

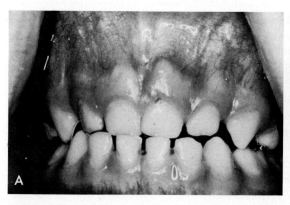 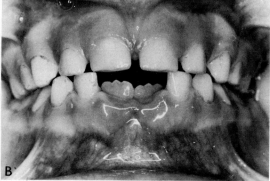

Figure 2–7. A, Primary dentition in a child 5 years of age. *B,* Eruption of central incisors in a child 6½ years of age. Note mamelons.

these primary teeth are in use and contributing to the health and well-being of the individual during the first years of greatest development, physically and mentally.

Premature loss of primary teeth, retention of primary teeth, congenital absence of teeth, dental anomalies, and insufficient space are considered important factors in the initiation and development of an abnormal occlusion. Premature loss of primary teeth from dental neglect is likely to cause a loss of arch length with consequent tendency for crowding of the permanent dentition.

The transition from primary to permanent dentition begins about 6 years of age with the eruption of the first permanent molars. The timing of the shedding of the primary teeth has an effect on the emergence of the permanent teeth, i.e., early shedding of primary teeth advances the emergence of the permanent teeth (Clements, 1957).

Permanent Dentition

The formation of the permanent dentition has been described by Schour and Massler (1940) as occurring in clusters. The first cluster consists of the first molar, the central and lateral incisors, and cuspids, which all begin formation during the first year; the second cluster forms during the ages of 2–4 years; and the third cluster forms during the same age group. The third cluster consists of the third molar, which forms some 5–6 years after the second molar, though its formation varies widely for various population groups.

The first teeth of permanent dentition to emerge through the gingiva are the first molars. Because eruption occurs at approximately 6 years of age (Table 2–1) the teeth are often called "6-year molars." They begin to calcify at about the time of birth (Table 2–1). These teeth emerge distal to the primary second molar (see Fig. 3–7) and are larger than any of the primary teeth.

The central incisor is the second permanent tooth to emerge into the oral cavity. Eruption time occurs quite close to that of the first molar; i.e., tooth emergence occurs between 6 and 7 years (Table 2–1). As with the first molar at 6 years 50 percent of the individuals have reached the stage considered to be the age of attainment of the stage or, more specifically, age of emergence for the central incisor. The mandibular permanent teeth tend to erupt before maxillary teeth. The mandibular central incisor usually erupts before the maxillary central incisor (Fig. 2–6, *B*) and may erupt simultaneously with, or even before, the mandibular first molar. The mandibular lateral incisor may erupt along with the central incisor.

Before the permanent central incisor can come into position, the primary central incisor must be exfoliated. This is brought about by the phenomenon called *resorption* of the deciduous roots. The permanent tooth in its follicle attempts to force its way into the position held by its predecessor. The pressure brought to bear against the primary root evidently causes resorption of the root, which continues until the primary crown has lost its anchorage, becomes loose, and is finally exfoliated (see Fig. 3–8). In the meantime, the permanent tooth has moved occlusally, so that when the primary tooth is lost, the permanent one is at the point of eruption and in proper position to succeed its predecessor.

The *follicles* of the developing *incisors* and *canines* are in a position lingual to the deciduous roots (see Figs. 2–8, 3–3 and 3–8). The developing *premolars* which are to take the place of deciduous molars are within the bifurcation of primary molar roots (Figs. 2–12 and 2–13). The permanent incisors, canines, and premolars are called *succedaneous teeth*, since they take the place of their primary predecessors.

Root resorption sometimes does not follow the routine procedure, with the result that

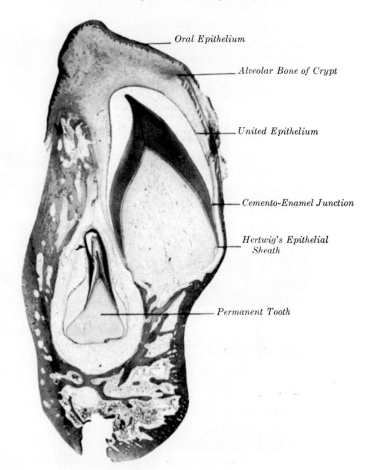

Oral Epithelium

Alveolar Bone of Crypt

United Epithelium

Cemento-Enamel Junction

Hertwig's Epithelial Sheath

Permanent Tooth

Figure 2–8. Section of mandible in a 9-month-old infant cut through unerupted primary canine and its permanent successor, which lies lingually and apically to it. The enamel of the primary canine crown is completed and lost because of decalcification. Root formation has begun. (Modified from Schour, I., and Noyes, H. J.: *Oral Histology and Embryology,* 8th ed. Philadelphia, Lea & Febiger, 1960.)

the permanent tooth cannot emerge or else is kept out of its normal place. The failure of the deciduous root to resorb may bring about prolonged retention of the deciduous tooth (Figs. 2–11 and 2–12).

Mandibular lateral incisors erupt very soon after the central incisors, often simultaneously. The *maxillary central incisors* erupt next in the chronological order, and the *maxillary lateral incisors* make their appearance about a year later (Table 2–1) and Figs. 2–1 and 2–2). The *first premolars* follow the maxillary laterals in sequence when the child is about 10 years old; the *mandibular canines* (cuspids) often appear at the same time. The *second premolars* follow during the next year, and then the *maxillary canines* follow. Usually, the second molars come in when the individual is about 12; they are posterior to the first molars and are commonly called "12-year molars." The maxillary canines occasionally erupt along with the second molars, but in most instances of normal eruption the canines precede them somewhat.

The *third molars* do not come in until the age of 17 years or later. Considerable jaw growth is required after the age of 12 to allow room for these teeth. Third molars are subject to many anomalies and variations of form. Insufficient jaw development for their accommodation complicates matters in the majority of cases. Individuals who have properly developed third molars in good alignment are very much in the minority. Third-molar anomalies and variations with the complications brought about by malalignment and subnormal jaw development comprise a subject too vast to be covered here.

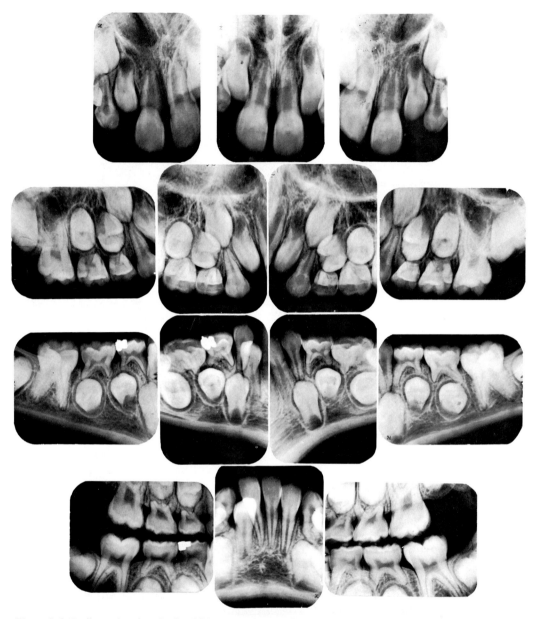

Figure 2–9. Radiographs of teeth of a child 8 years old. Maxillary teeth have crowns pointed downward, whereas mandibular teeth have crowns pointed upward. Some of the permanent teeth have erupted, while others may be seen forming above or below primary predecessors. Note the resorption of the roots of deciduous teeth.

Development of the Teeth

Apparently there are four or more *centers of formation* for each tooth. The formation of each center proceeds until there is a coalescence of all of them. Each of these centers (when referring to the crown portion) is called a *lobe*.

Although no lines of demarcation are found in the dentin to show this development, there are signs to be found on the surfaces of the crowns and roots; these are called *developmental grooves* (see Fig. 4–20).

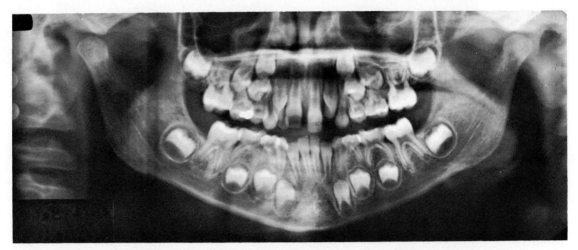

Figure 2–10. Panoramic radiograph of a child about 7 years old. This type of examination is of great value in registering an overall record of development. (From Pappas, G. C., and Wallace, W. R.: Panoramic sialography. Dent. Radiogr. Photogr., 43:27, 1970.)

After the *crown* of the tooth is formed, the *root portion* is begun. At the cervical border of the enamel, at the cervix of the crown, cementum starts to form as a root covering of the dentin. The *cementum* is hard tissue (similar in some ways to bone tissue) which covers the root of the tooth in a thin layer. The junction of enamel and cementum is called the *cementoenamel junction.* For descriptive purposes in dental anatomy, this is spoken of as the *cervical line,* forming a line of demarcation between the crown and root.

The development of the crown and root takes place within a bony crypt in the jaw bone. The development of the permanent teeth and resorption of the roots of deciduous teeth may be seen in periapical radiographs (Fig. 2–9) as well as panoramic radiographs (Fig. 2–10).

Figures 2–11 through 2–15 are photographs of the skull of a child who was probably in his tenth year. The skull has been dissected to show the positions of the remaining primary teeth and their root resorption as well as the positions and development of the permanent teeth. Figure 2–16 shows the position and development of third molars. Figure 2–17 shows maxillary and mandibular arches with a full complement of 32 teeth.

Figure 2–11. Front view of skull of child 9 or 10 years of age. Note the stages of development and eruption of the various teeth. The canines are lingual to the roots of predecessors. The relation and development of the teeth are normal except for the prolonged retention of the maxillary right lateral incisor, which is locked in a lingual relation to the mandibular teeth.

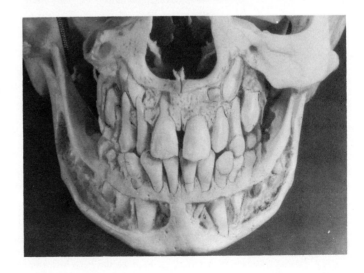

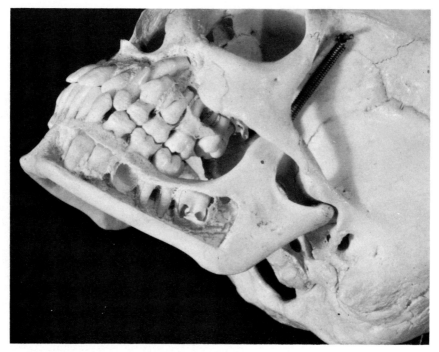

Figure 2–12. Left side of the skull shown in Figure 2–11. Note the placement of the permanent maxillary canine and the second premolar; also observe the position and stage of development of the maxillary second permanent molar. The bony crypt of the mandibular second permanent premolar is in full view, since the developing tooth was lost from the specimen. Observe the large openings in the developing roots of the mandibular second permanent molar.

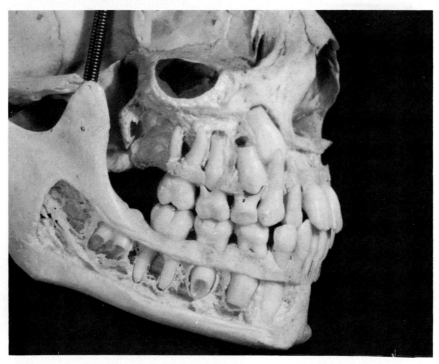

Figure 2–13. View of the right side of the skull shown in Figure 2–11. Note the amount of resorption of the roots of the primary maxillary molars which has taken place and the relation of the developing premolars above them. The roots of the first permanent molars have been completed. Note the open pulp chambers and the pulp canals in the developing mandibular teeth. The lingual inclination of the lower second premolar is common. The developing upper second molar has been lost from the specimen.

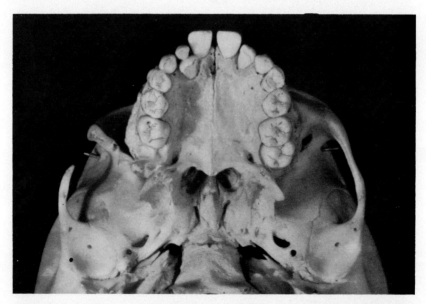

Figure 2–14. Occlusal view of the skull shown in Figures 2–11 through 2–13. Both maxillary lateral incisors have erupted, but the right lateral has come in lingually to the deciduous tooth because of prolonged retention of the latter. (Compare with Figure 2–11.) The primary canines and molars remain in position. The left maxillary second permanent molar is no longer covered by bone.

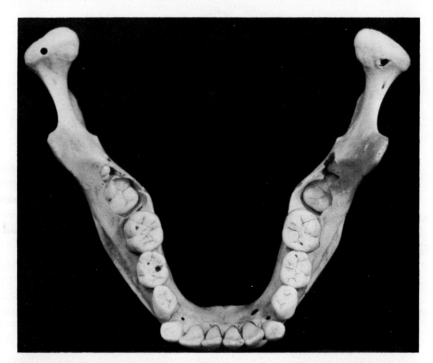

Figure 2–15. Occlusal view of the mandibular arch of the skull shown in Figure 2–14. The development is typical, with a distal inclination of the lower lateral incisors (permanent) and a labial inclination of the primary canines. Note the openings that have been started in the bone immediately lingual to the primary canines to facilitate the eruption of the permanent successors. Also note the developing second molars, typically located, and a tip of the developing third molar (right). The primary canines are approaching exfoliation. The primary molars remain in their normal positions with good contact relation.

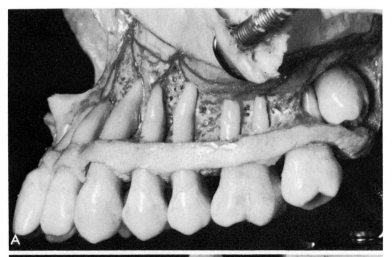

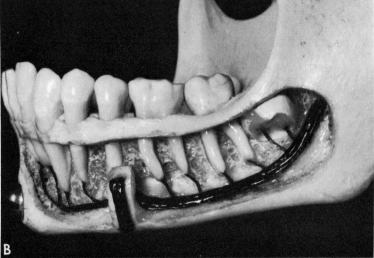

Figure 2–16. *A, B,* Development of maxillary and mandibular third molars.

After the crown and part of the root are formed, the tooth penetrates the mucous membrane and makes its entry into the mouth. Further formation of the root is supposed to be an active factor in pushing the crown toward its final position in the mouth. Eruption of the tooth is said to be completed when most of the crown is in evidence and when it has made contact with its antagonist or antagonists in the opposing jaw. Actually, eruption may and usually does continue after this; i.e., more of the crown may become exposed and the tooth may move farther occlusally to accommodate itself to new conditions.

Formation of root dentin and cementum continues after the tooth is in use. The *root* formation is about half finished when the tooth emerges. Ultimately, the root is completed. Cementum covers the root. The pulp tissue continues to function with its blood and nerve supply after the tooth is formed. The pulp cavity within the tooth has by this time become small in comparison with the tooth size. Its outline is similar to the outline of the crown and root, and the opening of the pulp cavity at the apex is constricted. This opening is called the *apical foramen.* The pulp keeps its tissue-forming function, in that it may form *secondary dentin* on occasion as a protection to itself.

Formation of the tooth is said to be *completed* when the apex of the root is formed; as a matter of fact, however, this process continues slowly throughout the life of the tooth. The

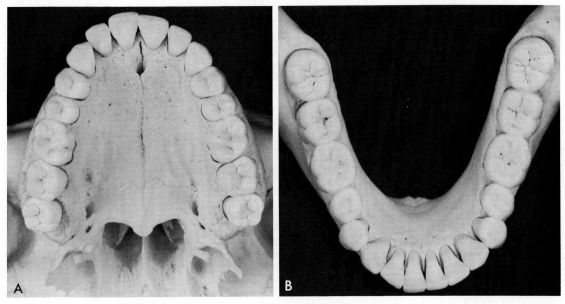

Figure 2–17. *A, B,* Maxillary and mandibular arches with full complement of 32 teeth.

pulp cavity becomes smaller and more constricted with age. Sometimes the pulp chamber within the crown is entirely obliterated, and in rare instances the entire pulp cavity has been found filled with secondary deposit. This process is not so extensive in deciduous teeth, since the years of their usefulness are fewer; nevertheless, the same powers are inherent in the primary pulp. Primary teeth will show secondary dentin in their pulp chambers as a result of the irritation produced by caries or excessive wear.

The *dental pulp* is a connective-tissue organ containing a number of structures, among which are arteries, veins, a lymphatic system, and nerves. Its primary function is to form the dentin of the tooth. When the tooth is newly erupted, the dental pulp is large; it becomes progressively smaller as the tooth is completed. The pulp is relatively large in primary teeth and also in young permanent teeth. For this reason, the teeth of children and young people are more sensitive than teeth of older people to thermal change and dental operative procedure.

References

Adler, P. (1958). Studies on the eruption of the permanent teeth. IV. The effect upon the eruption of the permanent teeth of caries in the deciduous dentition, and of urbanisation. Acta. Genet. (Basel) 8:78.

Alvàrez, J., Navia, J. M. (1989). Nutritional status, tooth eruption and dental caries: A review. Am. J. Clin. Nutr. 49:417.

Anderson, D. L., et al. (1976). Age of attainment of mineralization stages of the permanent dentition. J. For. Sci. 21:191.

Atkinson, S. R. (1949). Changing dynamics of the growing face. Am. J. Orthod. 35:815.

Atkinson, S. R. (1940). Growth and development of teeth and jaws. Am. J. Orthod. Oral Surg. 26:829.

Atkinson, S. R. (1943). The permanent maxillary lateral incisor. Am. J. Orthod. Oral Surg. 29:685.

Bosma, J. F. (1972). Third Symposium on Oral Sensation and Perception—The Mouth of the Infant. Springfield, Ill.: Charles C. Thomas.

Bosma, J. F. (1973). Fourth Symposium on Oral Sensation and Perception—Development in the Fetus and Infant. Washington, D.C., U.S. Government Printing Office.

Brauer, J. C., and Bahador, M. A. (1942). Variations in calcification and eruption of the deciduous and the permanent teeth. J. Am. Dent. Assoc. 29:1373.

Broadbent, B. H. (1937). The face of the normal child. Angle Orthod. 7:183.

Broomell, I. N., and Fischelis, P. (1923). Anatomy and Histology of the Mouth and Teeth, 6th ed. Philadelphia: Blakiston's.

Brown, T. (1978). Tooth emergence in Australian aboriginals. Ann. Hum. Biol. 5:41.

Cattell, P. (1928). *Dentition as a Measure of Maturity*. Harvard Monographs in Education No. 9. Cambridge, Mass.: Harvard University Press.

Clements, E. M. B., et al. (1957). Age at which deciduous teeth are shed. Brit. Med. J. 1:1508.

Demirjian, A. (1978). Dentition. In Falkner, F., and Tanner, J. H. (eds.), *Human Growth, Vol. 2: Postnatal Growth*. New York: Plenum.

Demirjian, A. (1986). Dentition. In Falkner, F., and Tanner, J. M. (eds)., *Human Growth, Vol. 2: A Comprehensive Treatise*, 2nd ed. New York: Plenum.

Demirjian, A., et al. (1973). A new system of dental age assessment. Human Biol. 45:211.

Demirjian, A., Levesque, G. Y.: (1980). Sexual differences in dental development and prediction of emergence. J. Dent Res. 59:1110.

Demisch, A., and Wartman, P. (1956). Calcification of the mandibular third molar and its relation to skeletal and chronological age in children. Child. Dev. 27:459.

Falkner, F. (1957). Deciduous tooth eruption. Arch. Dis. Child. 32:386.

Fanning, E. A., Moorrees, C. F. A. (1969). A comparison of permanent mandibular molar formation in Australian aborgines and caucasoids Arch. Oral Biol. 14:999.

Fanning, E. A., Brown, T. (1971). Primary and permanent tooth development. Aust. Dent. J. 16:41.

Fass, E. N. (1969). A chronology of growth of the human dentition. J. Dent. Child. 36:391.

Finn, S. B. (1962). *Clinical Pedodontics*, 2nd ed. Philadelphia; Saunders.

Garn, S. M., and Smith, B. H. (1980). Developmental communalities in tooth emergence timing. J. Dent. Res. 59:1178.

Garn, S. M., et al. (1965). Genetic, nutritional, and maturational correlates of dental development. J. Dent. Res. 44:228.

Garn, S. M., et al. (1958). Variability of tooth formation in man. Science 128:1510.

Garn, S. M., et al. (1959). Variability of tooth formation. J. Dent. Res. 38:135.

Gleiser, I., and Hunt, E. E. (1955). The permanent mandibular first molar: Its calcification, eruption, and decay. Am. J. Phys. Anthropol. 13:253.

Goldstein, H. (1979). *The Design and Analysis of Longitudinal Studies*. London: Academic Press.

Gregory, W. K., Hellman, M. (1927). Evolution of Dental Occlusion from Fish to Man. First International Orthodontic Congress. St. Louis, Mo.: Mosby.

Gron, A. M. (1962). Prediction of tooth emergence. J. Dent. Res. 41:573.

Gustafson, G., and Koch, G. (1974). Age estimation up to 16 years of age based on dental development. Odont. Revy. 25:297.

Haataja, J. (1965). Development of the mandibular permanent teeth of Helsinki children. Proc. Finn. Dent. Soc. 61:43.

Hagg, U., and Matsson, L. (1985). Dental maturity as an indicator of chronological age: The accuracy and precision of three methods. Eur. J. Orthod. 7:25.

Healy, M.J.R., and Goldstein, H. (1976). An approach to scaling of categorized attributes. Biometrika 63:219.

Hess, A., et al. (1932). A radiographic study of calcification of the teeth from birth to adolescence. Dental Cosmos 11:74.

Johanson, G. (1971). Age determinations from human teeth. Odont. Revy 22(Suppl.):1.

Kopsch, F. W. T. (1914–1916). *Rauber-Kopsch Lehrbuch der Anatomie des Menschen*, Vol. 3, 10th ed. (6 vols.) Leipzig: G. Thieme.

Korkhaus, G. (1929). Die erste Dentition und der Zahnwichsel im Lichte der Zwillingsforschung Vjschr. Zahynheilk H. 3.

Kraus, B. S. (1959). Calcification of the human deciduous teeth. J. Am. Dent. Assoc. 59:1128.

Kraus, B. S., and Jordan, R. E. (1965). The Human Dentition Before Birth. Philadelphia: Lea & Febiger.

Kronfeld, R. (1935). Development and calcification of the human deciduous and permanent dentition. Bur. 15:18.

Kronfeld, R., Schour, I. (1939). Neonatal dental hypoplasia. J. Am. Dent. Assoc. 26:18.

Levesque, G.-Y., et al. (1981). Sexual dimorphism in the development, emergence, and agenesis of the mandibular third molar. J. Dent. Res. 60:1735.

Lo, R. T., and Moyers, R. M. (1953). Studies in the etiology and prevention of malocclusion. Am. J. Orthod. 39:460.

Logan, W. H. G., and Kronfeld, R. (1933). Development of the human jaws and surrounding structures from birth of age fifteen. J. Am. Dent. Assoc. 20:379.

Lunt, R. C., and Law, D. B. (1974). A review of the chronology of deciduous teeth. J. Am. Dent. Assoc. 89:872.

Lysell, L. et al. (1962). Time and order of eruption of the primary teeth: a longitudinal study. Odont. Revy. 13:217.

Massler, M., et al. (1944). Developmental pattern of the child as reflected in the calcification pattern of the teeth. Am. J. Dis. Child. 63:33.

McCall, J. O., and Wald, S. S. (1947). *Clinical Dental Roentgenology*, 2nd ed. Philadelphia: Saunders.

Moorrees, C. F. A., et al. (1963a). Age variation of formation stages for ten permanent teeth. J. Dent. Res. 42:1490.

Moorrees, C. F. A., et al. (1963b). Formation and resorption of three deciduous teeth in children. Am. J. Phys. Anthropol. 21:205.

Moorrees, C. F. A., and Kent, R. L. (1981). Interrelations in the timing of root formation and tooth emergence. Proc. Finn. Dent. Soc. 77:113.

Nanda, R. S., and Chawla, T. N. (1966). Growth and development of dentitions in Indian children. I. Development of permanent teeth. Am. J. Orthod. 52:837.

Nolla, C. M. (1960). Development of the permanent teeth. J. Dent. Child. 27:254.

Nolla, C. M. (1952). The Development of Permanent Teeth. Doctoral thesis, University of Michigan, Ann Arbor.

Nomata, N. (March 1964). A chronological study on the crown formation of the human deciduous dentition. Bull. Tokyo. Med. Dent. Univ. 11:55.

Nystrom, M., et al. (1986). Dental maturity in Finnish children, estimated from the development of seven permanent mandibular teeth. Acta. Odontol. Scand. 44:193.

Olson, W. C., and Hughes, B. O. (1943). Growth of the child as a whole. In Barker, R. C. Kounin, J. S., and Wright, H. F. (eds.) *Child Behavior and Development*. New York: McGraw-Hill.

Orban, B. (1944). *Oral Histology and Embryology,* 2nd ed. St. Louis, Mo.: Mosby, Table VIII, p. 240.

Pappas, G. C., Wallace, W. R. (1970). Panoramic sialography. Dent. Radiogr. Photogr. 43:27.

Proffit, W. R., et al. (1986). *Contemporary Orthodontics*. St. Louis, Mo.: Mosby, p. 67.

Richards, L., and Brown, T. (1981). Dental attrition and age relationships in Australian aboriginals. Archaeol. Oceania 16:94.

Rönnerman, A. (1977). The effect of early loss of primary molars on tooth eruption and space conditions: A longitudinal study. Acta. Odontol Scand. 35:229.

Sato, S., and Ogiwara, Y. (1971). Biostatistic study of the eruption order of deciduous teeth. Bull. Tokyo. Dent. Coll. 12:45.

Schour, I., and Massler, M. (1940). Studies in tooth development: the growth pattern of human teeth, part II. J. Am. Dent. Assoc. 27:1918.

Schour, I., and Massler, M. (1941). The development of the human dentition. J. Am. Dent. Assoc. 28:1153.

Schour, I., and Noyes, H. J. (1960). *Oral Histology and Embryology,* 8th ed. Philadelphia: Lea & Febiger.

Sessle, B. J. (1979). Mastication in man: Comments and critique. In Bryant, P., Gale, E., and Rugh, J. (eds.), *Oral Motor Behavior: Impact on Oral Conditions and Dental Treatment*. Workshop Proceedings May 16–17, 1979, U.S. Dept. HEW, PHS, NIH Publication No. 79-1845.

Smith, H. B.: (1991). Standards of human tooth formation and dental age assessment. In Kelley, M. A. and Larsen, C. S. (eds.), *Advances in Dental Anthropology*. Wiley-Liss.

Smith, H. B., and Garn, S. M. (1987). Polymorphisms in eruption sequence of permanent teeth in American children. Am. J. Phys. Anthropol. 74:289.

Sunderland, E. P., et al. (1987). A histological study of the chronology of initial mineralization in the human deciduous dentition. Arch. Oral Biol. 32:167.

Tanner, J. M. (1986). Use and abuse of growth standards. In Falkner, F., and Tanner, J. M. (eds), *Human Growth: A Comprehensive Treatise,* Vol. III, 2nd ed. New York: Plenum, p. 95.

Ubelaker, D. H. (1976). Human Skeletal Remains. Chicago: Aldine.

van der Linden, F. P. G. M., and Duterloo, H. S. (1976). *Development of the Human Dentition: An Atlas*. Hagerstown, Md.: Harper & Row.

Watson, E. H., and Lowrey, G. H. (1954). *Growth and Development of Children,* 2nd ed. Chicago: Year Book Publishers.

Wolanski, N. (1966). A new method for the evaluation of tooth formation. Acta. Genet. (Basel) 16:186.

3 *The Primary (Deciduous) Teeth*

Life Cycle

After the eruption of the primary teeth, which is completed between 3 and 4 years of age, the period of stability of the teeth is short. Some of the teeth will be found to be missing at age 4, and by age 6 as many as 19 percent may be missing (Fulton and others, 1964). By the age of 10, only about 26 percent may be present. The second molars in both arches and the maxillary incisors appear to be the most unstable of the teeth.

Importance of Primary Teeth

The general order of eruption (Fig. 3–1) of the primary dentition is central incisor, lateral incisor, first molar, canine, and second molar, with the mandibular pairs preceding the maxillary teeth. The loss of the deciduous teeth tends to mirror the eruption sequence—incisors, first molars, canines, and second molars, with the mandibular pairs preceding the maxillary teeth. The high peak for caries attack occurs at age 13, when only 5 percent of the primary teeth remain. The susceptibility to dental caries is a function of exposure time to the oral environment and morphological type. The increase in prevalence of dental caries among tooth types reverses their order of eruption. However, the relative susceptibility of different tooth surfaces is a complex problem. Although dental caries of the primary dentition and loss of these teeth are sometimes thought of erroneously as only an annoyance, this belief fails to acknowledge the role of the primary teeth in mastication and their function in maintaining the space for eruption of the permanent teeth. A lack of space associated with premature loss of deciduous teeth is a significant factor in the development of malocclusion; the development of adequate spacing (Fig. 3–2) is a significant positive factor in the development of normal occlusal relations in the permanent dentition. Thus, there should be no question of the importance of preventing and treating dental decay and providing the child with a comfortable functional occlusion of the deciduous teeth.

Therefore, in this book the primary teeth will be described in advance of the permanent dentition so that they may be given their proper sequence in the study of dental anatomy and physiology. Alignment and occlusion will be under discussion also.

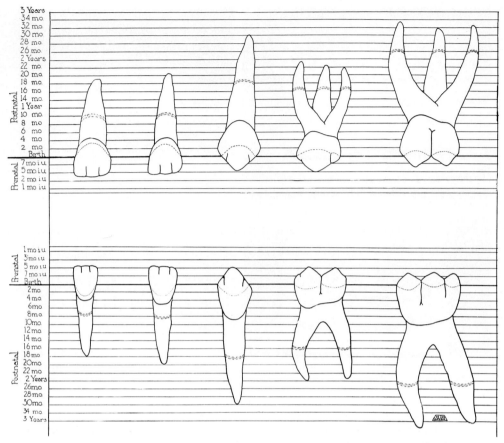

Figure 3–1. Diagrammatic representation of the chronology of the primary teeth. Eruption is completed at the approximate time indicated by the dotted area on the roots of the teeth. (Modified from McBeath, E. C.: New concept of the development and calcification of the teeth. J. Am. Dent. Assoc., 23:675, 1936; by Noyes, F. B., Schour, I., and Noyes, H. J.: *Dental Histology and Embryology,* 5th ed. Philadelphia, Lea & Febiger, 1938.)

Nomenclature

The process of exfoliation of the primary teeth takes place between the seventh and the twelfth years. This does not, however, indicate the period at which the root resorption of the deciduous tooth begins. For only a year or two after the root is completely formed and the apical foramen is established, resorption begins at the apical extermity and continues in the direction of the crown until resorption of the entire root has taken place and the crown is lost from lack of support.

The primary teeth are 20 (twenty) in number, 10 in each jaw, and they are classified as follows: four *incisors,* two *canines,* and four *molars* in each jaw. Beginning with the median line, the teeth are named in each jaw on each side of the mouth as follows: *central incisor, lateral incisor, canine, first molar,* and *second molar.*

The primary teeth have been called "temporary," "milk," and "baby" teeth. These terms are improper because they foster the implication that these teeth are useful for a short period only. It should be emphasized again that they are needed for many years of growth and physical development. Premature loss of primary teeth is to be avoided.

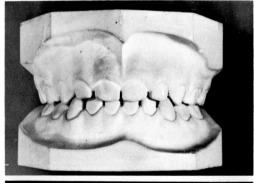

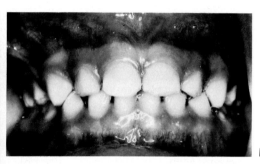

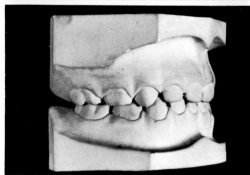

Figure 3–2. A, Cast of normally developed teeth of a child 5 years old, labial aspect. Note the form and occlusion of the teeth and their even separation. *B,* Clinical picture of a 5-year-old child showing spacing of teeth and wear of incisors, labial aspect. *C,* Cast of normally developed teeth of a child 6 years old, buccal aspect. Occlusal aspects of the casts depicted in *A* and *C* are shown in Figure 1–1.

The first permanent molar, commonly called the *6-year molar,* makes its appearance in the mouth *before any of the primary teeth are lost.* It comes in immediately distal to the primary second molar (see Fig. 3–7).

The primary dentition is complete at about 2½ years of age, and no obvious intraoral changes occur (Figs. 3–3 through 3–8) until the eruption of the first permanent molar. The position of the incisors is usually relatively upright with spacing frequently between them. Attrition occurs, and a pattern of wear may be present.

The primary molars are replaced by *permanent premolars.* There are no premolars in the primary set, and there are no teeth in the deciduous set that resemble the permanent premolar. However, the crowns of the *primary maxillary* first molars resemble the crowns of the permanent premolars as much as they do any of the permanent molars. Nevertheless, they have three well-defined roots, as do maxillary first permanent molars. The deciduous *mandibular* first molar is unique in that it has a crown form unlike that of any permanent tooth. It does, however, have two strong roots, one mesial and one distal—an arrangement similar to that of a mandibular permanent molar. These two primary teeth, the maxillary and mandibular first molars, differ from any teeth in the permanent set when crown forms are compared in particular. The primary first molars, maxillary and mandibular, will be described in detail later on.

Major Contrasts between Primary and Permanent Teeth

In comparison with their counterparts in the permanent dentition, the primary teeth are smaller in overall size and crown dimensions. They have markedly more prominent cervical ridges, are narrower at their "necks," are lighter in color, and have roots that are more widely flared; in addition, the buccolingual diameter of primary molar teeth is less

Figure 3–3. This is a picture of a remarkable specimen of a 5- to 6-year-old child. It was carefully prepared to show a full complement of primary teeth in place, the beginning of resorption of deciduous roots in some, and no apparent resorption in others. This straight front view shows the relative positions of the developing tooth crowns of the permanent anterior teeth. The maxillary central and lateral incisors and the canine are shown overlapped in a narrow space, waiting for future development of the maxilla that will allow them to develop roots and improve the alignment. See also Figures 3–4 and 3–5.

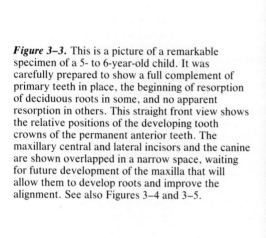

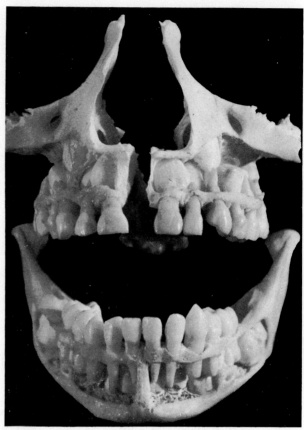

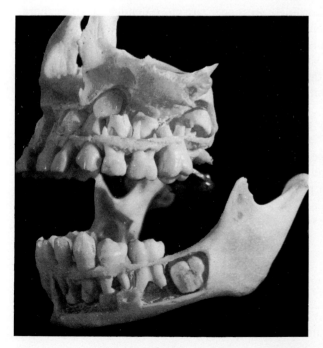

Figure 3–4. A view from the left of the specimen in Figure 3–3. Note the crowns of permanent maxillary premolars located between the roots of first and second primary molars, with their roots still intact. Another interesting observation is the well-developed first permanent maxillary molar entirely erupted with half its roots formed. Ordinarily, the mandibular first permanent molar comes in and takes its place first, the maxillary molar following. The specimen shows the mandibular molar still covered with bone and no roots in evidence. The maxillary second molar crown is well developed and located in a place that is about level with the present root development of the permanent maxillary first molar.

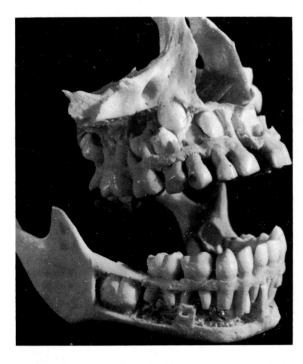

Figure 3–5. This picture of the specimen shown in Figure 3–3 was taken from the right side and slightly forward. It makes an interesting study from a different aspect. It does show the developing anterior maxillary crowns a little better. Unless they were lost in preparation, no development shows of mandibular permanent premolars. The tiny cusps formed at this age would be lost easily in preparation.

than that of permanent teeth. More specifically, in comparison with permanent teeth, the following differences are noted:

1. The crowns of primary anterior teeth are wider mesiodistally in comparison with their crown length than are the permanent teeth.
2. The roots of primary anterior teeth are narrower and longer comparatively. Narrow roots with wide crowns present an arrangement at the cervical third of crown and root that differs markedly from the permanent anterior teeth.
3. The roots of the primary molars accordingly are longer, are more slender, and flare more, extending out beyond projected outlines of the crowns. This flare allows more room between the roots for the development of permanent tooth crowns (see Figs. 3–24 and 3–25).
4. The cervical ridges of enamel of the anterior teeth are more prominent. These bulges must be considered seriously when they are involved in any operative procedure (see Fig. 3–17).
5. The crowns and roots of primary molars at their cervical portions are more slender mesiodistally.
6. The cervical ridges buccally on the primary molars are much more pronounced, especially on first molars, maxillary and mandibular (see Figs. 3–28 through 3–31).
7. The buccal and lingual surfaces of primary molars are flatter above the cervical curvatures than those of permanent molars, thereby narrowing the occlusal surfaces.
8. The primary teeth are usually less pigmented and are whiter in appearance than the permanent teeth.

Pulp Chambers and Pulp Canals

A comparison of sections of primary and permanent teeth demonstrates the shape and relative size of pulp chambers and canals (Fig. 3–9).

A   B

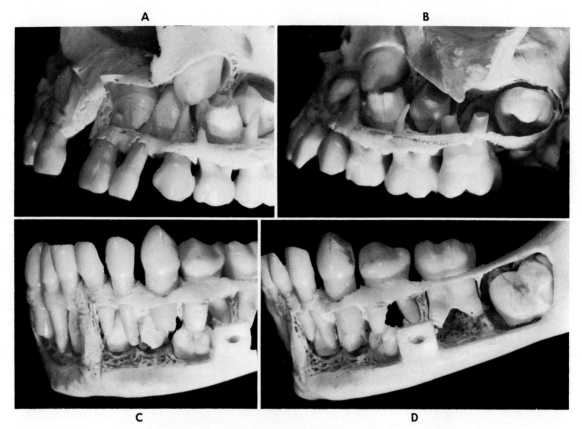

C   D

Figure 3–6. A, A sectional close-up of Figure 3–3. This section is somewhat anterior to the left side of the maxilla. The developing crowns of the central and lateral incisors, the canine and two premolars are clearly in view.

B, The left side of the maxilla of the specimen, taken from an angle posteriorly. The molar relationship, both deciduous and permanent, is accented here.

C, This angle of the specimen in Figure 3–3 presents a good view of the mandible anteriorly and to the left. Permanent central and lateral incisors and the canine may be seen. Notice that the permanent canine develops distally to the primary canine root.

D, Posteriorly, examination of the specimen mandible fails to find crown development of permanent premolars. However, the hollow spaces showing between the roots of primary molars may indicate a loss of material during the difficult process of dissection. The first permanent molar has progressed in crown formation, but the maturation of the whole tooth with alignment is far behind its opposition in the maxilla above it (see Fig. 3–4).

1. Crown widths in all directions are large in comparison with root trunks and cervices.
2. The enamel is relatively thin and has a consistent depth.
3. The dentin thickness between the pulp chambers and the enamel is limited, particularly in some areas (lower second deciduous molar).
4. The pulpal horns are high and pulp chambers are large (Fig. 3–10).
5. Primary roots are narrow and long when compared with crown width and length.
6. Molar roots of primary teeth flare markedly and thin out rapidly as the apices are approached.

It is well, at all times, to study the comparisons between the deciduous and the permanent dentitions (Figs. 3–11 and 3–12). Further variations between the macroscopic form of the deciduous and the permanent teeth will follow, with a detailed description of each deciduous tooth.

Text continued on page 56

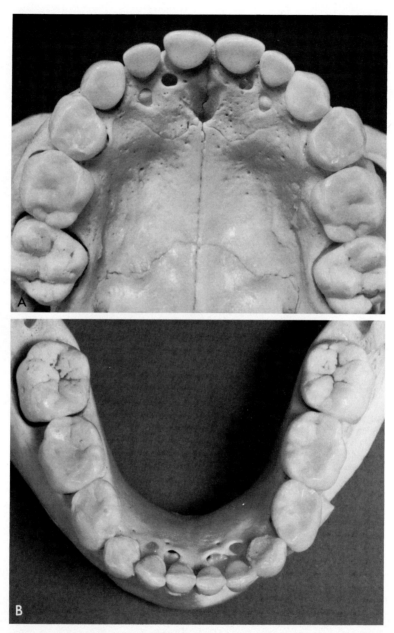

Figure 3–7. *A,* Maxillary teeth of child with full complement of primary teeth and first permanent molars. *B,* Mandibular teeth of same child with primary teeth and first permanent molars.

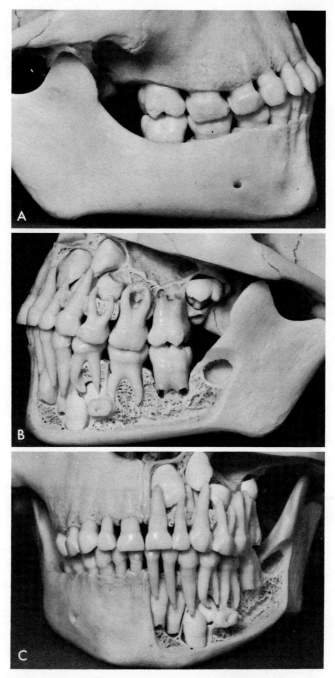

Figure 3–8. Same child as in Figure 3–7. *A*, From right side.
B, From front view with bone covering roots and developing
permanent teeth removed on left side. *C*, From left side showing
position of first and second permanent molars. Developing second
molar crown has been lost from its bony crypt during preparation
of the specimen.

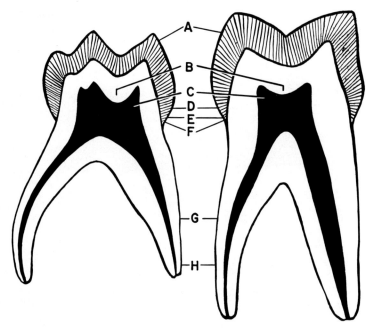

Figure 3–9. Comparison of maxillary, primary, and permanent second molars, linguobuccal cross section.

    A, The enamel cap of primary molars is thinner and has a more consistent depth.

    B, There is a comparatively greater thickness of dentin over the pulpal wall at the occlusal fossa of primary molars.

    C, The pulpal horns are higher in primary molars, especially the mesial horns, and pulp chambers are proportionately larger.

    D, The cervical ridges are more pronounced, especially on the buccal aspect of the first primary molars.

    E, The enamel rods at the cervix slope occlusally instead of gingivally as in the permanent teeth.

    F, The primary molars have a markedly constricted neck compared with the permanent molars.

    G, The roots of the primary teeth are longer and more slender in comparison with crown size than those of the permanent teeth.

    H, The roots of the primary molars flare out nearer the cervix than do those of the permanent teeth.
(From Finn, S. B.: *Clinical Pedodontics,* 2nd ed. Philadelphia, W. B. Saunders Company, 1957.)

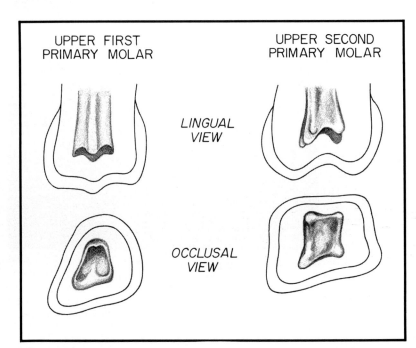

Figure 3–10. *A. See legend on opposite page*

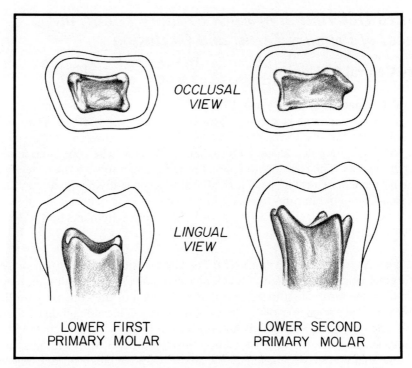

OCCLUSAL
VIEW

LINGUAL
VIEW

LOWER FIRST
PRIMARY MOLAR

LOWER SECOND
PRIMARY MOLAR

Figure 3–10. *A, B,* Pulp chambers in the primary molars. Note the contours of the pulp horns within them. (Modified from Finn, S. B.: *Clinical Pedodontics,* 2nd ed. Philadelphia, W. B. Saunders Company, 1957.)

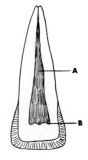

Figure 3–11. Permanent central incisor. This figure represents a sectioned central incisor of a young person. Although the pulp canal is rather large, it is smaller than the pulp canal shown in Figure 3–12 and it becomes more constricted apically. Note the dentin space between the pulp horns and the incisal edge of the crown. *A,* Pulp canal; *B,* pulp horn.

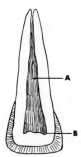

Figure 3–12. Primary central incisor. This figure represents a sectioned primary central incisor. The pulp chamber with its horns and the pulp canal are broader than those found in Figure 3–11. The apical portion of the canal is much less constricted than that of the permanent tooth. Note the narrow dentin space incisally. *A,* Pulp canal; *B,* pulp horns.

A Detailed Description of Each Primary Tooth, the Alignment of Primary Teeth, and Occlusion

Maxillary Central Incisor

Labial Aspect (Figs. 3–13 and 13–14). In the crown of the primary central incisor, the mesiodistal diameter is greater than the cervicoincisal length. (The opposite is true of permanent central incisors.) The labial surface is very smooth, and the incisal edge is nearly straight. Developmental lines are usually not seen. The root is cone-shaped with even, tapered sides. The root length is greater in comparison with the crown length than that of the permanent central incisor. It is advisable when studying the primary teeth, and also the permanent teeth later on, to make direct comparisons between the table of measurements of the primary teeth (Table 3–1) and the table of measurements for the permanent teeth (see also Table 1–1).

Lingual Aspect (Figs. 3–3 and 3–15). The lingual aspect of the crown shows well-developed marginal ridges and a highly developed cingulum. The cingulum extends up toward the incisal ridge far enough to make a partial division of the concavity on the lingual surface below the incisal edge, practically dividing it into a mesial and distal fossa.

The root narrows lingually and presents a ridge for its full length in comparison with a flatter surface labially. A cross section through the root where it joins the crown shows an outline that is somewhat triangular in shape, with the labial surface making one side of the triangle and mesial and distal surfaces making up the other two sides.

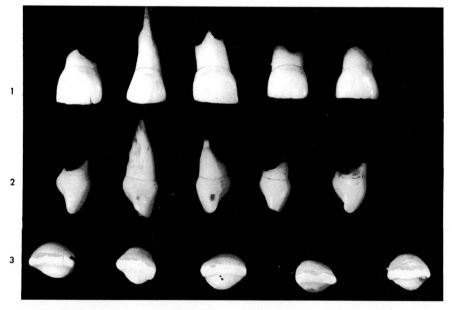

Figure 3–13. Primary maxillary central incisors (first incisors).
1, Labial aspect. Note the lack of character in the mold form; also note the mesiodistal width when compared with the shorter crown length. A little of the crown length was lost through abrasion before the date of extraction.
2, Mesial aspect. The cervical ridges are quite prominent labially and lingually, with the bulge much greater than that found on permanent incisors. This characteristic is common to each primary tooth to a varied degree. Normally, these curvatures are covered by gum tissue with epithelial attachment. (See Chapter 5.)
3, Incisal aspect.

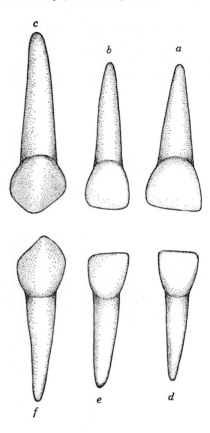

Figure 3–14. Primary right anterior teeth, labial aspect.
a, Maxillary central incisor. *b*, Maxillary lateral incisor.
c, Maxillary canine. *d*, Mandibular central incisor. *e*, Mandibular
lateral incisor. *f*, Mandibular canine.

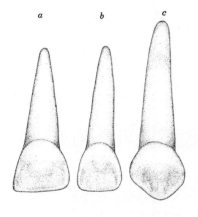

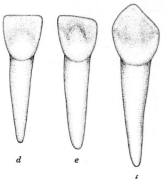

Figure 3–15. Primary right anterior teeth, lingual aspect. *a*, Maxillary central
incisor. *b*, Maxillary lateral incisor. *c*, Maxillary canine. *d*, Mandibular central
incisor. *e*, Mandibular lateral incisor. *f*, Mandibular canine.

Table 3–1. Table of Measurements of the Primary Teeth of Man (Averages Only)*

	Length Overall	Length of Crown	Length of Root	Mesio-distal Diameter of Crown	Mesio-distal Diameter at Cervix	Labio-lingual Diameter of Crown	Labio-lingual Diameter at Cervix
Upper Teeth							
Central Incisor	16.0†	6.0	10.0	6.5	4.5	5.0	4.0
Lateral Incisor	15.8	5.6	11.4	5.1	3.7	4.0	3.7
Canine	19.0	6.5	13.5	7.0	5.1	7.0	5.5
First Molar	15.2	5.1	10.0	7.3	5.2	8.5	6.9
Second Molar	17.5	5.7	11.7	8.2	6.4	10.0	8.3
Lower Teeth							
Central Incisor	14.0	5.0	9.0	4.2	3.0	4.0	3.5
Lateral Incisor	15.0	5.2	10.0	4.1	3.0	4.0	3.5
Canine	17.5	6.0	11.5	5.0	3.7	4.8	4.0
First Molar	15.8	6.0	9.8	7.7	6.5	7.0	5.3
Second Molar	18.8	5.5	11.3	9.9	7.2	8.7	6.4

* From Black, G. V.: *Descriptive Anatomy of the Human Teeth*, 4th ed. Philadelphia, S. S. White Dental Manufacturing Co., 1897.
† Millimeters.

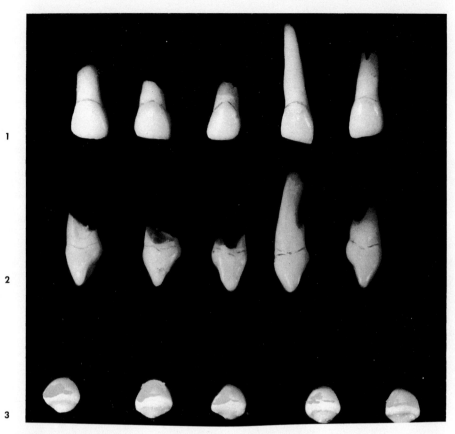

Figure 3–16. Primary maxillary lateral incisors (second incisors).
1, Labial aspect.
2, Mesial aspect.
3, Incisal aspect.

Mesial and Distal Aspects (Figs. 3–13 and 3–17). The mesial and distal aspects of the primary maxillary central incisors are similar. The measurement of the crown at the cervical third shows the crown from this aspect to be wide in relation to its total length. The average measurement will be only about 1 mm less than the entire crown length cervicoincisally. Because of the short crown and its labiolingual measurement, the crown appears thick at the middle third and even down toward the incisal third. The *curvature of cervical line,* which represents the *cementoenamel junction,* is distinct, curving toward the incisal ridge. However, the curvature is not as great as that found on its permanent successor. The cervical curvature distally is less than the amount of curvature mesially, a design that compares favorably with the permanent central incisor.

Although the root from this aspect appears more blunt than it did from the labial and lingual aspects, still it is of an even taper and is the shape of a long cone. It is, however, blunt at the apex. Usually the mesial surface of the root will have a developmental groove or concavity, whereas distally the surface is generally convex.

Note the development of the cervical ridges of enamel at the cervical third of the crown labially and lingually.

Incisal Aspect (Figs. 3–3 and 3–13). An important feature to note from the incisal aspect is the measurement mesiodistally as compared with the measurement labiolingually. The incisal edge is centered over the main bulk of the crown and is relatively straight. Looking

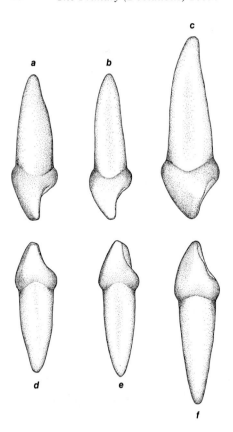

Figure 3–17. Primary right anterior teeth, mesial aspect. *a*, Maxillary central incisor. *b*, Maxillary lateral incisor. *c*, Maxillary canine. *d*, Mandibular central incisor. *e*, Mandibular lateral incisor. *f*, Mandibular canine.

down on the incisal edge, we see that the labial surface is much broader and also smoother than the lingual surface. The lingual surface tapers toward the cingulum.

The mesial and the distal surfaces of this tooth are relatively broad. The mesial and distal surfaces toward the incisal ridge or at the incisal third are generous enough to make good contact areas with the adjoining teeth, although this facility is used for a short period only because of rapid changes that take place in the jaws of children.

Maxillary Lateral Incisor (Figs. 3–14 through 3–18)

In general, the maxillary lateral is similar to the central incisor from all aspects, but its dimensions differ. Its crown is smaller in all directions. The cervicoincisal length of the lateral crown is greater than its mesiodistal width. The distoincisal angles of the crown are more rounded than those of the central incisor. Although the root has a similar shape, it is much longer in proportion to its crown than the central ratio indicates when a comparison is made.

Maxillary Canine (Fig. 3–19)

Labial Aspect (Fig. 3–14, *C*). Except for the root form, the labial aspect of the maxillary canine does not resemble either the central or the lateral incisor. The crown is more constricted at the cervix in relation to its mesiodistal width, and the mesial and distal

Figure 3–18. Primary right anterior teeth, incisal aspect. *a,* Maxillary central incisor; *b,* Maxillary lateral incisor; *c,* Maxillary canine; *d,* Mandibular central incisor; *e,* Mandibular lateral incisor; *f,* Mandibular canine.

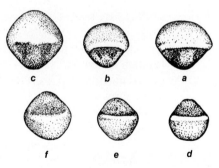

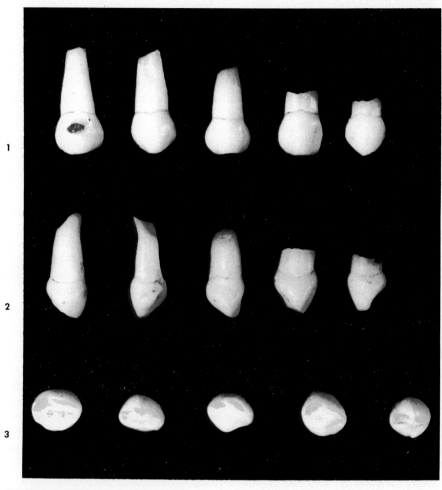

Figure 3–19. Primary maxillary canines.
1, Labial aspect.
2, Mesial aspect.
3, Incisal aspect.

surfaces are more convex. Instead of an incisal edge that is relatively straight, it has a long, well-developed, and sharp cusp.

Compared with that of the permanent maxillary canine, the cusp on the primary canine is much longer and sharper, and the crest of contour mesially is not as far down toward the incisal portion. A line drawn through the contact areas of the deciduous canine would bisect a line drawn from the cervix to the tip of the cusp. In the *permanent* canine, the contact areas are not at the same level. When the cusp is intact the mesial slope of the cusp will be longer than the distal slope.

The root of the primary canine is long, slender, and tapering and is more than twice the crown length.

Lingual Aspect (Fig. 3–15, *C*). The lingual aspect shows pronounced enamel ridges that merge with each other. They are the cingulum, mesial and distal marginal ridges, and incisal cusp ridges, besides a tubercle at the cusp tip, which is a continuation of the lingual ridge connecting the cingulum and the cusp tip. This lingual ridge divides the lingual surface into shallow mesiolingual and distolingual fossae.

The root of this tooth tapers lingually. It is usually inclined distally also above the middle third (Figs. 3–14, *C*, and 3–17, *C*.)

Mesial Aspect (Fig. 3–17, *C*). From the mesial aspect, the outline form is similar to that of the lateral and central incisors. However, there is a difference in proportion. The measurement labiolingually at the cervical third is much greater. This increase in crown dimension, in conjunction with the root width and length, permits resistance against forces the tooth must withstand during function. The function of this tooth is to punch, tear, and apprehend food material.

Distal Aspect. The distal outline of this tooth is the reverse of the mesial aspect. No outstanding differences may be noted except that the curvature of the cervical line toward the cusp ridge is less than on the mesial surface.

Incisal Aspect (Fig. 3–18, *C*). From the incisal aspect, we observe that the crown is essentially diamond-shaped. The angles that are found at the contact areas mesially and distally, at the cingulum on the lingual surface, and at the cervical third, or enamel ridge, on the labial surface are more pronounced and less rounded in effect than are those found on the permanent canines. The tip of the cusp is distal to the center of the crown, and the mesial cusp slope is longer than the distal cusp slope. This allows for intercuspation with the lower, or mandibular, canine, which has its longest slope distally (Fig. 3–14).

Mandibular Central Incisor (Fig. 3–20)

Labial Aspect (Fig. 3–14, *D*). The labial aspect of this crown has a flat face with no developmental grooves. The mesial and distal sides of the crown are tapered evenly from the contact areas, the measurement being less at the cervix. This crown is wide in proportion to its length in comparison with that of its permanent successor. The heavy look at the root trunk makes this small tooth resemble the permanent maxillary lateral incisor.

The root of the primary central incisor is long and is evenly tapered down to the apex, which is pointed. The root is almost twice the length of the crown.

Lingual Aspect (Fig. 3–15, *D*). On the lingual surface of the crown, the marginal ridges and the cingulum may be located easily. The lingual surface of the crown at the middle third and

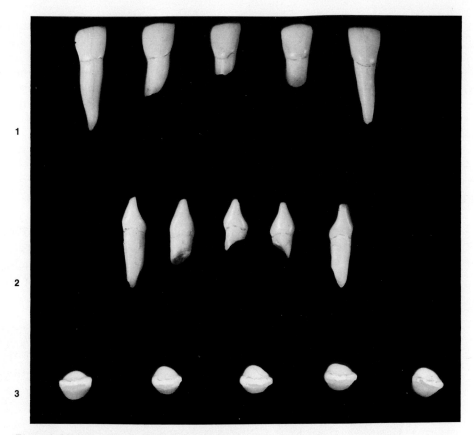

Figure 3–20. Primary mandibular central incisors.
1, Labial aspect.
2, Mesial aspect.
3, Incisal aspect.

the incisal third may have a flattened surface level with the marginal ridges, or it may present a slight concavity, called the *lingual fossa*. The lingual portion of the crown and root converges so that it is narrower toward the lingual than toward the labial surface.

Mesial Aspect (Fig. 3–17, *D*). The mesial aspect shows the typical outline of an incisor tooth even though the measurements are small. The incisal ridge is centered over the center of the root and between the crest of curvature of the crown, labially, and lingually. The convexity of the cervical contours labially and lingually at the cervical third is just as pronounced as in any of the other primary incisors and more pronounced by far than the prominences found at the same locations on a permanent mandibular central incisor. As mentioned before, these cervical bulges are important.

Although this tooth is small, its labiolingual measurement is only about a millimeter less than that of the primary maxillary central incisor. The primary incisors seem to be built for strenuous service.

The mesial surface of the root is nearly flat and is evenly tapered; the apex presents a more blunt appearance than is found when one observes the lingual or labial aspects.

Distal Aspect. The outline of this tooth from the distal aspect is the reverse of that found from the mesial aspect. There is little difference to be noted between these aspects except that the cervical line of the crown is less curved toward the incisal ridge than that found on the mesial surface. Often there is a developmental depression on the distal side of the root.

Incisal Aspect (Fig. 3–18, D). The incisal ridge is straight and bisects the crown labio-lingually. The outline of the crown from the incisal aspect emphasizes the crests of contour at the cervical third labially and lingually. There is a definite taper toward the cingulum on the lingual side.

The labial surface from this view presents a flat surface slightly convex, whereas the lingual surface presents a flattened surface slightly concave.

Mandibular Lateral Incisor (Figs. 3–14, 3–15, 3–17, 3–18)

The fundamental outlines of the primary mandibular lateral incisor (Fig. 3–21) are similar to those of the primary central incisor. These two teeth supplement each other in function. The lateral incisor is somewhat larger in all measurements except the labiolingual, where the two teeth are practically identical. The cingulum of the lateral incisor may be a little

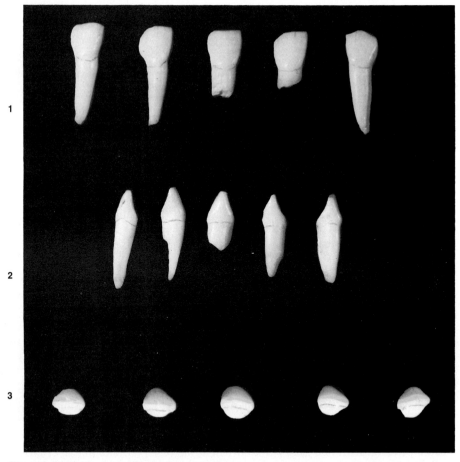

Figure 3–21. Primary mandibular lateral incisors.
1, Labial aspect.
2, Mesial aspect.
3, Incisal aspect.

more generous than that of the central incisor, and the lingual surface of the crown between the marginal ridges may be more concave. In addition, there is a tendency for the incisal ridge to slope downward distally. This design lowers the distal contact area apically in order that proper contact may be made with the mesial surface of the primary mandibular canine.

Mandibular Canine (Figs. 3–14, 3–15, 3–17, 3–18)

There is very little difference in functional form between this tooth and the maxillary canine. The difference is mainly in the dimensions. The crown is perhaps 0.5 mm shorter, and the root is at least 2 mm shorter; the mesiodistal measurement of the mandibular canine at the root trunk is greater when compared with its mesiodistal measurement at the contact areas than is the maxillary canine (Fig. 3–22). It is "thicker" accordingly at the "neck" of the tooth. The outstanding variation in size between the two deciduous canines is shown by the labiolingual calibration. The deciduous maxillary canine is much larger labiolingually (Fig. 3–17).

The cervical ridges labially and lingually are not quite as pronounced as those found on the maxillary canine. The greatest variation in outline form when one compares the two teeth is seen from the labial and lingual aspects; the distal cusp slope is longer than the mesial slope. The opposite arrangement is true of the maxillary canine. This makes for proper intercuspation of these teeth during mastication.

Figure 3–23 presents the primary mandibular canines.

Maxillary First Molar

Buccal Aspect (Fig. 3–24, A). The widest measurement of the crown of the maxillary first molar is at the contact areas mesially and distally. From these points, the crown converges toward the cervix, the measurement at the cervix being fully 2 mm less than the measure-

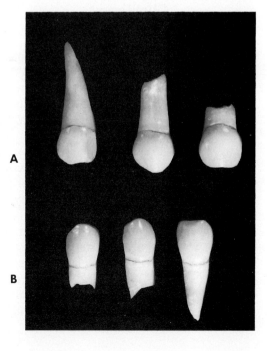

Figure 3–22. A comparison of primary canines, both in the size and shape of the crowns. Two of them have their roots intact and show no dissolution. *A,* Maxillary canines. *B,* Mandibular canines. Compare Figures 3–19 and 3–23.

A

B

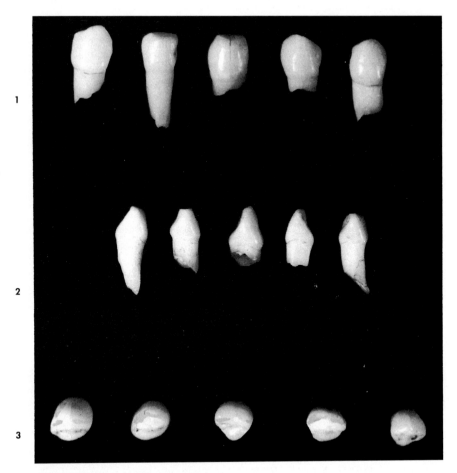

Figure 3–23. Primary mandibular canines.
1, Labial aspect.
2, Mesial aspect.
3, Incisial aspect.

ment at the contact areas. This dimensional arrangement furnishes a narrower look to the cervical portion of the crown and root of the primary maxillary first molar than that of the same portion of the permanent maxillary first molar. The occlusal line is slightly scalloped but with no definite cusp form. The buccal surface is smooth, and there is little evidence of developmental grooves. It is from this aspect that one may judge the relative size of the primary maxillary first molar when it is compared with the second molar. It is much smaller in all measurements than the second molar. Its relative shape and size suggest that it was designed to be the "premolar section" of the primary dentition. In function it acts as a compromise between the size and shape of the anterior primary teeth and the molar area; this area being held temporarily by the larger primary second molar. At 6 years of age, the large first permanent molar is expected to take its place distal to the second primary molar, which will complete a more extensive molar area for masticating efficiency.

The *roots* of the maxillary first molar are slender and long, and they spread widely. All three roots may be seen from this aspect. The distal root is considerably shorter than the mesial one. The bifurcation of the roots begins almost immediately at the site of the cervical line (cementoenamel junction). Actually, this arrangement is in effect for the entire root trunk, which includes a "trifurcation," and this is a characteristic of all primary molars, maxillary and mandibular.

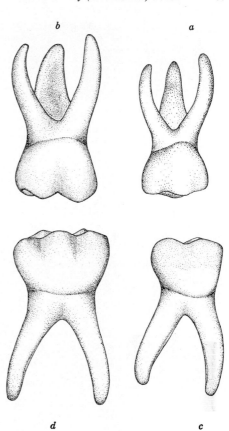

Figure 3–24. Primary right molars, buccal aspect. *a,* Maxillary first molar; *b,* Maxillary second molar; *c,* Mandibular first molar; *d,* Mandibular second molar.

This characteristic is not possessed by permanent molars. The root trunk on all permanent molars is much heavier, with a greater calibration between the cervical line and the points of bifurcation (see Figs. 11–7 and 11–8).

Lingual Aspect (Fig. 3–25, A). The general outline of the lingual aspect of the crown is similar to the buccal aspect. The crown converges considerably in a lingual direction, making the lingual portion calibrate less mesiodistally than the buccal portion.

The mesiolingual cusp is the most prominent cusp on this tooth. It is the longest and sharpest cusp. The distolingual cusp is poorly defined: it is small and rounded when it exists at all. From the lingual aspect, the distobuccal cusp may be seen, since it is longer and better developed than the distolingual cusp. There is a type of primary maxillary first molar that is not uncommon and that presents one large lingual cusp with no developmental groove in evidence lingually. This type is apparently a three-cusped molar (see Fig. 3–28, division 4, second from left).

All three roots may be seen from this aspect also. The lingual root is larger than the others.

Mesial Aspect (Fig. 3–26, A). From the mesial aspect, the dimension at the cervical third is greater than the dimension at the occlusal third. This is true of all molar forms, but it is more pronounced on primary teeth than on permanent teeth. The mesiolingual cusp is longer and sharper than the mesiobuccal cusp. There is a pronounced convexity on the buccal outline in the cervical third. This convexity is an outstanding characteristic of this tooth. Actually, it gives the impression of overdevelopment in this area when comparisons are made with

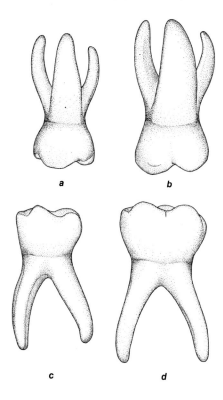

Figure 3–25. Primary right molars, lingual aspect. *a*, Maxillary first molar. *b*, Maxillary second molar. *c*, Mandibular first molar. *d*, Mandibular second molar.

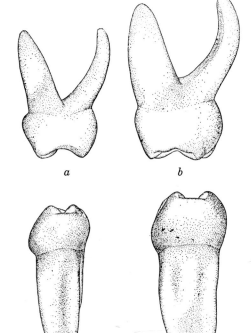

Figure 3–26. Primary right molars, mesial aspect. *a*, Maxillary first molar. *b*, Maxillary second molar. *c*, Mandibular first molar. *d*, Mandibular second molar.

any other tooth, primary or permanent, the mandibular first primary molar being a close contender. The cervical line mesially shows some curvature in the direction of the occlusal surface.

The mesiobuccal and lingual roots are visible only when we look at the mesial side of this tooth from a point directly opposite the contact area. The distobuccal root is hidden behind the mesiobuccal root. The lingual root from this aspect looks long and slender and extends lingually to a marked degree. It curves sharply in a buccal direction above the middle third.

Distal Aspect. From the distal aspect, the crown is narrower distally than mesially; it tapers markedly toward the distal (Fig. 3–27, *A*). The distobuccal cusp is long and sharp, and the distolingual cusp is poorly developed. The prominent bulge seen from the mesial aspect at the cervical third does not continue distally. The cervical line may curve occlusally, or it

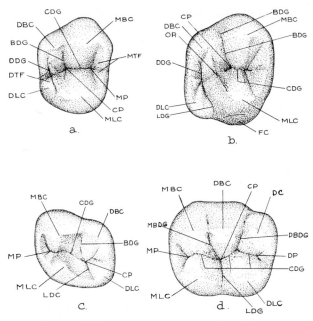

Figure 3–27. a, Maxillary first molar. *MBC,* Mesiobuccal cusp; *MTF,* mesial triangular fossa; *MP,* mesial pit; *CP,* central pit; *MLC,* mesiolingual cusp; *DLC,* distolingual cusp; *DTF, distal triangular fossa; DDG, distal developmental groove; BDG,* buccal developmental groove; *DBC,* distobuccal cusp; *CDG,* central developmental groove.

b, Maxillary second molar. *BDG,* Buccal developmental groove; *MBC,* mesiobuccal cusp; *CDG,* central developmental groove; *MLC,* mesiolingual cusp; *FC,* fifth cusp; *LDG,* lingual developmental groove; *DLC,* distolingual cusp; *DDG,* distal developmental groove; *OR,* oblique ridge; *DBC,* distobuccal cusp; *CP,* central pit.

c, Mandibular first molar. *CDG,* Central developmental groove; *DBC,* distobuccal cusp; *BDG,* buccal developmental groove; *CP,* central pit; *DLC,* distolingual cusp; *LDC,* lingual developmental groove; *MLC,* mesiolingual cusp; *MP,* mesial pit; *MBC,* mesiobuccal cusp.

d, Mandibular second molar. *DBC,* Distobuccal cusp; *CP,* central pit; *DC,* distal cusp; *DBDG,* distobuccal developmental groove; *DP,* distal pit; *CDG,* central developmental groove; *DLC,* distolingual cusp; *LDG,* lingual developmental groove; *MLC,* mesiolingual cusp; *MP,* mesial pit; *MBDG,* mesiobuccal developmental groove; *MBC,* mesiobuccal cusp.

may extend straight across from the buccal surface to the lingual surface. All three roots may be seen from this angle, but the distobuccal root is superimposed on the mesiobuccal root so that only the buccal surface and the apex of the latter may be seen. The point of bifurcation of the distobuccal root and the lingual root is near the cementoenamel junction as described heretofore as being typical.

Occlusal Aspect (Fig. 3–27, *A*). The calibration of the distance between the mesiobuccal line angle and the distobuccal line angle is definitely greater than the calibration between the mesiolingual line angle and the distolingual line angle. Therefore, the crown outline converges lingually. Also, the calibration from the mesiobuccal line angle to the mesio-lingual line angle is definitely greater than that found at the distal line angles. Therefore, the crown converges distally also. Nevertheless, these convergencies are not reflected entirely in the working occlusal surface because it is more nearly rectangular with the shortest sides of the rectangle represented by the marginal ridges. The occlusal surface is more nearly rectangular, with the shortest side of the rectangle represented by the marginal ridges.

The occlusal surface has a *central fossa*. There is a *mesial triangular fossa*, just inside the mesial marginal ridge, with a mesial pit in this fossa and a sulcus with its central groove connecting the two fossae. There is also a well-defined *buccal developmental groove* dividing the mesiobuccal cusp and the distobuccal cusp occlusally. There are supplemental grooves radiating from the pit in the mesial triangular fossa. These grooves radiate as follows: one buccally, one lingually, and one toward the marginal ridge, the last sometimes extending over the marginal ridge mesially.

Sometimes the primary maxillary first molar has a well-defined triangular ridge connecting the mesiolingual cusp with the distobuccal cusp. When well developed, it is called the *oblique ridge*. In some of these teeth, the ridge will be very indefinite and the central developmental groove will extend from the mesial pit to the *distal developmental groove*. This disto-occlusal groove is always seen and may or may not extend through to the lingual surface, outlining a distolingual cusp. The distal marginal ridge is thin and poorly developed in comparison with the mesial marginal ridge.

Summary of the Occlusal Aspect of This Tooth. The form of the maxillary first primary molar varies from that of any tooth in the permanent dentition. Although there are no premolars in the primary set, in some respects the crown of this primary molar resembles a permanent maxillary premolar. Nevertheless, the divisions of the occlusal surface and the root form with its efficient anchorage make it a molar, both in type and function. Figure 3–28 presents all the aspects of the primary maxillary first molars.

Maxillary Second Molar

Buccal Aspect (Figs. 3–24, *B*, and 3–29, *1*). The primary maxillary second molar has characteristics resembling the *permanent* maxillary first molar, but it is smaller (Fig. 3–3).

The buccal view of this tooth shows two well-defined buccal cusps with a buccal developmental groove between them. In line with all primary molars, the crown is narrow at the cervix in comparison with its mesiodistal measurement at the contact areas. This crown is much larger than that of the first primary molar. Although the roots, from this aspect, appear slender, they are much longer and heavier than those that are a part of the maxillary first molar. The point of bifurcation between the buccal roots is close to the cervical line of the crown. The two buccal cusps are more nearly equal in size and development than those of the primary maxillary first molar.

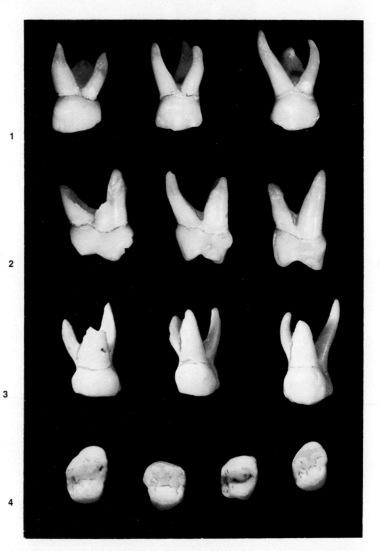

Figure 3–28. Primary maxillary first molars.

1, Buccal aspect. Note the flare of roots.

2, Mesial aspect. The cervical ridge on the buccal surface is curved to the extreme. Also note the flat or concave buccal surface above this bulge as it approaches the occlusal surface.

3, Lingual aspect.

4, Occlusal aspect. This aspect emphasizes the extensive width of the mesial portion of primary first molars.

The four specimens show size differentials even in deciduous teeth (see Fig. 3–27).

Lingual Aspect (Fig. 3–25, *B*). Lingually, the crown shows three cusps: (1) the mesiolingual cusp, which is large and well developed; (2) the distolingual cusp, which is well developed (more so than that of the primary first molar), and (3) a third supplemental cusp, which is apical to the mesiolingual cusp and which is sometimes called the *tubercle of Carabelli,* or the fifth cusp. This cusp is poorly developed and merely acts as a buttress or supplement to the bulk of the mesiolingual cusp. If the tubercle of Carabelli seems to be missing, some traces of developmental lines or "dimples" will remain (Fig. 3–29, division *3*). A well-defined developmental groove separates the mesiolingual cusp from the distolingual cusp and connects with the developmental groove, which outlines the fifth cusp.

All three roots are visible from this aspect; the lingual root is large and thick in comparison with the other two roots. It is approximately the same length as the mesio-buccal root. If it should differ, it will be on the short side.

Mesial Aspect (Fig. 3–26, *B*). From the mesial aspect, the crown has a typical molar outline that resembles that of the permanent molars very much. The crown appears short because of its width buccolingually in comparison with its length. The crown of this tooth is usually

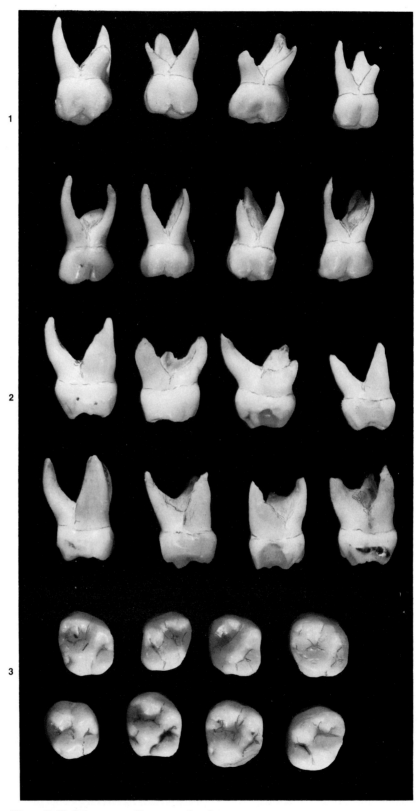

Figure 3–29. Primary maxillary second molars.
1, Buccal aspect.
2, Mesial aspect.
3, Occlusal aspect.

only about 0.5 mm longer than the crown of the first deciduous molar, but the buccolingual measurement is 1.5 to 2 mm greater. In addition, the roots are 1.5 to 2 mm longer. The mesiolingual cusp of the crown with its supplementary fifth cusp appears large in comparison with the mesiobuccal cusp. The mesiobuccal cusp from this angle is relatively short and sharp. There is very little curvature to the cervical line. Usually, it is almost straight across from buccal surface to lingual surface.

The mesiobuccal root from this aspect is broad and flat. The lingual root has somewhat the same curvature as the lingual root of the maxillary first deciduous molar.

The mesiobuccal root extends lingually far out beyond the crown outline. The point of bifurcation between the mesiobuccal root and the lingual root is 2 or 3 mm apical to the cervical line of the crown; this differs in depth on the root trunk from comparisons of this area in the recent discussion of primary molars. The mesiobuccal root presents itself as being quite wide from the mesial aspect. It will measure approximately two thirds the width of the root trunk, leaving one third for the lingual root. The mesiolingual cusp is directly below their bifurcation. Although the curvature lingually on the crown from this aspect is strong at the cervical portion, as on most deciduous teeth, the crest of curvature buccally at the cervical third is nominal and resembles the curvature found at this point on the permanent maxillary first molar. In this it differs entirely from the prominent curvature found on the primary maxillary first molars at the cervical third buccally.

Distal Aspect. From the distal aspect, it is apparent that the distal calibration of the crown is less than the mesial measurement but there is not the variation found on the crown of the deciduous maxilllary first molar. From both the distal and the mesial aspects, the outline of the crown lingually creates a smooth rounded line, whereas a line describing the buccal surface is almost straight from the crest of curvature to the tip of the buccal cusp. The distobuccal cusp and the distolingual cusp are about the same in length. The cervical line is approximately straight, as was found mesially.

All three roots are seen from this aspect, although only a part of the outline of the mesiobuccal root may be seen, since the distobuccal root is superimposed over it. The distobuccal root is shorter and narrower than the other roots. The point of bifurcation between the distobuccal root and the lingual root is more apical in location than any of the other points of bifurcation. The point of bifurcation between these two roots on the distal is more nearly centered above the crown than that on the mesial between the mesiobuccal and lingual roots.

Occlusal Aspect (Figs. 3–27, *B*; 3–29). From the occlusal aspect, this tooth resembles the permanent first molar. It is somewhat rhomboidal and has four well-developed cusps and one supplemental cusp: mesiobuccal, distobuccal, mesiolingual, distolingual, and fifth cusps. The buccal surface is rather flat, with the developmental groove between the cusps less marked than that found on the first permanent molar. Developmental grooves, pits, oblique ridge, and so forth, are almost identical. The character of the ''mold'' is constant.

The occlusal surface has a *central fossa* with a *central pit,* a well-defined *mesial triangular fossa,* just distal to the *mesial marginal ridge,* with a mesial pit at its center. There is, too, a well-defined developmental groove called the *central groove* at the bottom of a sulcus connecting the mesial triangular fossa with the central fossa. The *buccal developmental groove* extends buccally from the central pit, separating the triangular ridges, which are occlusal continuations of the mesio- and distobuccal cusps. Supplemental grooves often radiate from these developmental grooves.

The *oblique ridge* is prominent and connects the mesiolingual cusp with the distobuccal cusp. Distal to the oblique ridge one finds the *distal fossa,* which harbors the *distal developmental groove.* The distal groove has branches of supplemental grooves within the *distal triangular fossa*, which is rather indefinitely outlined just mesial to the distal marginal ridge.

The distal groove acts as a line of demarcation between the mesiolingual and distolingual cusps and continues on to the lingual surface as the *lingual developmental groove*. The *distal marginal ridge* is as well developed as the *mesial marginal ridge*. It will be remembered that the marginal ridges are not developed equally on the primary maxillary first molar.

Mandibular First Molar

This tooth does not resemble any of the other teeth, deciduous or permanent. Because it varies so much from all others, it appears strange and primitive.

Buccal Aspect (Figs. 3–24, *C* and 3–31, *A*). From the buccal aspect, the mesial outline of the crown of the primary mandibular first molar is almost straight from the contact area to the cervix, constricting the crown very little at the cervix. The outline describing the distal portion, however, converges toward the cervix more than usual, making the contact area extend distally to a marked degree.

The distal portion of the crown is shorter than the mesial portion, the cervical line dipping apically where it joins the mesial root.

The two buccal cusps are rather distinct, although there is no developmental groove between them. The mesial cusp is larger than the distal cusp. There is a developmental depression dividing them (not a groove), which extends over to the buccal surface.

The roots are long and slender, and they spread greatly at the apical third beyond the outline of the crown.

The strange primitive look of this tooth is emphasized by the *buccal aspect*. The primary first mandibular molar from this angle impresses one with the thought of the possibility that at some time in the dim past there was a fusion of two teeth that ended in a strange single combination. That thought seems particularly apropos when one is able to find a well-formed specimen of the tooth in question—one with its roots intact, showing no evidences of decalcification.

From the buccal aspect, if a line is drawn from the bifurcation of the roots to the occlusal surface, the tooth will be evenly divided mesiodistally. However, the mesial portion will represent a tooth with a crown almost twice as tall as the distal half and the root will be a third again as long as the distal one. Two complete teeth will be represented, but their dimensions will differ considerably (Figs. 3–25 and 3–28).

Lingual Aspect (Fig. 3–30). The *crown and root* converge lingually to a marked degree on the mesial surface. Distally the opposite arrangement is true of both crown and root. The distolingual cusp is rounded and suggests a developmental groove between this cusp and the mesiolingual cusp. The mesiolingual cusp is long and sharp at the tip, more so than any of the other cusps. The sharp and prominent mesiolingual cusp (almost centered lingually but in line with the mesial root) is an outstanding characteristic found occlusally on the primary first mandibular molar. It will be noted that the mesial marginal ridge is so well developed that it might almost be considered another small cusp lingually. Part of the two buccal cusps may be seen from this angle.

From the lingual aspect, the crown length mesially and distally is more uniform than it is from the buccal aspect. The cervical line is straighter.

Mesial Aspect (Fig. 3–31, *B*). The most noticeable detail from the mesial aspect is the extreme curvature buccally at the cervical third. Except for this detail, the crown outline of this tooth from this aspect resembles the mesial aspect of the primary second molar and that

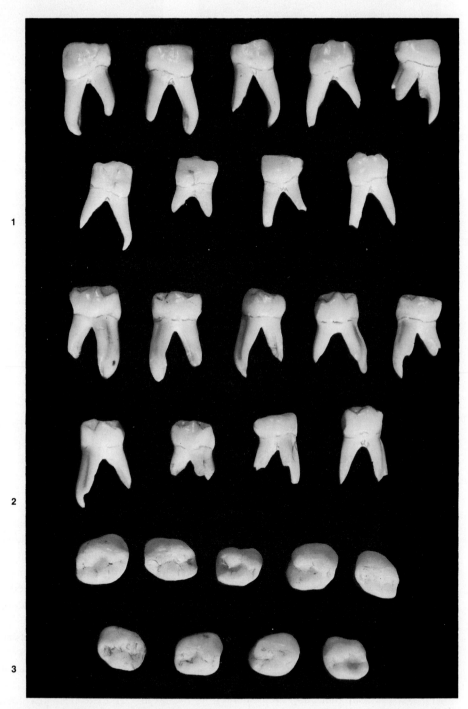

Figure 3–30. Primary mandibular first molars.
This tooth has characteristics unlike any other tooth in the mouth, primary or permanent.
1, Buccal aspect.
2, Lingual aspect.
3, Occlusal aspect.

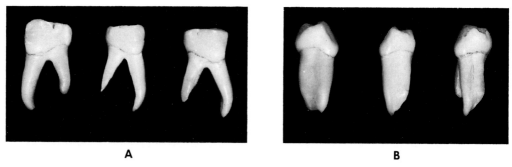

A   **B**

Figure 3–31. Three rare specimens of the primary mandibular first molars. *A,* Buccal aspect. *B,* Mesial aspect. These three specimens have their roots intact with little or no resorption showing. They enable the viewer to observe the actual shape and size of the mesial and distal roots. The mesial root is very broad, curved and long, with fluting down the center. This makes for tremendous anchorage. The distal root is much shorter, but it is heavy and also curved. It does its share in bracing the crown, being in partnership with the mesial root during the process.

aspect of the permanent mandibular molars. In this comparison, the buccal cusps are placed over the root base, and the lingual outline of the crown extends out lingually beyond the confines of the root base.

Both the mesiobuccal cusp and the mesiolingual cusp are in view from this aspect, as is the well-developed mesial marginal ridge. Since the mesiobuccal crown length is greater than the mesiolingual crown length, the cervical line slants upward buccolingually. Note the flat appearance of the buccal outline of the crown from the crest of curvature of the buccal surface at the cervical third to the tip of the mesiobuccal cusp. All of the primary molars have flattened buccal surfaces above this cervical ridge.

The outline of the mesial root from the mesial aspect does not resemble the outline of *any other primary tooth root.* The buccal and lingual outlines of the root drop straight down from the crown and are approximately parallel for over half their length, tapering only slightly at the apical third. The root end is flat and almost square. A developmental depression usually extends almost the full length of the root on the mesial side.

Distal Aspect. The distal aspect of the mandibular first molar differs from the mesial aspect in several ways. The cervical line does not drop buccally. The length of crown buccally and lingually is more uniform, and the cervical line extends almost straight across buccolingually. The distobuccal cusp and the distolingual cusp are not as long or as sharp as the two mesial cusps. The distal marginal ridge is not as straight and well defined as the mesial marginal ridge. The distal root is rounder and shorter and tapers more apically.

Occlusal Aspect (Fig. 3–30, 3). The general outline of this tooth from the occlusal aspect is rhomboidal. The prominence mesiobuccally is noticeable from this aspect, a fact that accents the mesiobuccal line angle of the crown in comparison with the distobuccal line angle, thereby accenting the rhomboidal form.

The mesiolingual cusp may be seen as the largest and the best developed of all the cusps, and it has a broad flattened surface lingually. The *buccal developmental groove* of the occlusal surface divides the two buccal cusps evenly. This developmental groove is short, extending from between the buccal cusp ridges to a point approximately in the center of the crown outline at a *central pit.* The *central developmental groove* joins it at this point and extends mesially, separating the mesiobuccal cusp and the mesiolingual cusp. The central groove ends in a *mesial pit* in the *mesial triangular fossa,* which is immediately distal to the *mesial marginal ridge.* Two supplemental grooves join the developmental groove in the center of the mesial triangular fossa; one supplemental groove extends buccally and the other extends lingually.

The mesiobuccal cusp exhibits a well-defined triangular ridge on the occlusal surface, which terminates in the center of the occlusal surface buccolingually at the *central developmental groove*. The *lingual developmental groove* extends lingually from this point, separating the mesiolingual cusp and the distolingual cusp. Usually, the lingual developmental groove does not extend through to the lingual surface but stops at the junction of lingual cusp ridges. There are some supplemental grooves immediately mesial to the *distal marginal ridge* in the *distal triangular fossa*, which join with the central developmental groove.

Mandibular Second Molar

The primary mandibular *second* molar has characteristics that resemble those of the *permanent* mandibular *first* molar, although its dimensions differ.

Buccal Aspect (Figs. 3–24, *D*, and 3–32, *1*). From the buccal aspect, the primary mandibular second molar has a narrow mesiodistal calibration at the cervical portion of the crown when compared with the calibration mesiodistally on the crown at contact level. The mandibular first *permanent* molar, accordingly, is wider at the cervical portion.

From this aspect also, it will be noted that mesiobuccal and distobuccal developmental grooves divide the buccal surface of the crown occlusally into three cuspal portions almost equal in size. This arrangement forms a straight buccal surface presenting a mesiobuccal, a buccal, and a distobuccal cusp. It differs, therefore, from the mandibular *first permanent* molar, which has an uneven distribution buccally, presenting two buccal cusps and one distal cusp.

The roots of the primary second molar from this angle are slender and long. They have a characteristic flare mesiodistally at the middle and apical thirds. The roots of this tooth may be twice as long as the crown.

The point of bifurcation of the roots starts immediately below the cementoenamel junction of crown and root.

Lingual Aspect (Figs. 3–25, *D*; 3–32, *2*). From the lingual aspect, one sees two cusps of almost equal dimensions. Between them is a short lingual groove. The two lingual cusps are not quite as wide as the three buccal cusps; this arrangement narrows the crown lingually. The cervical line is relatively straight, and the crown extends out over the root more distally than it does mesially. The mesial portion of the crown seems to be a little higher than the distal portion of the crown when viewed from the lingual aspect. It gives the impression of being tipped distally. A portion of each of the three buccal cusps may be seen from this aspect.

The roots from this aspect give somewhat the same appearance as from the buccal aspect. Note the length of the roots.

Mesial Aspect (Figs. 3–26, *D*; 3–32, *3*). From the mesial aspect, the outline of the crown resembles the permanent mandibular first molar. The crest of contour buccally is more prominent on the primary molar, and the tooth seems to be more constricted occlusally because of the flattened buccal surface above this cervical ridge.

The crown is poised over the root of this tooth in the same manner as all mandibular posteriors; its buccal cusp is over the root and the lingual outline of the crown extending out beyond the root line. The marginal ridge is high, a characteristic that makes the mesiobuccal cusp and the mesiolingual cusp appear rather short. The lingual cusp is longer, or extends higher at any rate, than the buccal cusp. The cervical line is regular, although it

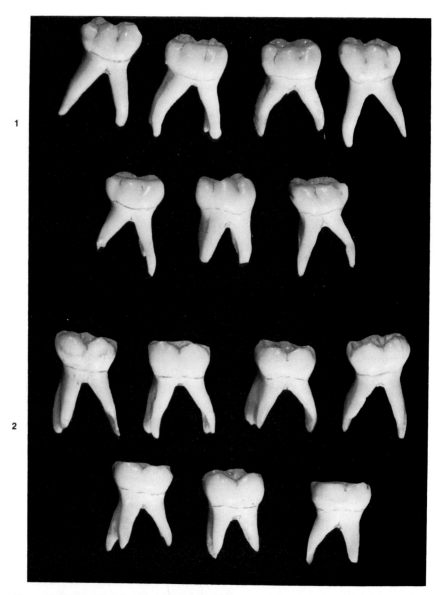

Figure 3–32. Primary mandibular second molars.
1, Buccal aspect.
2, Lingual aspect.
Illustration continued on opposite page

extends upward buccolingually, making up for the difference in length between the buccal and lingual cusps.

The mesial root is unusually broad and flat with a blunt apex that is sometimes serrated.

Distal Aspect. The crown is not as wide distally as it is mesially; therefore it is possible to see the mesiobuccal cusp as well as the distobuccal cusp from the distal aspect. The distolingual cusp appears well developed, and the triangular ridge from the tip of this cusp extending down into the occlusal surface is seen over the distal marginal ridge.

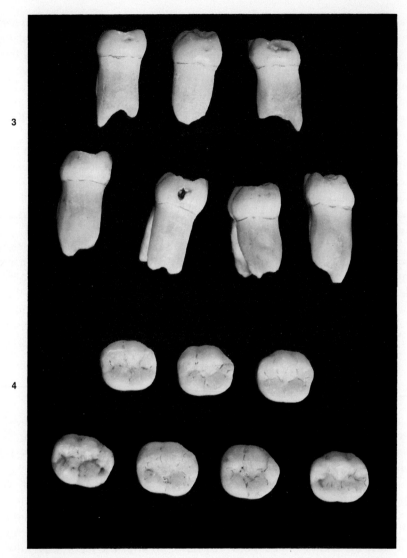

Figure 3–32. *Continued.*
3, Mesial aspect.
4, Occlusal aspect.

The distal marginal ridge dips down more sharply and is shorter buccolingually than the mesial marginal ridge. The cervical line of the crown is regular, although it has the same upward incline buccolingually on the distal as on the mesial.

The distal root is almost as broad as the mesial root, and it is flattened on the distal surface. The distal root tapers more at the apical end than does the mesial root.

Occlusal Aspect (Figs. 3–27, *D;* 3–32, *4*). The occlusal aspect of the primary mandibular second molar is somewhat rectangular. The three buccal cusps are similar in size. The two lingual cusps are also equally matched. However, the total mesiodistal width of the lingual cusps is less than the total mesiodistal width of the three buccal cusps.

There are well-defined triangular ridges extending occlusally from each one of these cusp tips. The triangular ridges end in the center of the crown buccolingually in a *central developmental groove* that follows a staggered course from the *mesial triangular fossa,* just inside the *mesial marginal ridge,* to the *distal triangular fossa,* just mesial to the *distal marginal ridge.* The distal triangular fossa is not so well defined as the mesial triangular fossa. Developmental grooves branch off from the central groove both buccally and lingually, dividing the cusps. The two *buccal grooves* are confluent with the buccal developmental grooves of the buccal surface, one *mesial* and one *distal,* and the single *lingual developmental groove* is confluent with the *lingual groove* on the lingual surface of the crown.

Scattered over the occlusal surface are supplemental grooves on the slopes of triangular ridges and in the mesial and distal triangular fossae. The mesial marginal ridge is better developed and more pronounced than the distal marginal ridge. The outline of the crown converges distally. An outline following the tips of the cusps and the marginal ridges conforms to the outline of a rectangle more closely than does the gross outline of the crown in its entirety.

A comparison occlusally between the deciduous mandibular second molar and the permanent mandibular first molar brings out the following points of difference: The deciduous molar has its mesiobuccal, distobuccal, and distal cusps almost equal in size and development. The distal cusp of the permanent molar is smaller than the other two. Because of the small buccal cusps, the deciduous tooth crown is narrower buccolingually, in comparison with its mesiodistal measurement, than is the permanent tooth.

The Occlusion of the Primary Teeth

The deciduous teeth are arranged in the jaws in the form of two arches: a maxillary and a mandibular. An outline following the labial and buccal surfaces of the maxillary teeth describes the segment of an ellipse and is larger than the segment following the same surfaces on the mandibular teeth (see Fig. 1–1, *A*).

The relation between the maxillary and mandibular primary teeth when in occlusion is such that each tooth, with the exception of the mandibular central incisor and the maxillary second molar, occludes with two teeth of the opposing jaw. The primary teeth should be in normal alignment and occlusion shortly after the age of 2, with all the roots fully formed by the time the child is 3 years old. A year or so after the teeth have fully erupted and have assumed their respective positions in the arches, the rapid development of the jaws is sufficient to create a slight space, or *diastema,* between some of them.

The anterior teeth separate and usually show greater separation as time goes on—a process that is caused by the growth of the jaws and the approach of the permanent teeth from the lingual side. This separation usually begins between the ages of 4 and 5 years. The canines and molars are supposed to keep their positive contact relation during all the jaw growth. However, some shifting and separation are seen quite often. Since the teeth do not hold their relative positions for long, they are worn off rapidly on incisal ridges and occlusal surfaces. As an example, when a primary canine is lost 8 years or more after its eruption, its long, sharp cusp has in most instances been worn down. If the deciduous teeth are in good alignment, the occlusion is most efficient during the time that these teeth are in their original positions (see Fig. 3–33). This situation exists for only a relatively short time.

After normal jaw growth has resulted in considerable separation, the occlusion is supported and made more efficient by the eruption and occlusion of the *first permanent molars* immediately *distal* to the *primary second molars.* The child is now approximately 6 *years* of age and will use some of the primary teeth for 6 *more years.*

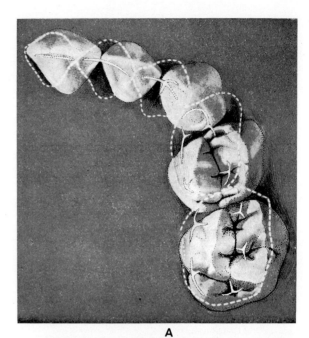

A

Figure 3–33. A, Occlusal surfaces of the maxillary primary teeth, with the outline of the opposing teeth superimposed in occlusion in a child 3 years old. *B,* Occlusal surface of the mandibular primary teeth, with the outlines of the opposing teeth superimposed in occlusion in a child 3 years old. (From Friel, S.: Occlusion: Observations on its development from infancy to old age. Int. J. Orthodont. Oral Surg., 13:322, 1927.)

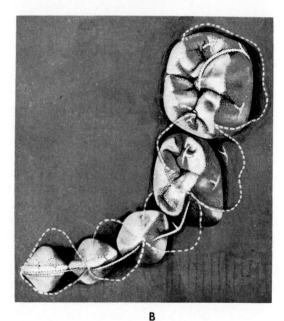

B

Details of Occlusion (Fig. 3–33)

The occlusion of deciduous teeth in a 3-year-old child will be described. After separation has begun, the migration of the teeth changes the occlusion. Nevertheless, if development is normal, the spacing of the teeth is rather uniform (Fig. 3–2). This biological change opens up contacts in the arch between teeth and increases occlusal wear. Nature seems to have anticipated the child's needs, however, because if normal healthy reactions are in effect, the child seldom suffers from mechanical irritations during this severe adjustment period.

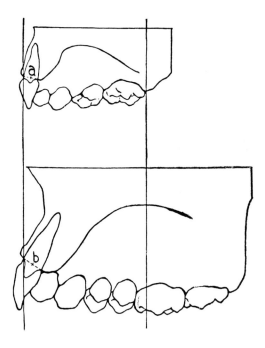

Figure 3–34. Drawing of a sagittal section through the permanent and primary maxillary incisors. The labial surface at the cervical margin is oriented in the same plane. Note that the midalveolar point of the permanent incisors (*b*) is more lingual than the midalveolar point of the primary incisor (*a*) but that the incisal edge of the permanent incisors is more labial than that of the primary incisors. (From Friel, S.: Occlusion: Observations on its development from infancy to old age. Int. J. Orthodont. Oral Surg., 13:322, 1927.)

Normal occlusion of primary teeth at the age of 3 years is as follows:

1. Mesial surfaces of maxillary and mandibular central incisors are in line with each other at the median line.
2. The maxillary central incisor occludes with the mandibular central incisor and the mesial third of the mandibular lateral incisor. The mandibular anterior teeth strike the maxillary anterior teeth lingually above the level of the incisal ridges.
3. The maxillary lateral incisor occludes with the distal two thirds of the mandibular lateral incisor and that portion of the mandibular canine which is mesial to the point of its cusp.
4. The maxillary canine occludes with that portion of the mandibular canine distal to its cusp tip and the mesial third of the mandibular first molar (that portion mesial to the tip of the mesiobuccal cusp).
5. The maxillary first molar occludes with the distal two thirds of the mandibular first molar and the mesial portion of the mandibular second molar, which portion is represented by the mesial marginal ridge and the mesial triangular fossa.
6. The maxillary second molar occludes with the remainder of the mandibular second molar, the distal surface of the maxillary molar projecting slightly over the distal portion of the mandibular second molar.

The interrelation of cusps and incisal ridges of the opposing arches of primary teeth may be studied in the illustration (Fig. 3–33) by Sheldon Friel. The relation in size of deciduous and permanent arches is also illustrated in Figure 3–34 (see also Fig. 1–1).

References

Barker, B. C. (1975). Anatomy of root canals: IV. Deciduous teeth. Aust. Dent. J. 20:101.
Baume, L. J. (1950). Physiologic tooth migration and its significance for the development of occlusion. I. The biogenetic course of the deciduous dentition. J. Dent. Res. 29:123.

Broadbelt, A. G. (1941). On the growth pattern of the human head, from the third month to the eighth year of life. Am. J. Anat. 68:209.

Carlsen, O., and Andersen, J. (1966). On the anatomy of the pulp chamber and root canals in human deciduous teeth. Tandlaegebladet. 70:93–115, 181–98, 421–42, 529–61.

Carlsen, O. (1968). Carabelli's structure on the human maxillary deciduous first molar. Acta. Odontol. Scand. 26:395.

de Campos Russo, M., et al. (1974). Observations on the pulpal floor of human deciduous teeth and possible implications in endodontic treatment. Rev. Fac. Odontal. Aracatuba. 3:61.

Fanning, E. A. (1962). Effect of extraction of deciduous molars on the formation and eruption of their successors. Angle Orthod. 32:44.

Finn, S. B. (1957). *Clinical Pedodontics*, 2nd ed. Philadelphia: Saunders.

Friel, S. (1927). Occlusion—Observations on its development from infancy to old age. Int. J. Orthod. Oral Surg. 13:322.

Friel, S. (1954). The development of ideal occlusion of the gum pads and the teeth. Am. J. Orthod. 40:196.

Fulton, J. T., Hughes, J. T., and Mercer, C. V. (1964). *The life cycle of the human teeth*. Dept. of Epidemiology, School of Public Health, University of North Carolina, Chapel Hill.

McBeath, E. C. (1936). New concept of the development and calcification of the teeth. J. Am. Dent. Assoc. 23:675.

Moorrees, C. F. A., and Chadha, M. (1962). Crown diameters of corresponding tooth groups in the deciduous and permanent dentition. J. Dent. Res. 41:466.

Richardson, A. S., and Castaldi, C. R. (1967). Dental development during the first two years of life. J. Canad. Dent. Assoc., 33:418.

Van der Linden, F. P. G. M., and Duterloo, H. S. (1976). *Development of the Human Dentition: An Atlas*. Hagerstown, Md.: Harper & Row.

Woo, R. K., et al. (1981). Accessory canals in deciduous molars. J. Int. Assoc. Dent. Child. 12:51.

4 General Considerations in the Physiology of the Permanent Dentition

Form and Function

The relationship between the form of the teeth and function is usually discussed in terms of type of food in the diet of humans, jaw movements, and protection of the periodontium and stimulation of the gingiva. It is also recognized that the teeth not only contribute to the digestion of food but also are important in speech and personal appearance.

The primary function of the teeth is to prepare food for swallowing and to facilitate digestion. The teeth have their respective forms to facilitate prehension, incision, and trituration of food. The dentition, joints, and muscles in humans have the form and alignment to enable the mastication of both animal and vegetable foods. This type of dentition is referred to as *omnivorous*. The shapes of incisal and occlusal surfaces of the teeth are related not only to the function they perform but also to the movements of the mandible required to carry out chewing of a variety of foods. In contrast to the facts regarding many animals, only up-and-down jaw closure is possible because of the interlocking conical form of the teeth, temporomandibular joint (TMJ) morphology, and lack of muscles to carry out lateral movements. In order to understand more completely the form and function of teeth, the protective aspects of form will be considered and the functional relationships will be considered in terms of what might be thought of as evolutionary teleology and comparative anatomy.

Alignment, Contacts, and Occlusion

When the teeth in the mandibular arch come into contact with those in the maxillary arch in any *functional relation,* they are said to be *in occlusion. Occlusion* is also used to designate the anatomic alignment of the teeth and their relationship to the rest of the masticatory system. *Malocclusion* is a term usually used to describe deviations in intramaxillary and/or intermaxillary relations of the teeth and/or jaws.

In proper alignment the teeth are arranged in arches in each jaw and placed in strong contact with their neighbors (Fig. 4–1). If, in addition, each tooth in the arch is placed at its

84

A

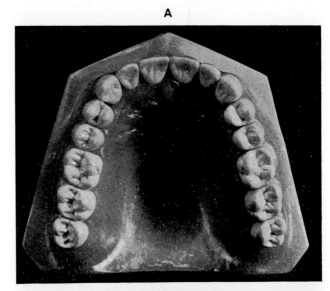

Figure 4–1. Model teeth placed in "ideal" alignment and contact relation. *A,* Maxillary arch. *B,* Mandibular arch.

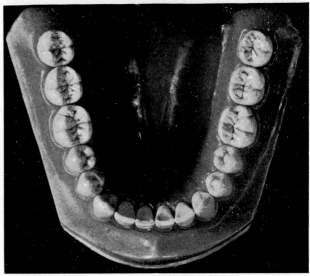

B

most advantageous angle to withstand forces brought to bear upon it, each tooth is more efficient, and the arches are stabilized by the collective action of the teeth in supporting each other (Figs. 4–2 and 4–3). Present evidence suggests that tangential loading results in reduced chewing forces and that negative feedback from receptors in the periodontium mediate chewing forces. Receptor thresholds for axially directed forces appear to be higher than those for tangentially directed forces and suggest a positive feedback control on axially directed tooth forces.

Contact of each tooth with its fellows in the arch protects the *gingiva* between them in the *interproximal spaces* (Figs. 4–4 and 4–5). The gingiva is the soft tissue in the mouth that covers the alveolar bone and surrounds the teeth.

The buccal and lingual contours of the teeth have an influence on the way in which food is directed to and away from the gingival tissues. When a tooth is normally positioned, the

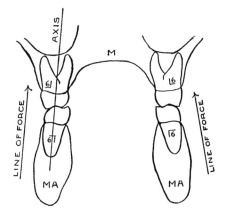

Figure 4–2. Outline of a cross section through the maxilla and mandible at the site of the first molars. The line of force exerted when the teeth come into contact should be parallel to the long axis of the teeth.

gingival margin and sulcus will have a physiologic relationship to the tooth in function. Food impaction, impinging trauma from tough foods, accumulation of dental plaque may be the consequence of malposed teeth or over- or undercontouring of restorations involving buccolingual surfaces. The exact relationship between contouring of restorations and gingival health is not clear. Ideas concerning the relationship of faulty buccal contours (undercontoured) to the initiation of gingivitis have been challenged. Plaque control by toothbrushing may be more important than simple deviations of the contour. However, over- and undercontoured restorations should be avoided.

Interproximal Form

The interproximal space between the teeth is a triangular region, normally filled with gingival tissue, which is bounded by the two proximal surfaces of contacting teeth and the alveolar bone between the teeth, which acts as the base of the triangle.

The gingiva within this space is called the *gingival,* or *interdental papilla* (see Fig. 5–35). Normally, the gingiva covers part of the cervical third of the tooth crowns and fills the interproximal spaces (Figs. 4–4 and 5–17). The *gingival line* follows the curvature but

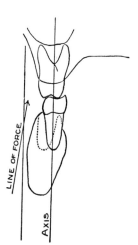

Figure 4–3. Diagram of the first mandibular molar out of normal position. Its axis is not parallel to the line of force. A buccally tipped molar causes higher oral-facial forces and reduced axial forces.

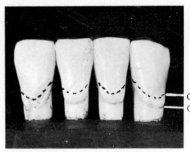

Figure 4–4. The mandibular centrals and laterals contact each other at the incisal third. The form of each tooth, plus the location of the contact areas, creates narrow pointed spaces between the teeth that differ from other interproximal spaces in other segments of the arches. *CL,* cervical line as established by the cementoenamel junction; *GL,* variable gingival line representing the gingival level.

GL
CL

not necessarily the level of the cervical line. The cervical line is defined as the "cemento-enamel junction of crown and root." The gingival line and the cervical line must not be thought of as being identical; although they normally follow a similar curvature, they are seldom at the same level on the tooth. The cervical line is a stable anatomic demarcation, whereas the gingival line merely represents the gingival level on the tooth at any one period in the individual's life, and this level is variable. Malalignment of the teeth will change the gingival line—something that may not be conducive to the health of the tissue (Fig. 4–6).

Even though the teeth are in good alignment, unless the proper relation is kept between the *width* of each tooth *at the cervix* and the width *at the point of contact* with neighboring teeth, the spacing interdentally will be changed. This is an important point to observe in clinical examinations.

When considering the tooth form from the mesial and distal aspects, it is possible to observe a curvature on the crowns at the cervical third above the cervical line, labially or buccally and lingually. It is called the cervicoenamel ridge (Figs. 1–15 and 1–16), or merely cervical ridge, with the location added (buccocervical ridge, and so forth).

Root Form

The *length* and *shape of the root* (or roots) of each tooth must be considered important: the canine, for instance, because of its position and the work required of it, would be torn out of its socket, or at least displaced, by forces brought to bear upon it, if the root were not of extra size and length. Fracture would be imminent if the root were not larger than that of other single-rooted teeth. The root form, therefore, is associated with the *overall form* of the tooth and the *work* it has to do.

The *angle* at which the incisal and occlusal surfaces of the tooth crowns are placed with respect to the root bases is also important. The mesial view of an anterior tooth will

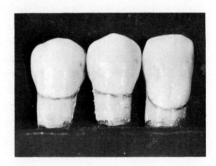

Figure 4–5. Contact design and interproximal (sometimes called interdental) spaces illustrated by the mandibular canine and first and second premolars. Note the variation in contact areas in relation to crown length.

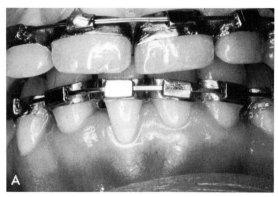

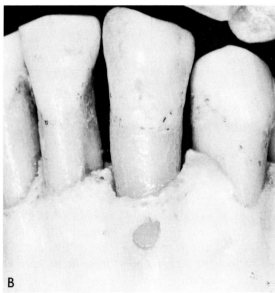

Figure 4–6. Influence of malalignment of teeth on form of gingiva and bone. *A*, Change in gingival line (free gingival margin) of central incisor. *B*, Absence of bone over root of tooth in labioversion (fenestration).

show that the incisal ridge or cusp is centered over the root (see Fig. 1–15). The mesial view of an upper first molar, which is a multicusped tooth, demonstrates the same principle. The points on the occlusal surface that are contacted by opposing teeth will prove to be well within the confines of the root base of the crown. The measurement from cusp tip to cusp tip buccolingually is much less than the buccolingual diameter of the root base (Fig. 1–16). Note the flare of roots for stabilization.

Occlusal Curvature

Close observation indicates that the occlusal and incisal surfaces of all the crowns taken together in either arch would not contact a flat plane. Looking at the teeth from a point opposite the first molars buccally, we see that a line following the occlusal and incisal surfaces describes a curve.

This arrangement of natural teeth was described originally in the German literature in 1890 by F. Graf von Spee, and it is called the *curve of Spee* (Fig. 4–7). There is no acceptable scientific evidence that the occlusion should be spherical, i.e., that each cusp and incisal edge touch or conform to a segment of the surface of a sphere. However, it has been suggested that the composite arrangement of the occlusal surfaces of all of the teeth in each dental arch and their approximate conformation to a segment of a sphere gives the curvature three-dimensional quality (Fig. 4–8). This curvature is reflected in the lingual inclination of the mandibular molars and is the basis for the curve of Wilson; i.e., the curvature of the mandibular teeth is concave and that of the maxillary teeth convex (Fig. 4–9). The occlusal surface of a maxillary molar makes an acute angulation mesially with the long axis of its roots.

The length and shape of the roots, the angle at which the incisal and occlusal surfaces are placed with respect to the roots, sufficient dimensions for strength, and an efficient design for thorough work with resistance against lines of force suggest their importance to occlusal stability.

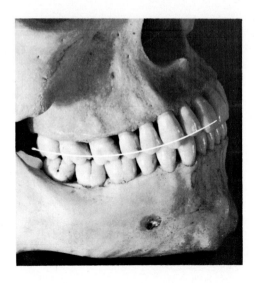

Figure 4–7. Centric occlusion. The occlusion of natural teeth is seldom if ever "ideal." This illustration shows normal occlusion. Note the "curve of Spee." Also note the margin of the alveolar bone in its relation to the cervical line of the teeth. (Observe a fourth mandibular molar, an anomaly.)

Comparative Dental Anatomy

To understand the human dentition, it is helpful to compare the dentitions of other vertebrates. In doing so, it should become clear that the dentition in humans is different in many ways from other vertebrates in form and function. However, it should be equally clear that the presence of related characteristics in a wide range of vertebrates suggests a plan common to all.

Only a superficial summary of the topic is presented here, starting with the primordial form of tooth, the single cone or lobe that was the forerunner of combinations of lobes forming the more complicated teeth found in highly developed animals and in the human being today. Additional material on the subject may be found in the references.

Figure 4–10 graphically illustrates with a schematic drawing the four stages of tooth development:

1. The Reptilian stage (Haplodont).
2. Early Mammalian stage (Triconodont).
3. Triangular stage (Tritubercular molar).
4. Quadritubercular molar.

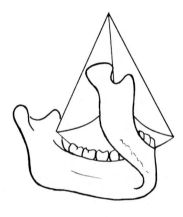

Figure 4–8. A segment of a sphere placed on the occluding surfaces of the mandibular teeth, showing their compensating occlusal curvature.

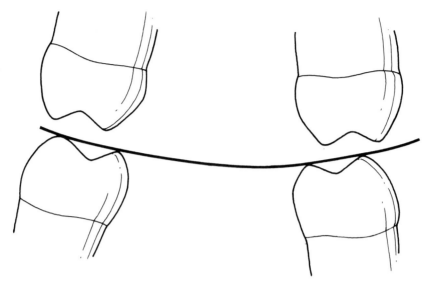

Figure 4–9. Curve of Wilson.

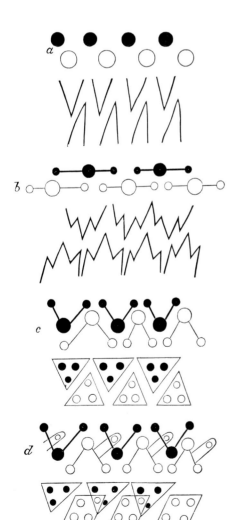

Figure 4–10. Phyletic history of the molar cusps.
a. The Reptilian stage (Haplodont).
b. Early Mammalian stage (Triconodont).
c. Triangular stage (Tritubercular molar).
d. Quadritubercular molar.
The solid black dots represent the cusps of the upper molars; the circles represent those of the lower molars. (After Osborn, H. F.: Evolution of mammalian molar teeth. In Gregory, W. K. (ed.): *Biological Studies and Addresses,* vol. 1. New York, The MacMillan Company, 1907; illustration from Thompson, A. H.: The teeth of vertebrates. In *Comparative Dental Anatomy,* 2nd ed., revised by Martin Dewey. St. Louis, C. Mosby, 1915, p. 65.)

The *Reptilian* or *Haplodont* stage is represented by the simplest form of tooth, the single cone (Fig. 4–11). This type of dentition usually includes many teeth in both jaws that limit jaw movement. There is no occlusion of the teeth in this class, the teeth being used mainly for prehension or combat. Their main function is the procurement of food. The limitation of jaw relation is confined to that of a simple hinge movement. Jaw movements are related to and governed by tooth form in all cases.

The *Early Mammalian* or *Triconodont* stage exhibits three cusps in line in the development of posterior teeth. The largest, or anthropologically the original cusp, is centered with a smaller cusp located anteriorly and another posteriorly. Today examples are not seen with a purely triconodont dentition. Some of the teeth in some breeds of dogs and other carnivores have some teeth that certainly indicate a triconodont background (Fig. 4–12). Nevertheless, the dog and other animals carnivorous by nature are considered to be in the third category, namely, the *Tritubercular* class (Figs. 4–13 through 4–15).

According to the recognized theories explaining evolutionary tooth development, the triconodont line of three changed to a three-cornered shape, with the teeth still bypassing each other more or less when the jaw opened or closed. The next stage of development created projections on the triangular form that finally occluded with an antagonist in the opposing jaw. As this development progressed, occlusion was established and the *Quadritubercular stage* had arrived. During these eons of time and as an accommodation to the changes in tooth form, the anatomy and articulation of the jaws changed accordingly.

The animals with a dentition similar to that of humans are anthropoid apes. This group of animals includes the chimpanzee, gibbon, gorilla, and orangutan (Figs. 4–16 and 4–17). The shapes of individual teeth in these animals are amazingly close to their counterparts in the human mouth. Nevertheless, the development of the canines, the arch form, and the jaw development are quite different.

The multiplication and fusion of lobes during tooth development are demonstrated graphically when human teeth are viewed from the mesial or distal aspects. Anterior teeth, which are used for incising or apprehending food, reflect the single cone, whereas the posterior or multicusp teeth, which are used for grinding food in addition to a shearing action, appear to be two or more cones fused (Fig. 4–18). Although the schematic form of the teeth from the mesial or distal aspects is that of a single cone in anteriors, or what seems to be an indication of a fusion of two or more cones in posteriors, close observation causes one to come to the conclusion that each tooth crown, regardless of location, will appear to be a combination of four or more lobes. Each lobe represents a primary center of formation.

All anterior teeth show traces of four lobes, three labially and one lingually, the lingual lobe being represented by the cingulum. Each labial lobe of the incisor terminates incisally in rounded eminences known as *mamelons*. These mamelons are prominent in newly erupted incisors. Soon after eruption they are worn down by use unless through malalignment, they escape incisal wear. Maxillary central incisors often show traces of the fusion of

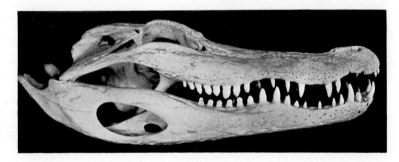

Figure 4–11. The Mississippi alligator. An interesting commentary on the anatomy of the alligator: because of the alligator's physical problems, the upper jaw is the mobile one. The lower jaw, closer to the ground, is static. (From Kronfeld, R.: *Dental Histology and Comparative Dental Anatomy.* Philadelphia, Lea & Febiger, 1937.)

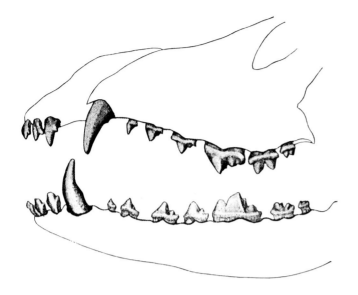

Figure 4–12. Permanent dentition of *Canis familiaris*. (Modified from Tims, H. W. Marett: Notes on the dentition of the dog. Anat. Anz. Bd., 11:537, 1896.)

three lobes on the labial face by visible markings in the enamel called *labial grooves* (Fig. 4–19, *A*. See also Figures 4–20 and 4–21).

In the anterior teeth, the four lobes are called the *mesial, labial, distal,* and *lingual lobes.* In *premolars* they are called *mesial, buccal, distal,* and *lingual lobes,* or, as in the case of the mandibular second premolar, which often has two lingual cusps, the *mesial, buccal, distal, mesiolingual,* and *distolingual lobes,* making five in all (Fig. 10–17).

The *molar lobes* are named the same as the cusps, e.g., *mesiobuccal lobe.* The tip of each cusp represents the primary center of formation of each lobe.*

It is possible, of course, to find a variation in the number of lobes in molars. Tubercles of enamel may be found in addition to the primary lobes. When present, they are usually smaller than, and supplementary to, the major lobes.

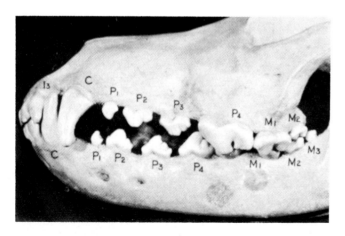

Figure 4–13. Jaws of a dog (collie). The premolars are tritubercular and widely spaced; the upper carnassial (fourth premolar, P_4) articulates with the lower carnassial (first molar, M_1). (From Kronfeld, R.: *Dental Histology and Comparative Dental Anatomy,* Philadelphia, Lea & Febiger, 1937.)

* *Tables of development of the teeth will be given under the complete description of each tooth. The description of the formation of the teeth histologically, however, will not be included. For this refer to a work on dental histology and embryology. See also Figs. 2–2 and 2–3.*

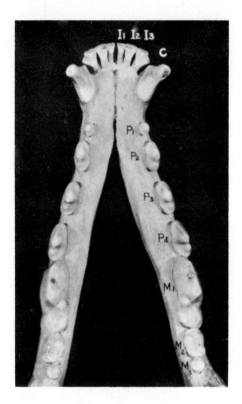

Figure 4–14. Occlusal view of the mandible of a dog (collie). The mandible is long and slender. The cutting edges of the four premolars and three molars are arranged in a sagittal plane. (From Kronfeld, R.: *Dental Histology and Comparative Dental Anatomy*. Philadelphia, Lea & Febiger, 1937.)

Tooth Form and Jaw Movements

In general terms, the primates are *bunodont* and relatively *isognathous* and consequently have limited lateral movement. Bunodont refers to tooth-bearing conical cusps. Isognathous means equal-jawed, and anisognathus refers to unequal jaws. Humans are not perfectly isognathus; i.e., the maxillary arch overlaps horizontally the mandibular arch. The shape of the glenoid cavity also is correlated with tooth form and jaw movements. A number of living and extinct species demonstrate a chain of dental forms, gradually departing from the bunodont type and passing into the selenodont, accompanied by an

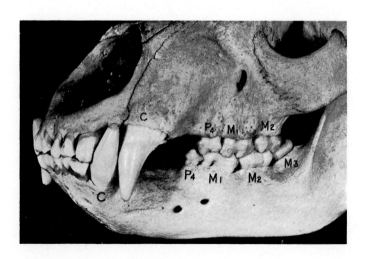

Figure 4–15. The bear. The extent of development of teeth and jaws and occlusion is often used to rate animal forms. Compare with Figure 4–19. (From Kronfeld, R.: *Dental Histology and Comparative Dental Anatomy*. Philadelphia, Lea & Febiger, 1937.)

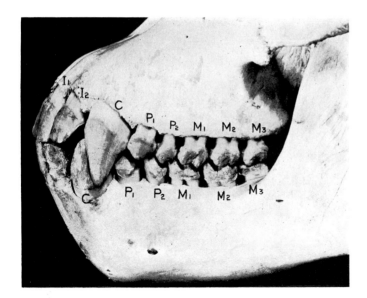

Figure 4–16. The ape. (From Kronfeld, R.: *Dental Histology and Comparative Dental Anatomy.* Philadelphia, Lea & Febiger, 1937.)

increased mobility of the mandible in a lateral direction and increased anisognathism. When the incisal point is viewed from the front during mastication, the mandible moves up and down without lateral deviation in dogs, cats, pigs, and all other bunodonts. Lateral movement increases in a number of animals to the extreme lateral excursion seen in the giraffe, camel, and ox. In relation to the latter type of movement, it has been proposed that where the condyle is greatly elongated transversely and very flat, there is great lateral movement during mastication with selenodont molars and a great degree of anisognathism. Also of interest is the general correlation between ridge and groove direction or curvature of the cross crests and intervening valleys of molars and a radius drawn to the center of the glenoid fossa. In contrast to such biaxial molars in some genera and in humans, no such correlation between ridge and groove direction and the center of rotation of the condyle

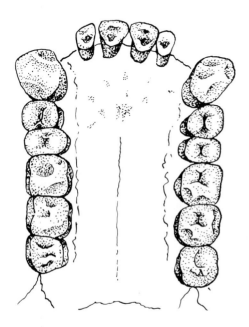

Figure 4–17. Occlusal view of the upper jaw of an orangutan. The arch is square, and the canines, premolars, and molars stand in a straight sagittal line. Note the diastema between lateral incisor and canine. (Modified from Kronfeld, R.: *Dental Histology and Comparative Dental Anatomy.* Philadelphia, Lea & Febiger, 1937.)

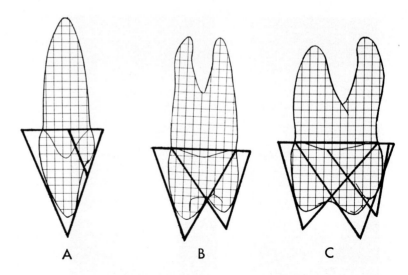

Figure 4–18. The functional form of the teeth when outlined schematically from the mesial or distal aspects is that of the fusion of two or three cones. *A*, Maxillary incisor. *B*, Maxillary premolar. *C*, Maxillary first molar. Note that the major portion of the incisor in view is made up of one cone or lobe.

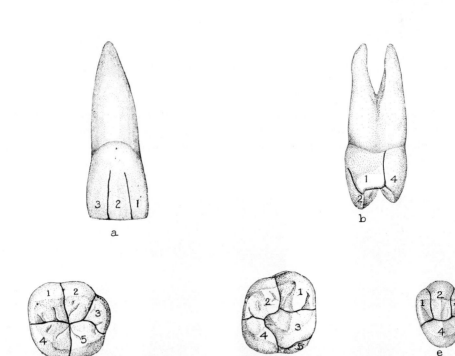

Figure 4–19. General outlines of some of the lobes.

   a, Labial aspect of maxillary central incisor, showing the labial grooves marking the division of the lobes. *1*, Mesial lobe; *2*, labial lobe; *3*, distal lobe. The lingual lobe, or cingulum, is not in view. (See Figure 4–20, A-4.)

   b and *e*, Mesial and occlusal aspects of maxillary first premolar. *1*, Mesial lobe; *2*, buccal lobe; *3*, distal lobe; *4*, lingual lobe.

   c, Occlusal aspect of mandibular first molar. *1*, Mesiobuccal lobe; *2*, distobuccal lobe; *3*, distal lobe; *4*, mesiolingual lobe; *5*, distolingual lobe. Lobes on molars are named the same as cusps.

   d, Occlusal aspects of maxillary first molar. *1*, Mesiobuccal lobe; *2*, distobuccal lobe; *3*, mesiolingual lobe; *4*, distolingual lobe; *5*, fifth lobe (fifth cusp).

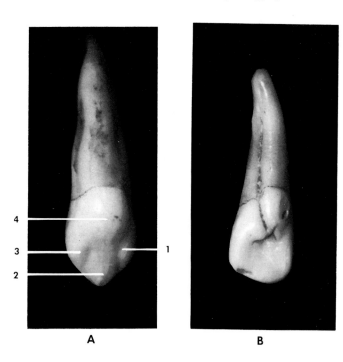

Figure 4–20. *A*, Lingual aspect of maxillary canine, with primary centers marked. *1*, Mesial lobe; *2*, central lobe (cusp); *3*, distal lobe; *4*, lingual lobe (cingulum).

B, Incomplete formation demonstrated by a developmental groove distolingually on a maxillary lateral incisor. This groove will sometimes harbor fissures at various points along its length, especially in the coronal portion. A tooth with this handicap is more subject to caries.

exists because the center is midway between the condyles or glenoid cavities and thus uniaxial.

It has been suggested that the earliest and simplest type of jaw movement is opening and closing without lateral excursion and coexistent with the simple bunodont molar. And with increasing complexity of movement, there has been an apparent increase in the complexity of enamel folding, ridges, and crests. Such changes appear to follow correla-

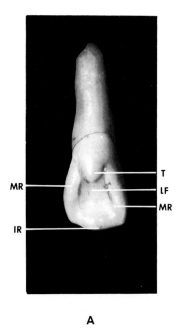

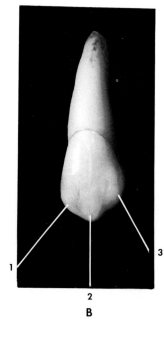

Figure 4–21. *A*, Maxillary lateral incisor, which shows prominences at the centers of calcification. *T*, Tubercle, prominence equal to a small cusp at the cingulum; *LF*, lingual fossa; *MR*, marginal ridges; *IR*, incisal ridge with a prominent enamel rise.

B, Maxillary canine showing evidences of lobe formation. *1*, Mesial lobe; *2*, labial lobe; *3*, distal lobe.

tively with the shape of the mandibular articulation and the skull. Thus the forms of the teeth, joints, muscles, skull, bones, and jaw movement are all related in function.

A Geometric Concept of Crown Outlines

In a general way, all aspects of each tooth crown except the incisal or occlusal aspects may be outlined schematically within three geometric figures: a *triangle,* a *trapezoid,* and a *rhomboid.* To one unfamiliar with dental anatomy, it may seem an exaggeration to say that curved outlines of tooth crowns can be included within geometric figures. Nevertheless, to one who realizes the problems involved in crown design it seems very plausible to consider fundamental outlines schematically to assist in visualization.

Facial and Lingual Aspects of All Teeth

The outlines of the facial and lingual aspects of all the teeth may be represented by *trapezoids* of various dimensions. The shortest of the uneven side represent the bases of the crowns at the cervices, and the longest of the uneven sides represent the working surfaces, or the incisal and occlusal surfaces, the line made through the points of contact of neighboring teeth in the same arch (Fig. 4–22). Disregarding the overlap of anterior teeth and the cusp forms of the cusped teeth in the schematic drawing, we can easily see the fundamental plan governing the form and arrangement of the teeth from this aspect.

   The occlusal line that forms the longest uneven side of each of the trapezoids represents the approximate point at which the opposing teeth come together when the jaw is closed. The viewer must not become confused at this point and think that the teeth actually occlude level with their points of contact. The illustration is made to help in visualizing the fundamental shape of the teeth from the labial and buccal aspects. (See Fig. 4–23.)

   This arrangement brings out the following *fundamentals* of form:

1. Interproximal spaces may accommodate interproximal tissue.
2. Spacing between the roots of one tooth and those of another allows sufficient bone tissue for investment for the teeth and a supporting structure required to hold up gingival tissue

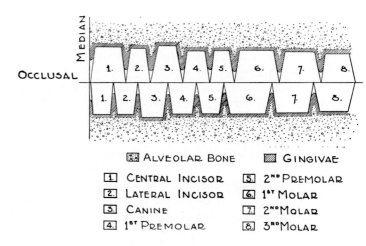

Figure 4–22. Schematic drawing of facial (labial and buccal) aspects of the teeth only, illustrating the teeth as trapezoids of various dimensions. Note the relations of each tooth to its opposing tooth or teeth in the opposite arch. Each tooth has two antagonists except number *1* below and number *8* above.

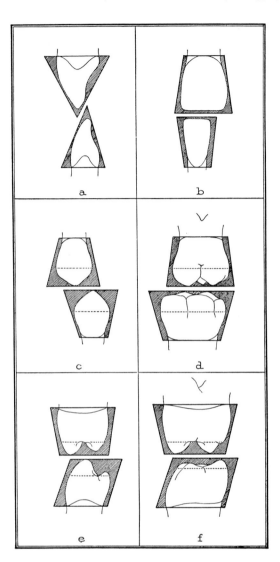

Figure 4–23. Outlines of crown forms within geometric outlines—triangles, trapezoids, and rhomboids. The upper figure in each square represents a maxillary tooth, the lower figure a mandibular tooth. Note that the trapezoid outline will not include the cusp form of posteriors actually. It does include the crowns from cervix to contact point or cervix to marginal ridge, however. This schematic drawing is intended to emphasize certain fundamentals.

    a, Anterior teeth, mesial or distal. (triangle)
    b, Anterior teeth, labial or lingual. (trapezoid)
    c, Premolars, buccal or lingual. (trapezoid)
    d, Molars, buccal or lingual. (trapezoid)
    e, Premolars, mesial or distal. (rhomboid)
    f, Molars, mesial or distal. (rhomboid)

to a normal level. Sufficient circulation of blood to the parts would be impossible without this spacing.

3. Each tooth crown in the dental arches must be in contact at some point with its neighbor, or neighbors, to help protect the interproximal gingival tissue from trauma during mastication. The contact of one tooth with another in the arch tends to ensure their respective positions by mutual support.

4. Each tooth in each dental arch has two antagonists in the opposing arch excepting the mandibular central incisor and the maxillary third molar. In the event of loss of any tooth, this arrangement tends to prevent elongation of antagonists and helps stabilize the remaining teeth over a longer period than would be likely if each tooth had but a single antagonist.

Mesial and Distal Aspects of the Anterior Teeth

The mesial and distal aspects of the anterior teeth, central incisors, lateral incisors, and canines, maxillary and mandibular, may be included within *triangles*. The base of the triangle is represented by the cervical portion of the crown, and the apex by the incisal ridge (Fig. 4–23, *a*).

The fundamentals portrayed here are:

1. A wide base to the crown for strength.
2. A tapered outline labially and lingually, narrowing down to a relatively thin ridge which facilitates the penetration of food material.

Mesial and Distal Aspects of Maxillary Posterior Teeth

The outlines of the mesial and distal aspects of all maxillary posterior teeth (premolars and molars) can be included within *trapezoidal* figures. Naturally, the uneven sides of the premolar figures are shorter than those of the molars (Fig. 4–23, *e* and *f*). Notice that in this instance the trapezoidal figures show the longest uneven side representing the *base* of the crown instead of the *occlusal line,* as was the case in showing the same teeth from the buccal or lingual view. In other words, the schematic outline used to represent the buccal aspect of premolars or molars is turned upside down to represent the mesial or distal aspects of the same teeth. (In Fig. 4–23, compare maxillary figures *c* and *d* with *e* and *f*.)

The fundamental considerations to be observed when reviewing the mesial or distal aspects of maxillary posterior teeth are:

1. Because the occlusal surface is constricted, the tooth can be forced into food material more easily.
2. If the occlusal surface were as wide as the base of the crown, the additional chewing surface would multiply the forces of mastication; then, too, the tooth would be less "self-cleansing" during the process.

It has been found necessary to emphasize the fundamental outlines of these aspects through the medium of schematic drawings because the correct anatomy is overlooked so often. The tendency is to take for granted that the tooth crowns are narrowest at the cervix *from all angles,* which is not true. The measurement of the cervical portion of a posterior tooth is smaller than that of the occlusal portion when viewed from buccal or lingual aspects only; when it is observed from the mesial or distal aspects, the comparison is just the reverse; the occlusal surface tapers from the wide root base. (Compare Fig. 4–23, *e* and *f*, with *c* and *d*.)

Mesial and Distal Aspects of Mandibular Posterior Teeth

Finally, the mandibular posterior teeth, when approached from the mesial or distal aspects, are somewhat *rhomboidal* in outline (Fig. 4–23, *e* and *f*). The occlusal surfaces are constricted in comparison with the bases—similar to the maxillary posterior teeth. The rhomboidal outline inclines the crowns lingual to the root bases, bringing the cusps into proper occlusion with the cusps of their maxillary opponents. At the same time, the axes of crowns and roots of the teeth of both jaws are kept parallel (Figs. 4–2 and 4–3). If the mandibular posterior crowns were to be set on their roots in the same relation of crown to root as that of the maxillary posterior teeth, the cusps would clash with one another. This would not allow the intercusp relations necessary for proper function.

Summary of Schematic Outlines

Outlines of the tooth crowns, when viewed from the labial or buccal, lingual, mesial, and distal aspects, are described in a general way by triangles, trapezoids, or rhomboids (Fig. 4–23, *a* through *f*).

>   Triangles
>   *Six anterior teeth*, maxillary and mandibular
>   1. Mesial aspect
>   2. Distal aspect
>   Trapezoids
>   A. Trapezoid with longest uneven side toward occlusal or incisal surface
>   1. *All anterior teeth*, maxillary and mandibular
>   a. Labial aspect
>   b. Lingual aspect
>   2. *All posterior teeth*
>   a. Buccal aspect
>   b. Lingual aspect
>   B. Trapezoid with shortest uneven side toward occlusal surface
>   1. *All maxillary posterior teeth*
>   a. Mesial aspect
>   b. Distal aspect
>   Rhomboids
>   *All mandibular posterior teeth*
>   1. Mesial aspect
>   2. Distal aspect

References

Ash, M. M. (1954). Physiology of the mouth. In Bunting, R. W. (ed.), *Oral Hygiene,* 3rd ed. Philadelphia: Lea & Febiger.

Barker, B. C. (1973). Dental anthropology: Some variations and anomalies on human tooth form. Aust. Dent. J. 18:132.

Cooke, W. P. (1923). Value and use of temporary teeth. Br. J. Dent. Sci. 66:267.

Cope, E. E. (1888). On the tritubercular molar in human dentition. J. Morphol. 2:7.

Farer, J. W., and Isaacson, D. (1974). Biologic contours. J. Prev. Dent. 1:4.

Ferguson, M. W. (1981). Review of the value of the American alligator (Alligator mississippensis) as a model for research in craniofacial development. J. Craniofac. Genet. Dev. Biol. 1:123.

Graf, H. (1975). Occlusal forces during function. In *Occlusion: Research in Form and Function*. Ann Arbor, University of Michigan, Symposium report.

Gregory, W. K. (1906). *The Origin and Evolution of Human Dentition.* Baltimore, Md.: Williams and Wilkins.

Hellman, M. (1920). The relationship of form to position in teeth and its bearing on occlusion. Dent. Items Interest 42:161.

Humphreys, H. F. (1921). Function in the evolution of man's dentition. Br. Dent. J. 42:939.

Kronfeld, R. (1937). *Dental Histology and Comparative Dental Anatomy.* Philadelphia: Lea & Febiger.

Lindhe, J., and Wicen, P. O. (1969). The effects on the gingiva of chewing fibrous foods. J. Periodont. Res. 4:193.

Osborn, H. F. (1907). Evolution of mammalian molar teeth. In Gregory, W. K. (ed.). *Biological Studies and Addresses,* Vol. 1. New York: Macmillan.

Perel, M. L. (1971). Periodontal considerations of crown contours. J. Prosthet. Dent. 26:627.

Ramfjord, S. P., and Ash, M. M. (1979). *Periodontology and Periodontics*. Philadelphia: Saunders.

Russell, E. S. (1917). *Form and Function*. New York: Dutton.

Ryder, J. A. (1878). On the mechanical genesis of tooth-forms. *Natural Sciences of Philadelphia,* p. 45.

Shaw, D. M. (1917). Form and function of teeth: A theory of maximum shear. J. Anat. Physiol. 13:97.

Thompson, A. H. (1915). *Comparative Dental Anatomy,* 2nd ed., revised by Martin Dewey. St. Louis, Mo.: Mosby.

Tims, H. W. Marett (1896). Notes on the dentition of the dog. Anat. Anz. Bd. 11:537.

Wheeler, R. C. (1961). Complete crown form and the periodontium. J. Prosthet. Dent. 11:722.

Wortman, J. L. (1902). Origin of the tritubercular molar. Am. J. Sci. 13:93.

Youdelis, R. A., Weaver, J. D., and Sapkos, S. (1973). Facial and lingual contours of artificial complete crown restorations and their effect on the periodontium. J. Prosthet. Dent. 19:61.

5 Physiologic Form of the Teeth and the Periodontium

Fundamental Curvatures

The form of the teeth is consistent with the function they are to perform and with their position and arrangement in the structures involved in oral motor behavior, especially mastication. To attempt to relate form and function in all the structures involved in such functions is beyond the scope of this book, and the reader is referred to several of the references provided at the end of this chapter. However, it is assumed that the form of the teeth and their arrangement are related to incising or crushing food without causing damage to the supporting structures, to be otherwise might be inconsistent with the survival of the species. Some of the form must also relate to that of the jaws and face and to occlusal forces that dictate that the teeth be at various angles and positions in the dental arches. And beyond assumptions or teleological approaches to morphology of the teeth, the relationships of tooth form to the form of the supporting structures (including the gingiva) must be considered in terms of clinical significance. Thus, food impaction may occur as a result of gingival enlargement as well as the result of driving food between the teeth because of improper marginal ridges and/or contact areas, irrespective of teleological considerations of tooth morphology.

Although there has been a great deal said about the relationship of the health of the gingiva to the contours of the teeth (as indicated in the references included at the end of this chapter), such appraisals are generally descriptive, involve restorations, and are retrospective observations. And to conclude that the gingival tissues around a tooth—natural or restored—need neither stimulation nor protection suggests that the true significance of buccolingual crown contours has not been evaluated. In no instance has the influence of axial contours (which begin with the height of contour of buccal and lingual surfaces) been tested in relation to such functions as chewing efficiency or occlusal stability. And even though the significance of buccolingual crown contours to gingival health relative to gingival stimulation, self-cleansing mechanisms, and gingival protection has been seriously questioned, the significance of other contours has also been questioned. Dental plaque accumulates on teeth in the absence of adequate oral hygiene, and gingivitis occurs in spite of ''self-cleansing'' mechanisms. The influence of a primitive diet does not appear to prevent gingivitis. However, plaque formation and gingivitis may be related more to bacterial attachment mechanisms and bacterial toxins and food substrates than physical form. But it should not be concluded from such observations that curvatures have nothing to do with function and health of the masticatory system. The effect of over- or undercontouring of surfaces of the teeth may be related more to occlusal mechanisms than to self-cleansing mechanisms and of more significance to the self-cleansing efficiency of food and/or musculature in one patient than another. The role of protective reflexes in relation to contours of the teeth is not known. Even though the significance of tooth forms has yet to be clarified, ideas about form and function that have been held should be understood and liberties with form avoided. To be considered are:

1. Proximal contact areas
2. Interproximal spaces (formed by proximal surface in contact)
3. Embrasures (spillways)
4. Labial and buccal contours at the cervical thirds (cervical ridges) and lingual contours at the middle thirds of crowns
5. Curvatures of the cervical lines on mesial and distal surfaces (cementoenamel junction)

These headings include the form, which has been considered to have a direct or primary bearing on the protection of the periodontium. Many other details of tooth form may have an indirect bearing on the stability of the teeth through their contribution to the maintenance of efficiency during function. Some of these details are cusp forms, the proportions of various measurements of the crowns and roots, root form, and anchorage and angles at which teeth are set in the jaws. It has been suggested that when well-formed teeth are in normal alignment with normal gingival contour (Figs. 5–1 and 5–2), the efficient use of the toothbrush during home care of the teeth is enhanced.

Proximal Contact Areas

Soon after the alignment of all of the teeth in their respective positions in the jaws takes place, there should be a positive contact relation mesially and distally of one tooth with another in each arch (Fig. 5–3). Except for the last molars (third molars, if present), each

Figure 5–1. Clinical appearance of gingiva. *A*, Attached gingiva above and interdental papilla below. *B*, Mucogingival line separating attached gingiva from mucosa. *C*, Free gingival margin. *D*, Posterior vestibular fornix. *E*, Anterior vestibular fornix or mucobuccal fold. *F*, Frenum area.

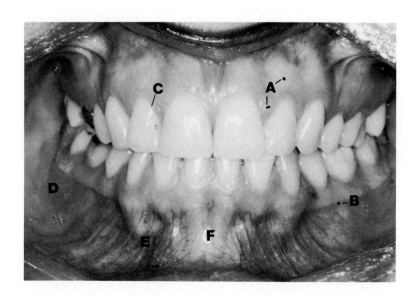

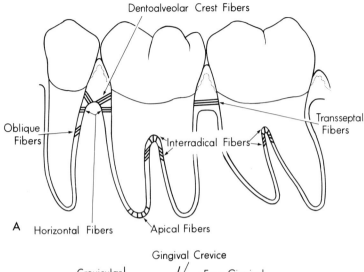

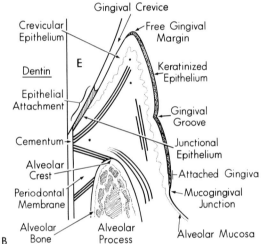

Figure 5–2. A, Principal fibers of the supporting structures. *B,* Schematic representation of periodontal structure at the junction of the enamel, cementum, and dentin showing attachment of gingival tissue to the tooth via the junctional epithelium. (From Ramfjord, S. R., and Ash, M. M.: *Periodontology and Periodontics.* Philadelphia, W. B. Saunders Company, 1979.)

Figure 5–3. Proximal "contacts" vary in size in relation to type of teeth and wear of these areas. Note flat contacts in molar region compared with absence of flattening in relation to space between canine and premolar. The form of the interproximal spaces is altered by wear of contact areas, extrusion of teeth, or tipping of teeth.

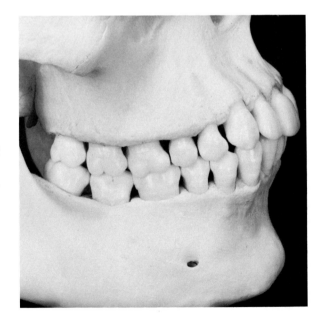

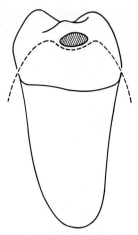

Figure 5–4. Schematic representation of form of gingiva in relation to contact area.

tooth has *two* contacting members adjoining it. The last molar is in contact only with the tooth mesial to it. Although the areas of contact are still very circumscribed, especially on anterior teeth, these are *areas* and not mere *points* of contact (Fig. 5–4). Actually, the term "contact point," which is often used to designate the contact of teeth in the same arch, is a misnomer. When the individual is quite young and the teeth are newly erupted, some of the teeth come close to having point contacts only when the contacting surfaces are nearly perfect curvatures. Examples of the few contacts made by such rounded surfaces are located distally on canines and mesially on first premolars, maxillary and mandibular.

The proper contact relation between neighboring teeth in each arch is important for the following reasons: It serves to keep food from packing between the teeth, and it helps to stabilize the dental arches by the combined anchorage of all the teeth in either arch in positive contact with each other (Figs. 5–3, 5–5, and 5–6). Except for the third molars, each tooth in the arch is supported in part by its contact with two neighboring teeth, one mesial and one distal. The third molars (and the second molars as well if there is no third molar) are prevented from drifting distally where there is no contacting tooth by the angulation of their occlusal surfaces with their roots and by the angle of the direction of the occlusal forces in their favor. This will be explained more fully in later chapters.

If for any reason food is forced between the teeth past the contact areas, the result may be pathologic. The gingival tissue, which normally fills the interdental spaces, may become inflamed (*gingivitis*) and ultimately involve deeper peridontal structures with loss of bone and attachment (periodontitis).

Excessive occlusal forces on an individual tooth may occur when normal forces are no longer distributed over several teeth, as may happen with loss of teeth, or when normal forces become excessive with loss of supporting structures as a result of periodontal diseases.

Contact areas must be observed from *two aspects* in order to obtain the proper perspective for locating them: the labial or buccal aspect, and the incisal or occlusal aspect (Figs. 5–12 and 5–14).

The *labial* or *buccal* view will demonstrate the relative positions of the contact areas cervicoincisally or cervico-occlusally. The center of the area from this aspect is gauged by its relation to the length of the crown portion of the tooth (Fig. 5–7).

The *incisal* or *occlusal* view will show the relative position of the contact areas labiolingually or buccolingually. In this instance, the center of the area may be located in its relation to the labiolingual or buccolingual measurement of the crown (Figs. 5–13, 5–14 and 5–15). The point at which the contact area is bisected will also depend upon the outline of

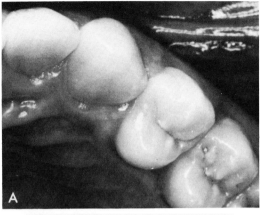

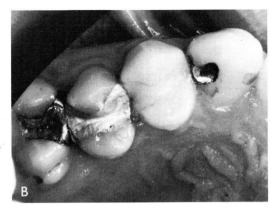

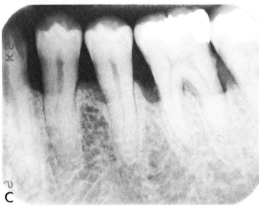

Figure 5–5. Contact areas. *A,* "Contacts" without evidence of dysfunction. *B,* "Restored" contact areas associated with dysfunction from food impaction. *C,* Loss of contacts associated with bone loss due to periodontal disease.

the form of the crown from the incisal or occlusal aspect. This outline is governed by the *alignment* of the tooth in the arch and also by the *occlusal relation* with its antagonists in the opposing arch. The mandibular first molar is an excellent example (Figs. 5–13 and 5–16). The contact and embrasure design for this tooth will be explained later when the incisal and occlusal aspects of the teeth are considered.

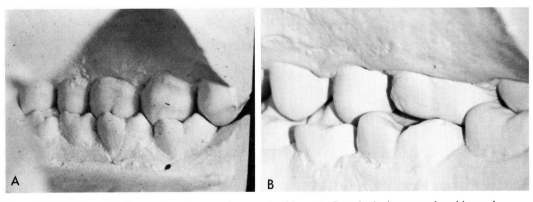

Figure 5–6. Relationship of cusps to embrasures in some dentitions. *A,* Casts in the intercuspal position and teeth in "normal" occlusion. *B,* Other casts in intercuspal position with alignment of the teeth preventing normal contact relations between cusps and embrasure areas.

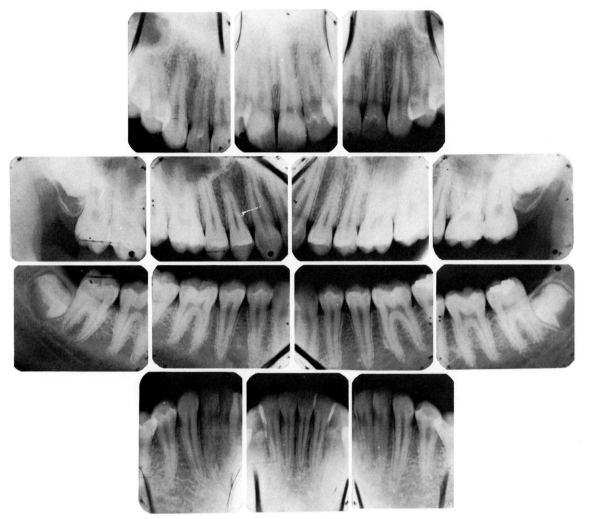

Figure 5–7. Radiograph demonstrating form of alveolar crest, contact areas, and relation to form of the crown.

Interproximal Spaces (Formed by Proximal Surfaces in Contact)

The interproximal spaces between the teeth are triangularly shaped spaces normally filled by *gingival tissue* (*gingival papillae*). The base of the triangle is the alveolar process; the sides of the triangle are the proximal surfaces of the contacting teeth, and the apex of the triangle is in the area of contact. The form of the interproximal space will vary with the form of the teeth in contact and will depend also upon the relative position of the contact areas (Figs. 5–3, 5–8, 5–9, and 5–11). There is normally a separation of 1 to 1½ mm between the enamel and alveolar bone. Thus, the distance from the cementoenamel junction (cervical line, CEJ) to the crest of the alveolar bone as seen radiographically (Fig. 5–7) is 1 to 1½ mm in a normal occlusion in the absence of disease.

Proper contact and alignment of adjoining teeth will allow proper spacing between them for the normal bulk of gingival tissue attached to the bone and teeth. This gingival tissue is a continuation of the gingiva covering all of the alveolar process. The surface

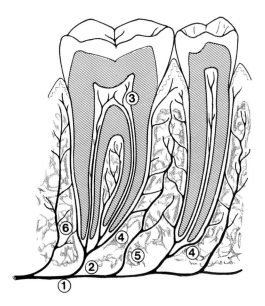

Figure 5–8. Schematic drawing of distribution of the periodontal blood vessels and interdental papillae. *1*, Inferior alveolar artery; *2*, dental arteriole; *3*, pulpal branches; *4*, periodontal ligament arteriole; *5, 6*, interalveolar arteriole. (From Ramfjord, S. R., and Ash, M. M.: *Periodontology and Periodontics.* Philadelphia, W. B. Saunders Company, 1979.)

Figure 5–9. The form of the gingiva is related to the form of the teeth, contact areas, spacing between the teeth, and effects of periodontal disease and dental caries. *A,* Interdental papillae do not fill the interproximal areas in several places because of spacing between the teeth. *B,* Clinically normal gingivae; the form is different because of the form of the teeth, including contact areas.

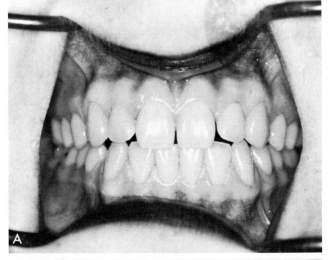

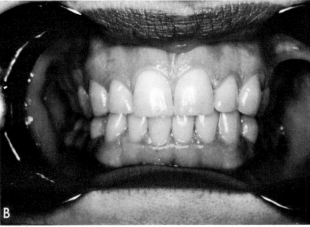

keratinization of the gingiva and the density and elasticity of the gingival tissues help to maintain these tissues against trauma during mastication and invasion by bacteria.

Since the teeth are narrower at the cervix mesiodistally than they are toward the occlusal surfaces and since the outline of the root continues to taper from that point to the apices of the roots, considerable spacing is created between the roots of one tooth and the roots of adjoining teeth. This arrangement allows sufficient bone tissue between one tooth and another, anchoring the teeth securely in the jaws. It also simplifies the problem of space for the blood and nerve supply to the surrounding alveolar process and other investing tissues of the teeth (Fig. 5–8).

The *type of tooth* also has a bearing upon the interproximal space. Some individuals have teeth that are wide at the cervices, constricting the space at the base. Others have teeth that are more slender at the cervices than usual; this type of tooth widens the space. Teeth that are oversize or unusually small will likewise affect the interproximal spacing. Nevertheless, this spacing will conform to a plan that is fairly uniform, provided that the anatomic form is normal and the teeth are in good alignment.

Embrasures (Spillways)

When two teeth in the same arch are in contact, their curvatures adjacent to the contact areas form spillway spaces called *embrasures*. The spaces that widen out from the area of contact labially or buccally and lingually are called *labial* or *buccal* and *lingual interproximal embrasures*. These embrasures are continuous with the interproximal spaces between the teeth (Fig. 5–13). Above the contact areas incisally and occlusally, the spaces, which are bounded by the marginal ridges as they join the cusps and incisal ridges, are called the *incisal* or *occlusal embrasures*. These embrasures, and the labial or buccal and lingual embrasures, are continuous (Figs. 5–10 and 5–14). The curved proximal surfaces of the contacting teeth roll away from the contact area at all points, occlusally, labially or buccally, and lingually and cervically, and the embrasures and interproximal spaces are continuous, as they surround the areas of contact.

This embrasure form serves two purposes: (1) It makes a spillway for the escape of food during mastication, a physiologic form which reduces forces brought to bear upon the teeth during the reduction of any material that offers resistance; and (2) It prevents food

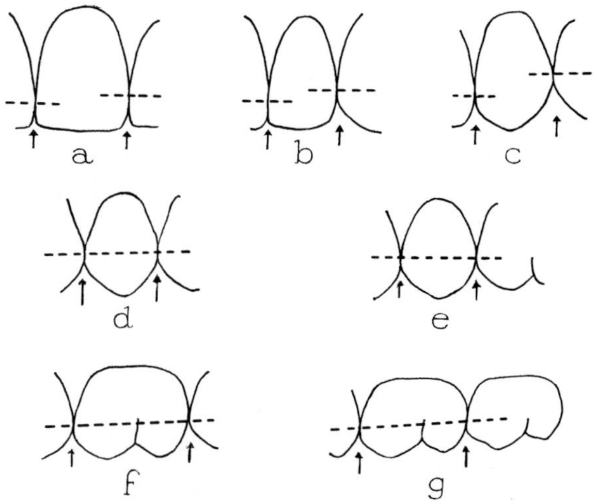

Figure 5–10. Outline drawings of the maxillary teeth in contact, with dotted lines bisecting the contact areas at the various levels as found normally. Arrows point to embrasure spaces.

    a, Central and lateral incisors.
    b, Central and lateral incisors and canine.
    c, Lateral incisor, canine and first premolar.
    d, Canine, first and second premolars.
    e, First and second premolars and first molar.
    f, Second premolar, first molar and second molar.
    g, First, second, and third molars.

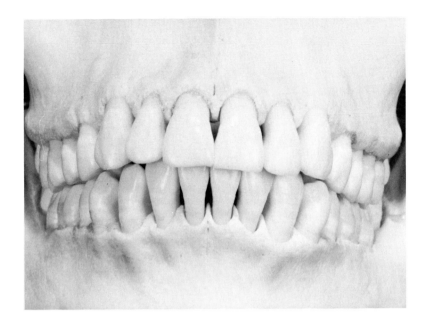

Figure 5–11. The form of the teeth, position and wear of contact areas, type of teeth, and level of eruption of the teeth determine the form of the interproximal "spaces." These factors also determine the interproximal shape of the crest of alveolar bone.

from being forced through the contact area. When teeth wear down to the contact area so that no embrasure remains, especially in the incisors, food is pushed into the contact area even when teeth are not mobile.

The design of contact areas, interproximal spaces and embrasures varies with the form and alignment of the various teeth; each section of the two arches will show similarity of form. In other words, the contact form, the interproximal spacing, and the embrasure form seem rather constant in sectional areas of the dental arches. These sections are named as follows: the maxillary anterior section, the mandibular anterior section, and the maxillary posterior and the mandibular posterior sections. All embrasure spaces are reflections of the form of the teeth involved. Maxillary central and lateral incisors will exhibit one embrasure form, the mandibular incisors another, and so on.

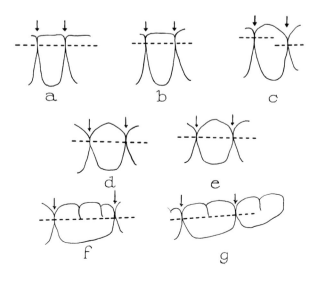

Figure 5–12. Contact levels found normally on mandibular teeth. Arrows point to embrasure spaces.

    a, Central and lateral incisors.
    b, Central and lateral incisors and canine.
    c, Lateral incisor, canine and first premolar.
    d, Canine, first and second premolars.
    e, First and second premolars and first molar.
    f, Second premolar, first and second molars.
    g, First, second and third molars.

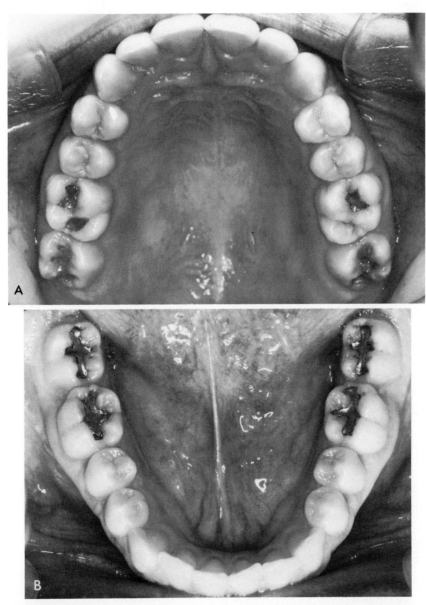

Figure 5–13. Contact relations in a patient with "normal" occlusion. *A*, Maxillary arch, *B*, Mandibular arch.

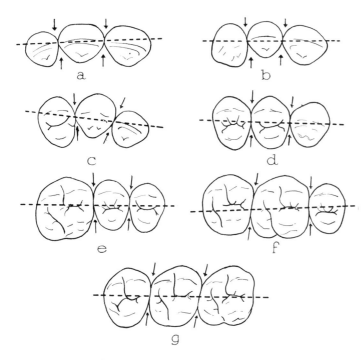

Figure 5–14. Outline drawings of the maxillary teeth from the incisal and occlusal aspects with broken lines bisecting the contact areas. These illustrations show the relative positions of the contact areas labiolingually and buccolingually. Arrows point to embrasure spaces.

a, Central incisors and lateral incisor.

b, Central and lateral incisor and canine.

c, Lateral incisor, canine and first premolar.

d, Canine, first premolar and second premolar.

e, First molar, second premolar and first molar.

f, Second premolar, first molar and second molar.

g, First, second and third molars.

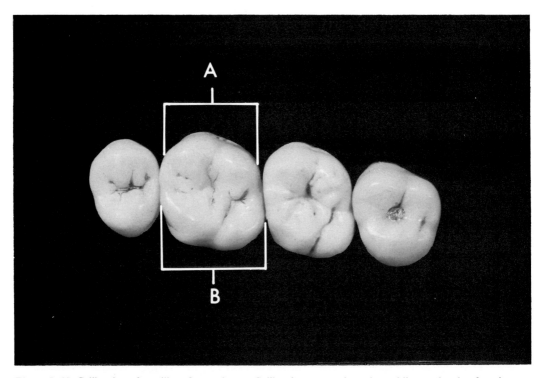

Figure 5–15. Calibration of maxillary first molar. *A,* Calibration at prominent buccal line angles that functions by deflecting food material during mastication. *B,* Calibration of lingual contour from contact area mesially to contact area distally. There are no prominent line angles, but the development of the mesiolingual cusp has widened the rounded lingual form. Thus, the two lingual embrasures are kept similar in size, even though the tooth makes contact with two teeth that are dissimilar lingually. This way, the lingual gingival tissue interproximally is properly protected by the equalization of lingual embrasures.

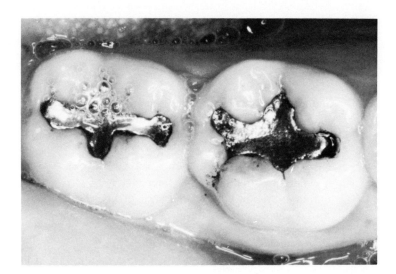

Figure 5–16. Broad contact areas of the mandibular first and second molars in a young adult 21 years old.

Maxillary posteriors and mandibular posteriors apparently require an embrasure design geared for their sections. In some cases, the constancy has to be attained by a tooth form adaptation (Fig. 5–15). The canines, for instance, are shaped so that they act as a catalyst in these matters between anterior and posterior teeth. A line bisecting the labial portion of either canine seems to create an anterior half mesially that resembles half of an anterior tooth and a posterior half that resembles a posterior tooth. The mesial contact is at one level for contact with the lateral incisor, but the distal contact form must be at a level consistent with the contact form of the first premolar whether maxillary or mandibular (Fig. 5–10,*c*).

Contact Areas and Incisal and Occlusal Embrasures from the Labial and Buccal Aspect

It is advisable to refer continually to the illustrations of contacts and embrasures during the reading of the descriptions which follow. Locate the illustration of interest (i.e., Fig. 5–10,*a*) while reading the details concerning contact area levels in the following paragraphs.

Maxillary Teeth

Central Incisors. The contact areas mesially on both central incisors are located at the incisal third of the crowns. Since the mesioincisal third of these teeth approaches a right angle, the incisal embrasure is very slight.

Central and Lateral Incisors. The distal outline of the central incisor crown is rounded. The lateral incisor has a shorter crown and has a more rounded mesioincisal angle than the central incisor. The form of these two teeth coming into contact with each other, therefore, opens up an embrasure space distal to the central larger than the small one mesial to central incisors. A line bisecting the contact areas distal to the central incisor and mesial to the lateral approaches the junction of the middle and incisal thirds of each crown.

Lateral Incisor and Canine. The distal contact area on the lateral incisor is approximately at the middle third. The mesial contact area on the canine is at the junction of the incisal and middle thirds. The form of these teeth creates an embrasure that is more open than the two previously described.

Canine and First Premolar. The canine has a long distal slope to its cusp, which puts the distal crest of curvature at the center of the middle third of the crown. The contact area is, therefore, at that point. This is a very important observation to be made clinically. As mentioned, it is at this point in the dental arch that the canine, situated between the anterior and posterior segments, becomes a part of both (Fig. 5–10, *b* and *c*).

The first premolar has a long cusp form also, which puts its mesial contact area rather high up on the crown. Usually it is just cervical to the junction of the occlusal and middle thirds. The embrasure between these teeth has a wide angle.

First and Second Premolars. The contact areas of these teeth are similar to those just mentioned—usually a little cervical to the junction of the occlusal and middle thirds of the crowns. The form of these teeth creates a wide occlusal embrasure.

It should be noted that the design of the interproximal spaces changes also with the form and dimensions of the teeth in contact.

Second Premolar and First Molar. The position of the contact areas cervico-occlusally is about the same as that found between the premolars.

First and Second and Second and Third Molars. These two contact and embrasure forms may be described together, since they are similar. The distal outline of the first molar is round—a fact that puts the contact area approximately at the center of the middle third of the crown. Here again, it must be emphasized that contact levels on maxillary molars (and even on premolars to some extent) tend to be centered in the middle third of the anatomical crown.

The mesial contact area of the second molar also approaches the middle third of the crown. The occlusal embrasure is generous as a consequence, even though the cusps are not long.

The contact and embrasure design of the second and third molars is similar to those of the first and second molars. The molars become progressively shorter from the first through the third. Again, the dimensions of the tooth crowns will affect the contact and embrasure design.

Mandibular Teeth

Central Incisors. The mesial contact areas on the mandibular central incisors are located at the incisal third of the crowns. At the time of the eruption of these teeth, the mesial and distal incisal angles are slightly rounded and the mamelons are noticeable on the incisal ridges. Soon, however, incisal wear reduces the incisal ridge to a straight surface and the mesial and distal angles approach right angles in sharpness. This is due partly to wear at the contact areas (Figs. 5–11 and 5–12). In many instances, the contact areas extend to the mesioincisal angle. There will, therefore, be a small incisal embrasure mesially between the mandibular central incisors unless wear through usage obliterates it.

Central and Lateral Incisors. The distal contact areas and the incisal embrasures on the central incisors and the mesial contact areas and incisal embrasures on the lateral incisors are similar to those just described. Since the mandibular central and lateral incisors are small mesiodistally and supplement each other in function, the design of their crowns brings about similar contact and embrasure forms.

Note the slender gothic archlike spaces that circumscribe the interproximal spaces between the mandibular anterior teeth.

Lateral Incisor and Canine. The positions of the contact areas distally on the lateral incisor and mesially on the canine are approximately the same, cervicoincisally, as the other two just described. The teeth are in contact at the incisal third close to the incisal ridges. However, the mesioincisal angle of the canine is more rounded than the others, which form opens up a small incisal embrasure at this point.

The interproximal spacing between lateral and canine is very similar in outline to the two interproximal spaces just described.

Canine and First Premolar. The distal slope of the cusp of the mandibular canine is pronounced and long, which places the distal contact area on this tooth somewhat cervical to the junction of its incisal and middle thirds.

The first premolar has a long buccal cusp, and although its crown is shorter than the canine, the mesial contact area has about the same relation cervico-occlusally as that found distally on the canine—just cervical to the junction of the occlusal and middle thirds. Thus, the whole arrangement places these contact areas level with each other.

The occlusal embrasure is quite wide and pronounced because of the cusp forms of the two teeth. The interproximal space has been reduced by the lowering of the contact areas cervically, comparing favorably to the design for posterior mandibular teeth.

First and Second Premolars. From the buccal aspect, the crowns of these two teeth are similar. The buccal cusp of the second premolar is not quite as long as that of the first premolar. The contact of these teeth is nearly level with that of the canine and first premolar. The slope of the cusps creates a large occlusal embrasure. The interproximal space is a little smaller than that between the canine and first premolar.

Second Premolar and First Molar. The contact and embrasure design for these teeth is similar to that just described for the premolars. The mesiobuccal cusp of the first molar is shorter and more rounded than the cusp of the second premolar, which varies the embrasure somewhat, and since the crown of the molar is a little shorter, it reduces the interproximal space to that extent.

First and Second and Second and Third Molars. These two contact and embrasure designs may be described together, since they are similar.

The proximal surfaces are quite round; that is, the distal surface of the first molar, mesial surface of the second molar, distal surface of the second molar, and mesial surface of the third molar. The occlusal embrasures are, therefore, generous above the points of contact even though the cusps are short and rounded.

Because the molars become progressively shorter from the first to the third, the centers of the contact areas drop cervically also. A line bisecting the contact areas of the second and third molars is located approximately at the center of the middle thirds of the crowns.

The interproximal spaces have been reduced considerably because of their shortened form.

Contact Areas and Labial, Buccal, and Lingual Embrasures from the Incisal and Occlusal Aspects*

To study the relative positions of contact areas and the related labial, buccal, and lingual embrasures, and also to get proper perspective, the eye must be directed at the incisal surfaces of anterior teeth and directly above the surface of each tooth being examined in series. Posterior teeth are examined in the same manner. Look down on each tooth or group of teeth by facing the occlusal surfaces on a line with the long axis.

The problem at this point is to discover the relative positions of contacts in a labio- or buccolingual direction and to observe the embrasure form facially and lingually created by the tooth forms and their contact relations.

A generalization may be established in locating contact areas faciolingually. Anterior teeth will have their contacts centered labiolingually, whereas posterior teeth will have contact areas slightly buccal to the center buccolingually. This buccal inclination must be carefully studied and must not be overemphasized.

Except for the maxillary first molar, all crowns converge more lingually than facially from contact areas. The maxillary first molar is the only tooth wider lingually than bucally. Its formation makes a necessary adjustment of the mesiolingual embrasure when the tooth form of maxillary posteriors changes from the maxillary premolar form to the purely rhomboidal form of maxillary second and third molars. This situation will be discussed more fully later on (Fig. 5–15).

The narrower measurement lingually rather than facially causes wider embrasures lingually compared with facial embrasures. Compare the two types of embrasures displayed by maxillary central and lateral incisors.

Maxillary Teeth (Figs. 5–13, A, and 5–14)

Central Incisors. The contact areas of these teeth are centered labiolingually. The labial embrasure is a V-shaped space created by the labial form of these crowns. The lingual embrasure widens out more than the labial embrasure because of the lingual convergence of the crowns (Fig. 5–13, A). Note the centering of the labioincisal edge in respect to the crown outline of these teeth, and the narrowness of the lingual surfaces in comparison with the broad labial faces.

Central and Lateral Incisors. The contact areas of these teeth are centered labiolingually also.

Lateral Incisor and Canine. The contact area is centered labiolingually on both canine and lateral incisors. The lingual embrasure is similar to that of the central and lateral incisors, but the labial embrasure is changed somewhat by a definite convexity at the mesiolabial line angle of the canine.

Canine and First Premolar. The contact area is centered on the distal surface of the canine but is a little buccal to center on the mesial surface of the first premolar. The embrasure design lingually is marked by a concavity in the region of the distolingual line angle of the canine and by a developmental groove crossing the mesial marginal ridge of the first premolar.

---

* *Refer to Figures 5–13, 5–14, 5–16, and 5–17.*

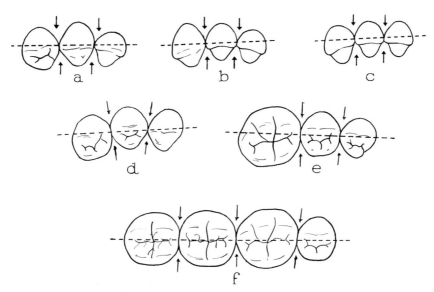

Figure 5–17. Contact relation of mandibular teeth labiolingually and buccolingually when surveyed from the incisal and occlusal aspects. Arrows point to embrasure spaces.

    a, Central incisors and lateral incisor.
    b, Central and lateral incisor and canine.
    c, Lateral incisor, canine, and first premolar.
    d, Canine, first premolar, and second premolar.
    e, First premolar, second premolar, and first molar.
    f, Second premolar and first, second, and third molars.

First and Second Premolars. The contact areas are nearly centered buccolingually. The embrasures buccally and lingually are regular in outline although slightly different in design.

    The prominence of the mesio- and distobuccal line angles of the premolars is in direct contrast to the even taper of these teeth lingually, as viewed from the occlusal aspect. This form demonstrates a slight variation between buccal and lingual embrasures.

Second Premolar and First Molar. As usual, a line bisecting the contact areas of these teeth will be nearly centered on the distal surface of the second premolar. The area on the mesial surface of the first molar will be located farther buccally than other contact areas on the maxillary posterior teeth. The contact areas are wider on molars because of the greater width buccolingually of the molar teeth.

    The buccal embrasure between these teeth and the location of the mesial contact area of the first molar are influenced by the prominence of the mesiobuccal line angle of the maxillary first molar and the matching prominence of the distobuccal line angle of the maxillary second premolar. The lingual embrasure is kept standard for the molar area by the enlargement of the mesiolingual cusp of the first molar. Occasionally, this cusp will carry a small conformation lingually as part of the change in form (fifth cusp, or cusp of Carabelli). Usually, the mesiolingual cusp of the maxillary first molar will be rounded out, with no more than a developmental groove showing that an extra cusp formation may have been intended.

    The mesiolingual lobe of this tooth is always large, however, causing the tooth to be wider lingually from its mesiolingual line angle to its distolingual line angle than it is from the mesiobuccal line angle to the distobuccal line angle. If it were not for this fact, the rhomboid form of the first molar in contact with the tapered form of the second premolar would open up a lingual embrasure of extremely large proportions. The large mesiolingual lobe makes up for the change in occlusal outline from premolar form to molar form, keeping the conformity of the lingual embrasures (Fig. 5–15).

First and Second and Second and Third Molars. These contact and embrasure forms may be described together, since they are similar. Although the mesiobuccal line angles of the second and third molars are not as sharp as that of the first molar, they are prominent nevertheless.

The distobuccal line angles of all the maxillary molars are indistinct and rounded, so that the buccal embrasure forms are shaped and characterized mainly by the prominent mesiobuccal line angle. The mesiolingual line angles of the second and third molars are rounded and in conjunction with the rounded distolingual line angles; the lingual embrasures between first, second, and third molars present a regular and open form (Fig. 5–14, *f* and *g*).

The contact areas are broad and centered buccolingually. The embrasures are uniform. Note the generous proportions of the buccal embrasures.

Mandibular Teeth (Figs. 5–13, *B*, 5–16, and 5–17)

Central Incisors and Central and Lateral Incisors. These contact areas and embrasures may be described together, since they are similar.

Although these teeth are narrow mesiodistally, their labiolingual measurements are not much less than those of the maxillary central and lateral incisors. The mandibular central incisors will come within a millimeter or so of having the same labiolingual diameter as that of the maxillary central incisors; the *mandibular* lateral incisors will have a labiolingual diameter as great if not greater than that of the *maxillary* lateral incisors.

The contact areas are centered labiolingually and the embrasures are uniform. Although the mesiodistal dimensions are less, the outline form of the incisal aspects of the mandibular central and lateral incisors is similar to that of the maxillary central and lateral incisors in that the lingual outlines have a rounded taper in comparison with broader, flattened labial faces.

Lateral Incisor and Canine. The contact areas are centered, and the lingual embrasure is similar to those just described. The labial embrasure is influenced by the prominance of the mesiolabial line angle of the canine. It will be remembered that the maxillary canine presents the same characteristic.

Canine and First Premolar. The contact areas are approximately centered, and the buccal embrasure is smooth and uniform in outline. The lingual embrasure is opened up somewhat by a slight concavity on the canine distolingually and by a characteristic developmental groove across the marginal ridge of the first premolar mesiolingually.

First and Second Premolars. The contact areas are nearly centered buccolingually but are broader than those found mesial to them because the distal curvature of the first premolar describes a larger arc than the mesial curvature and the mesial contacting surface of the second premolar is relatively broad and describes a shallower curved surface than that of the distal surface of the first premolar.

Because of the lingual convergence of the first premolar and the narrow lingual cusp form, the lingual embrasure is as wide as the one mesial to it.

Second Premolar and First Molar. The contact areas are wide and almost centered. The extent of the contact areas is sometimes increased by a slight concavity in the outline of the mesial surface of the first molar below the marginal ridge. The mesial contact area of the first molar is located farther buccally than any of the other contact areas on mandibular posterior teeth. It must be remembered that the same situation holds true in the upper dental arch when describing the contacts of maxillary first molars and second premolars.

The prominence of the first molar at the mesiobuccal line angle is readily apparent. The mesial outline of the crown tapers to the lingual, forming a generous lingual embrasure in conjunction with the smooth curvature of the second premolar distolingually.

First and Second Molar. The contact areas are nearly centered buccolingually, although they are not so broad as the contact just described. This variation is brought about by the design of the first molar distally. The distal contact area of the first molar is confined to the distal cusp, which does not present the broad surface for contact with the second molar that was found mesially in contact with the second premolar. This form, along with the rounded outline at the distobuccal line angle, opens up both embrasures wider than those found immediately mesial.

The outline of the first molar crown just lingual to the distal contact area presents a straight line and occasionally a concavity.

The second molar outline buccally and lingually on both sides of the mesial contact area is uniformly rounded.

Second and Third Molars. The contact areas are broad, and they are nearly centered buccolingually. When the third molar is normally developed, it is similar in outline to the second molar from the occlusal aspect. The buccal and lingual embrasures between these teeth are almost alike in form and extent.

A straight line may be drawn through the contact areas of the second premolar and the three molars, and it will come very near to bisecting all of the contact areas. These four mandibular teeth are set in a line that is almost straight (Figs. 5–13, *B,* and 5–17*f*).

Facial and Lingual Contours at the Cervical Thirds (Cervical Ridges) and Lingual Contours at the Middle Thirds of Crowns*

The teeth are unique in that their static outside form is physiologic. Even the maxillary teeth, which are firmly set in their alveoli, when moving through food material activated by mandibular movement change their functional crown form from a static to a dynamic form. All details of tooth form will have some effect upon the stabilization of the tooth in the arch.

Examinations will show that all tooth crowns, when viewed from mesial or distal aspects, have rather uniform curvatures at the cervical thirds and at the middle thirds labially or buccally or lingually, depending upon the teeth being examined (Fig. 5–18, *a, d,* and *e*). As has already been discussed briefly, concepts about the importance of these contours in relation to protection and stimulation of the gingiva have been challenged. However, the evidence does not contradict the possibility of food impaction or trauma occurring as the result of "faulty" contours (undercontoured). It is, rather, that inflammatory periodontal disease is caused primarily by bacterial plaque and that buccal and lingual contours do not appear to be related to plaque removal during mastication. Thus in the

* *All are protective contours. See Figures 5–19 through 5–23.*

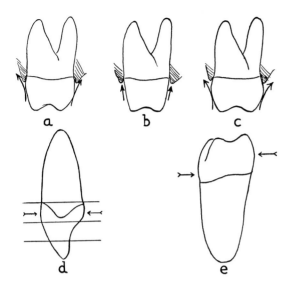

Figure 5–18. Schematic drawings of curvatures labially, buccally and lingually.

  a, Normal curvatures as found on maxillary molar. Arrow shows theoretical path of food during mastication.

  b, If molar shows little or no curvature, there is possibility for food impaction.

  c, Molar with curvature in excess of normal. The significance of such an excess in curvature has not been firmly established.

  d, Normal cervical curvatures as found on maxillary incisors. The crests of curvature are opposite each other labiolingually.

  e, Curvatures as found on mandibular posterior teeth.

absence of oral hygiene measures, the self-cleansing mechanisms of the musculature and suggested cleansing action of coarse food are not adequate to remove plaque sufficiently well to prevent gingivitis. However, the relative importance of contour on trauma, food impaction, and occasionally, the initiation of a localized inflammatory response cannot be overlooked. The buccal and lingual contours can deflect food material away from the gingival margins during mastication (Fig. 5–18, *a*). Undercontoured surfaces can lead to food impaction (Fig. 5–18, *b*), but the significance of overcontouring (Fig. 5–18, *c*) has yet to be clarified, although overcontouring does not appear to be beneficial. Marginal adaption and oral hygiene are of far greater significance for gingival health.

The cervical third formation of the crowns is the area of soft tissue attachment. The *epithelial attachment* of soft tissue to the teeth, soon to be described more fully, is entirely within the area of the cervical third of the crowns. The cervical curvatures are often spoken of as *cervical ridges*. However, cervical *curvatures* is a more descriptive term because few of these areas are pronounced enough to be called "ridges" and yet rarely will a normal tooth be seen with no curvature at all.

In young people, and some older ones, most of the curvature lies beneath the gingival crest. In older persons, the cementoenamel line may be visible or may be just under the gingival crest, with most of the prominent curvature exposed.

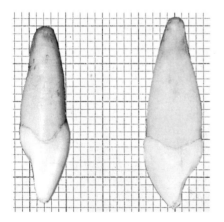

Figure 5–19. The maxillary central incisor exhibits a curvature of approximately 0.5 mm labially and somewhat less lingually at the cervical third of the crown. Many specimens will show equal curvature on the two sides. The maxillary canine exhibits approximately the same curvature. Note the limitation of the curvature at the cingulum area above the cervical line.

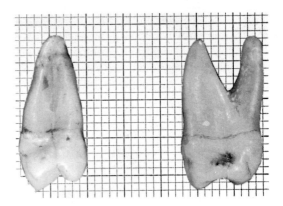

Figure 5–20. The maxillary first premolar has a curvature of approximately 0.5 mm buccally and lingually. The crest of curvature buccally is located at the cervical third of the crown and lingually at the middle third. The maxillary first molar has curvatures of the same degree at similar points on both sides.

Gradual recession of the gingivae throughout life may be a normal procedure. However, root exposure may lead to cemental caries, cervical sensitivity, and abrasion with improper toothbrushing.

All protective curvatures are most functional when the teeth are in proper alignment. *It should be quite plain that when teeth are malposed, their curvatures are displaced and may be ineffective.*

The curvatures are rather uniform at the cervical third or lingual third of all of the maxillary teeth and on the buccal portion of mandibular posterior teeth (Figs. 5–19 through 5–21).

The normal curvature from the cementoenamel junction to the crest of contour is approximately 0.5 mm in extent. When the long axis of the tooth is placed vertically, it is found that this curvature is fairly constant and may be recognized as average or normal for the maxillary teeth, labially or buccally and lingually, and for the mandibular posterior teeth on the buccal surfaces. The curvature, lingually, of mandibular posterior teeth extends about a millimeter beyond the cervical line. Here, however, the extreme curvature does not contribute to the stasis of food material at the cervix because of the activity of the tongue in keeping the lingual surfaces of these teeth clean.

Figure 5–19 shows that the maxillary central incisor and canine have curvatures, labially and lingually, that are almost identical. *Because the canines have a more massive development of the cingulum, clinical observation only gives an impression of greater curvature. This is an optical illusion that is dispelled when the outline of the canine is properly compared with other teeth on a graph.*

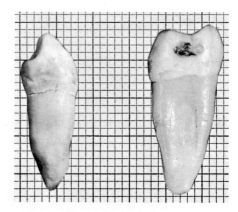

Figure 5–21. Mandibular first premolar and first molar. Both teeth have a curvature of approximately 0.5 mm buccally at the cervical third of the crown and a curvature of approximately 1 mm lingually, with the crest of curvature at the middle third.

The maxillary premolar and molar show the same limited curvatures. The crest of curvature, lingually, on all posterior teeth is at or near the middle third of the crowns.

When curvatures are found that are greater in extent than 0.5 mm, rarely is the curvature as much as 1 mm, except lingually on mandibular posterior teeth and often lingually on maxillary posterior teeth. In these instances, the crest of contour will be found at the middle third of the crowns instead of at the cervical third (Fig. 5–21). These crests are always lingual.

The eye is easily confused at times when viewing certain aspects of the teeth because of the abrupt sweep of curvatures as they travel from the cervical line toward occlusal and incisal surfaces; i.e., the buccal surfaces of mandibular posterior teeth, the lingual surfaces of posterior maxillary teeth, or the lingual surfaces of canines. When the actual photographs are placed on a background of squares (Fig. 5–22), with the long axis of each tooth held vertically, we readily see that the extent of curvature from the cervical line to the crest of curvature facially or lingually is slight. Quite often, in restorative procedures, it is *greatly overestimated and reproduced.*

Figure 5–23 shows a mandibular central incisor and canine from the mesial aspect. Here the curvature at the cervical third is less than that of the other teeth in the mouth, occasionally appearing so slight that it is hardly distinguishable. The canine often has very little more curvature immediately above the cervical line than the mandibular central or lateral incisor.

Summary of Physiologic Contours of Tooth Crowns, Facially and Lingually

All tooth crowns will exhibit some curvature above the cervical line. Again, this slight bulge at the cervical third is sometimes called the *cervical ridge*. Although the extent of curvature will vary in different individuals, apparently it is not normal for the curvatures on permanent teeth to extend out as much as 1 mm beyond the cervical line; usually the curvature will be less.

The curvatures on the labial, buccal, and lingual surfaces of all maxillary teeth and on the buccal surfaces of mandibular posterior teeth will be rather uniform; the average curvature as mentioned before is about 0.5 mm.

Mandibular posterior teeth will have a lingual curvature of approximately 1 mm, with the crest of curvature at the *middle third* of the crown instead of at the cervical third. Occasionally *maxillary posterior* teeth will have similar curvatures on the lingual aspect. (Compare the lingual curvatures in Figures 5–20 and 5–21.)

Mandibular anterior teeth will show less curvature on the crown above the cervical line than any of the other teeth. Usually, it is less than 0.5 mm, and, occasionally, it is so slight that it is hardly distinguishable. The mandibular canines may show a little more curvature than central and lateral incisors.

Regardless of whether or not theories explaining the functional significance of these contours are correct, there is little doubt that they are important. If this were not so, there would be more variance in the presence or the extent of curvature. The curvatures as described seem to be as standard and as constant as any anatomical detail can be.

The Height of Epithelial Attachment—Curvatures of the Cervical Lines (Cementoenamel Junction) Mesially and Distally

The *epithelial attachment* seals the soft tissue to the tooth. It is a remarkable system capable of adjustment to local physiologic changes, but it is vulnerable to physical injury. Careless treatment can cause breaks in the attachment, making the tooth liable to further

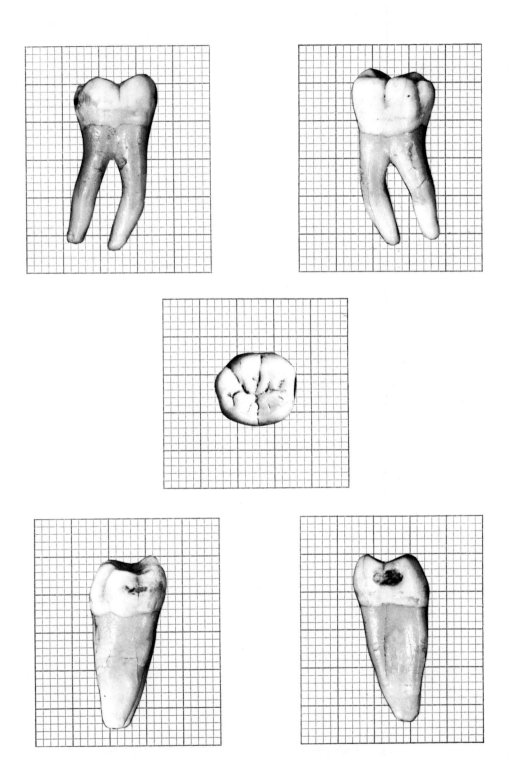

Figure 5–22. Photographs of a natural specimen of a mandibular first molar, taken with a lens capable of two diameter registrations. Cut-outs of these photos were placed on graphs depicting squared millimeters. The result is an accurate graph in millimeters of tooth outlines from five aspects.

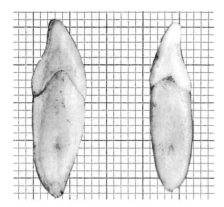

Figure 5–23. Mandibular central incisor and canine. The central incisor curvature labially and lingually is less than 0.5 mm in extent, and the crest of curvature is near the cervical line. The canine also exhibits less than 0.5-mm curvatures, although the crest of curvature is higher up on the crown; however, it is still within the confines of the cervical third.

physical or pathologic injury. The teeth can be injured by careless probing during clinical examination, by improper scaling during prophylactic treatment, by tooth preparation techniques in operative procedures, and so forth.

The height of normal gingival tissue, mesially and distally on approximating teeth, is directly dependent upon the heights of the epithelial attachment on these teeth. Normal attachment follows the curvature of the cementoenamel junction if the teeth are in normal alignment and contact. This does not mean that the cementoenamel junction and the epithelial attachment are at the same level, but it does mean that they tend to follow the same curvature even though the epithelial attachment may be higher on the crown on its enamel surface (Fig. 5–24). A comparison of the curvatures of the cementoenamel junction mesially and distally on the teeth is therefore in order. Measurement and comparisons are shown in Figures 5–25 and 5–26; see also Table 1–1.

The extent of curvature seems to depend upon the height of the contact area above the crown cervix and also upon the diameter of the crown labiolingually or buccolingually. The crowns of anterior teeth, which are narrower and longer from these aspects, show the greatest curvature (Fig. 5–25). In using the words ''height'' and ''above,'' the supposition is made that in either the maxillary or the mandibular arch the occlusal surfaces of the teeth are above the cervices. Any point approaching the incisal edge or occlusal surface of a crown is considered above the cervix, and the height is increased as it approaches occlusal levels.

Periodontal attachment that follows the curvature of the cementoenamel junction mesially and distally seems to be about as high on *mandibular* anterior teeth as on their counterparts that are larger in the maxillary arch. Although the crowns of the mandibular anterior teeth average 1 mm less in labiolingual diameter (the lateral incisors excepted), the

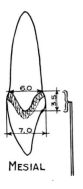

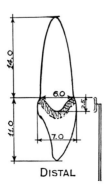

MESIAL   DISTAL

Figure 5–24. Curvatures of the cervical line (cementoenamel junction) mesially and distally on the maxillary central incisor, demonstrating the points of measurement in determining the relation between the curvatures of the cervical line mesially and distally. Other points of measurement of the crown and root, when one observes the mesial and distal aspects, are outlined and are considered average measurements for a mandibular central incisor. The shaded area in the form of a band on the enamel follows the cervical curvature and represents the epithelial attachment of gingival tissue to the enamel of the crown.

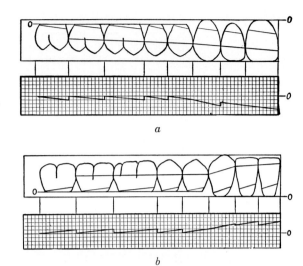

Figure 5–25. Schematic drawings of the crowns of maxillary and mandibular teeth with associated graphs of the average extent of curvatures of the cervical line mesially and distally. *a,* Maxillary teeth. *b,* Mandibular teeth. Compare the graph of cervical curvatures with a line drawn through the center of contact areas. Note that the graph tends to run somewhat parallel to this line.

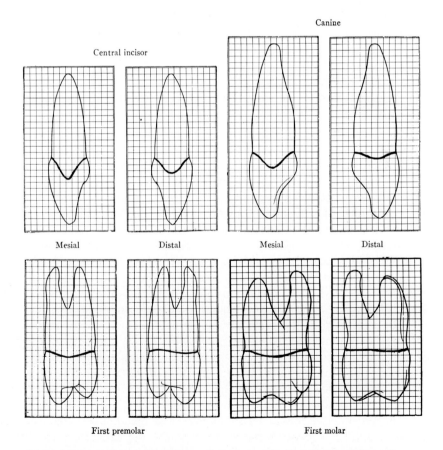

Figure 5–26. Graphs of typical forms of maxillary teeth accenting the outlines of cervical lines mesially and distally.

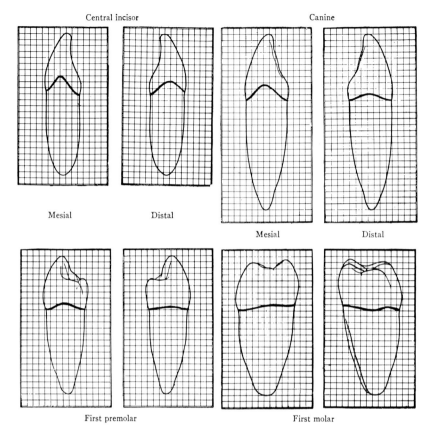

Figure 5–27. Graphs of typical forms of mandibular teeth accenting the outlines of cervical lines mesially and distally.

contact areas are higher accordingly, being near the incisal edges on centrals and laterals. Consequently, measurements will usually show less than 1 mm variation in mesial and distal curvatures between maxillary and mandibular anterior teeth.

Posterior teeth will show little variation in either arch. Figure 5–25 is a diagrammatic drawing of the outlines of the teeth on one side of the arch when viewed from the labial and buccal aspects. These outlines have been placed so that a direct comparison can be made with the graphs below them. The graphs demonstrate the relative height of individual attachments in the average normal case. They are based on cases having upper central incisors with crowns 10.5 to 11 mm in length. Unless the teeth were very large or very small, the graphs would not vary from those illustrated by more than 0.5 mm.

The curvature of the cervical line of most teeth (cementoenamel junction) will be approximately 1 mm less distally than mesially. The greater curvature will be found at the median line on central incisors, maxillary and mandibular. The height of attachment is dependent upon the height of the contact areas of the two teeth creating the interproximal space. If the mesial curvature of the central incisor is calibrated at 3.5 mm, the distal curvature will be about 1 mm less, or 2.5 mm.

The six anterior teeth, both maxillary and mandibular, when compared with posteriors, exhibit the greatest curvature. Because the canine crowns function distally as posterior teeth, their curvatures distally represented by the cementoenamel junction are slight, being about 1 to 1.5 mm on the average. Premolars and molars have rather uniform but slight curvatures. The contact levels are low in relation to total crown length; consequently, these teeth do not have high periodontal attachments interproximally. The average premolar or molar has a curvature mesially of only 1 mm or less, with no curvature, or even a "minus" curvature distally (Fig. 5–27).

From the operator's point of view, anterior teeth especially must be carefully approached (when attachment is normal) as, for example, in preparing them for restoration Posterior teeth have curvatures that are less critical.

A summary of the height of periodontal attachment interproximally indicates the attachment to be highest at the median line on central incisors. In distal progression the height of attachment decreases along with the decrease in curvature of cementoenamel junctions until the mesial surface of the first premolar is reached. From this point distally through third molars, curvatures are slight.

The possibility of injury to mesial and distal periodontal attachment during tooth preparation should be considered. The height of attachment must be ascertained by careful probing and by the continuous observation of landmarks during the operation. Careless manipulation of band impressions must be avoided also.

To secure scientific data regarding comparative curvatures, it was necessary to examine many tooth specimens. It was found that, usually, a graph of the cementoenamel curvatures from the median line distally could be staggered, as in Figure 5–25. It will be noticed that in the posterior teeth, the variation in curvature is slight and the amount of curvature is minor, the variance ranging from 1 mm mesially toward the occlusal surface to a slight curvature in the opposite direction. (Note the distal aspect of the mandibular first molar, Fig. 5–27.)

Figures 5–26 and 5–27 are graphs of maxillary and mandibular teeth demonstarting typical cervical curvatures mesially and distally.

References

Ash, M. M., and Karring, T. (1988). Periodontal and occlusal considerations in operative dentistry. In Hörsted-Bindslev P., and Mjör, I. A. (eds.), Modern Concepts in Operative Dentistry. Copenhagen: Munksgaard.

Beaudreau, D. E. (1973). Tooth form and contour. J. Am. Soc. Psychosom. Dent. Med. 3:36.

Becker, C. M., and Kaldahl, W. B. (1981). Currrent theories of crown contour, margin placement and pontic design. J. Prosthet. Dent. 45:268.

Butler, P. M., and Joysey, K. A. (eds.). (1978). *Development, Function and Evolution of Teeth.* New York: Academic Press.

Eissman, H. F., Radke, R. A., and Noble, W. H. (1971). Physiologic design criteria for fixed dental restorations. Dent. Clin. North Am. 15:543.

Farer, J., and Isaacson, D. (1974). Biologic contours. J. Prev. Dent. 1:4.

Herdlanda, R. E., et al. (1962). Forms and contours and extensions of full coverage in occlusal reconstruction. Dent. Clin. N. Am. 147 (March).

Lindhe, J., and Wicen, P. O. (1969). The effects on the gingivae of chewing fibrous foods. J. Periodont. Res. 4:193.

Morris, M. (1962). Artifical crown contours and gingival health. J. Prosthet. Dent. 12:1146.

Perel, M. L. (1971). Periodontal considerations of crown contours. J. Prosthet. Dent. 26:627.

Ramfjord, S. P., and Ash, M. M. (1989). *Periodontology and Periodontics.* St. Louis, MO: Ishiyaku Euro America, p. 69.

Ryder, J. A. (1878). On the mechanical genesis of tooth forms. Proc. Acad. Natl. Sci. Phila., p. 45.

Sackett, B. P., and Gildenhuys, R. R. (1976). The effect of axial crown over-contour on adolescents. J. Periodont. 47:320.

Volchansky, A. (1979–1980). The role of clinical crown height and gingival margin position in oral disease. Diastema 7:17.

Wade, A. B. (1971). Effect on dental plaque of chewing apples. Dent. Pract. 21:194.

Wheeler, R. C. (1961). Complete crown form and the periodontium. J. Prosthet. Dent. 11:722.

Youdelis, R. A., Weaver, J. D., and Sapkos, S. (1973). Facial and lingual contours of artifical complete crown restorations and their effects on the periodontium. J. Prosthet. Dent. 29:61.

6 *The Permanent Maxillary Incisors*

The maxillary incisors are *four* in number. The maxillary *central* incisors are centered in the maxilla, one on either side of the median line, with the mesial surface of each in contact with the mesial surface of the other. The maxillary and mandibular central incisors are the only neighboring teeth in the dental arches with mesial surfaces in contact. The right and left maxillary *lateral* or *second* incisors are distal to the central incisors.

The maxillary central incisor is larger than the lateral incisor. These teeth supplement each other in function, and they are similar anatomically. The incisors are shearing or cutting teeth. Their major function is to punch and cut food material during the process of mastication. These teeth have incisal *ridges* or *edges* rather than cusps such as are found on the canines and posterior teeth.

It might be well at this point to differentiate between the two terms, "incisal *ridge*" and "incisal *edge*." The incisal ridge is that portion of the crown which makes up the complete incisal portion. When an incisor is newly erupted, the incisal portion is rounded and merges with the mesio- and distoincisal angles and the labial and lingual surfaces. This ridge portion of the crown is called the *incisal ridge*. The term "edge" implies an angle formed by the merging of two flat surfaces. Therefore, an incisal edge does not exist on an incisor until occlusal wear has created a flattened surface linguoincisally, which surface forms an angle with the labial surface. The *incisal edge* is formed by the junction of the linguoincisal surface, sometimes called the "incisal surface," and the labial surface (Fig. 6–1).

Preceding the description of each tooth in this and subsequent chapters, the chronology of *calcification* and *eruption* of the tooth will be given as in the table following. A table of measurements as suggested by the author for carving technique will follow. Knowing the proportions of the individual tooth helps one learn the proportions of one tooth to another.

Outline drawings of the five aspects of the teeth, and following that tooth carving, are explained more fully in *An Atlas of Tooth Form* (W. B. Saunders Company, Philadelphia). *Atlas of Tooth Form* will be of interest not only to undergraduates in dentistry but also to dental ancillaries who are to be trained to work with graduate dental organizations.

Maxillary Central Incisor

The maxillary central incisor is the widest mesiodistally of any of the anterior teeth (Table 6–1). The labial face is less convex than the maxillary lateral incisor or canine, which gives the central incisor a squared or rectangular appearance. From this aspect, the crown nearly

128

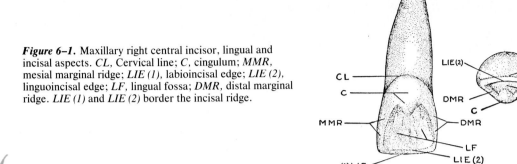

Figure 6–1. Maxillary right central incisor, lingual and incisal aspects. *CL,* Cervical line; *C,* cingulum; *MMR,* mesial marginal ridge; *LIE (1),* labioincisal edge; *LIE (2),* linguoincisal edge; *LF,* lingual fossa; *DMR,* distal marginal ridge. *LIE (1)* and *LIE (2)* border the incisal ridge.

always looks symmetrical and regularly formed, having a nearly straight incisal edge, a cervical line with even curvature toward the root, a mesial side with straight outline, the distal side more curved. The mesial incisal angle is relatively sharp, the distal incisal angle rounded (Fig. 6–2).

Although the *labial* surface of the crown is usually convex, especially toward the cervical third, some central incisors will be flat at the middle and incisal portions. The enamel surface is relatively smooth. When the tooth is newly erupted or if little wear is evident, mamelons will be seen on the incisal ridge. The middle one is the smallest. The developmental lines on the labial surface which divide the surface into three parts are most noticeable at the middle portion if they can be distinguished at all (see Fig. 4–22).

Lingually, the surface form of the maxillary central incisor is more irregular. The largest part of the middle and incisal portions of the lingual area is concave. The concavity is bordered by mesial and distal marginal ridges, the lingual portion of the incisal ridge, and the convexity rootwise of the cingulum. The lingual topography gives a scooplike form to the crown (Fig. 6–3).

The maxillary central incisor usually develops normally. One anomaly that sometimes occurs is a short root. Another variation is an unusually long crown (see Fig. 6–12, specimens *4* and *5*).

The maxillary central incisors are the most prominent teeth in the mouth. There are two basic forms: The first is relatively wide at the cervix when viewed from the labial aspect, in comparison with the mesiodistal width at the contact areas (see Fig. 6–9, specimens *1* and *4*); the second form is relatively narrow at the cervix, where the root joins the crown, in comparison with the mesiodistal width at the contact areas (Fig. 6–9, specimens *5, 7,* and *9*).

In the description of the central incisor, an attempt will be made to strike an average between the extremes of the two forms.

Detailed Description of the Maxillary Central Incisor from All Aspects

Figures 6–1 through 6–12 illustrate the maxillary central incisor in various aspects.

Labial Aspect (Figs. 6–2 and 6–9)

The crown of the average central incisor will be 10 to 11 mm long from the highest point on the cervical line to the lowest point on the incisal edge. The mesiodistal measurement will

Table 6–1. Maxillary Central Incisor

First evidence of calcification   3 to 4 months
Enamel completed   4 to 5 years
Eruption   7 to 8 years
Root completed   10 years

Measurement Table

	Cervico-incisal Length of Crown	Length of Root	Mesiodistal Diameter of Crown	Mesiodistal Diameter of Crown at Cervix	Labio-or Bucco-lingual Diameter of Crown	Labio-or Bucco-lingual Diameter at Cervix	Curvature of Cervical Line—Mesial	Curvature of Cervical Line—Distal
Dimensions suggested for carving technique	10.5*	13.0	8.5	7.0	7.0	6.0	3.5	2.5

* In millimeters.

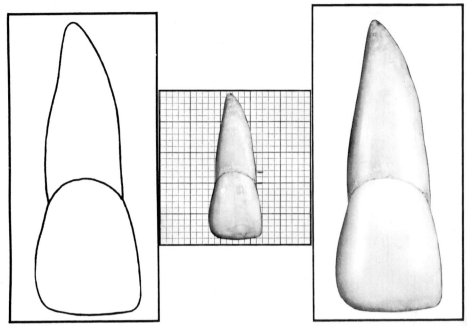

Figure 6–2. Maxillary right central incisor, labial aspect.

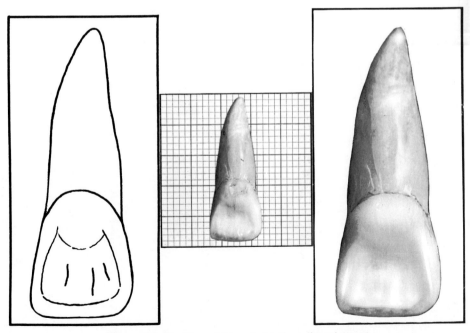

Figure 6–3. Maxillary right central incisor, lingual aspect.

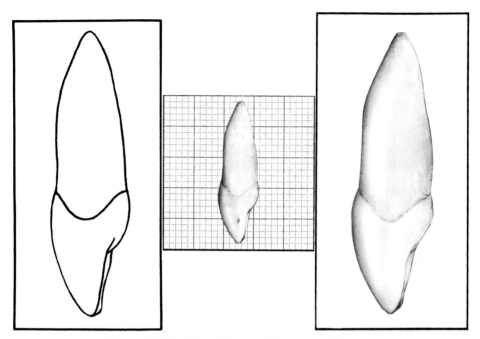

Figure 6–4. Maxillary right central incisor, mesial aspect.

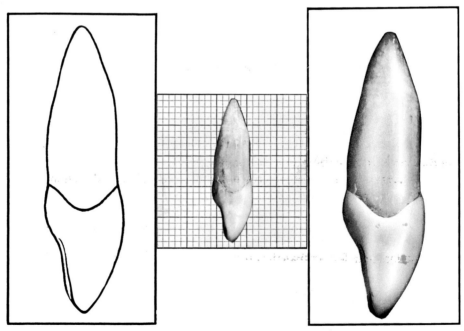

Figure 6–5. Maxillary right central incisor, distal aspect.

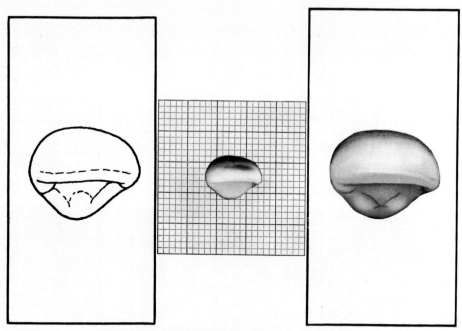

Figure 6–6. Maxillary right central incisor, incisal aspect.

be 8 to 9 mm wide at the contact areas. The mesiodistal measurement, where the root joins the crown, will be 1.5 to 2 mm less. The crests of curvature mesially and distally on the crown represent the areas at which the central incisor contacts its neighbors. Any change in the position of this crest of contour affects the level of the contact area (Fig. 5–10, *a*).

The mesial outline of the crown is only slightly convex, with the crest of curvature (representing the contact area) approaching the mesioincisal angle (See "Proximal Contact Areas," Chapter 5.)

The distal outline of the crown is more convex than the mesial outline, the crest of curvature being higher toward the cervical line. The distoincisal angle is not so sharp as the mesioincisal angle, the extent of curvature depending upon the typal form of the tooth.

The incisal outline is usually regular and straight in a mesiodistal direction after the tooth has been in function long enough to obliterate the mamelons. The incisal outline tends to curve downward toward the center of the crown outline, making the crown length greater at the center than at the two mesial angles.

The cervical outline of the crown follows a semicircular direction with the curvature rootwise, from the point at which the root outline joins the crown mesially to the point at which the root outline joins the crown distally.

The root of the central incisor from the labial aspect is cone-shaped, in most instances with a relatively blunt apex, the outline mesially and distally being regular. The root is usually 2 or 3 mm longer than the crown, although it varies considerably. (See illustrations of typical central incisors and those of variations from the labial aspects (Figs. 6–9 and 6–12).

A line drawn through the center of the root and crown of the maxillary central incisor tends to parallel the mesial outline of the crown and root.

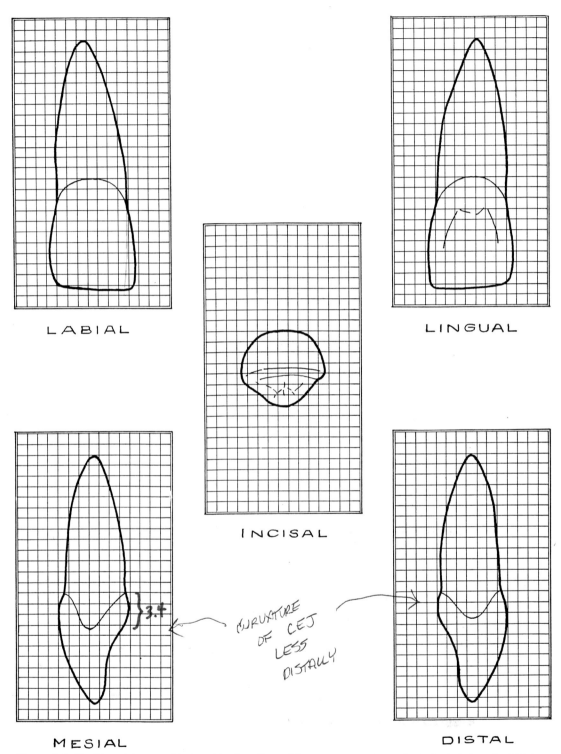

LABIAL

LINGUAL

INCISAL

MESIAL

DISTAL

CURVATURE OF CEJ LESS DISTALLY

Figure 6–7. Maxillary right central incisor. Graph outlines of five aspects are shown. In the incisal view, the labial aspect is at top of drawing.

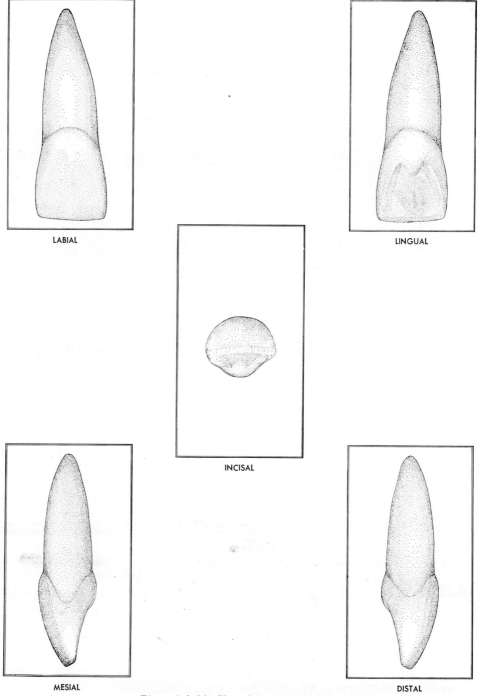

LABIAL

LINGUAL

INCISAL

MESIAL

DISTAL

Figure 6–8. Maxillary right central incisor.

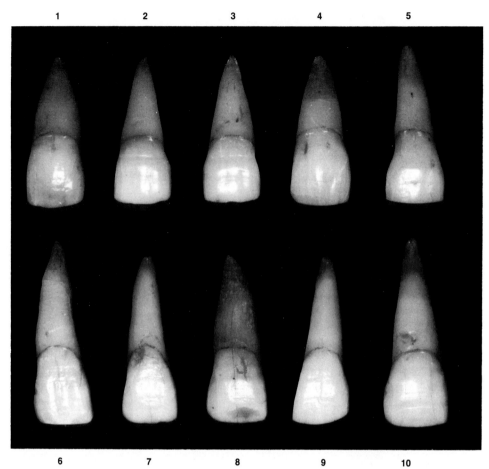

Figure 6–9. Maxillary central incisor, labial aspect. Ten typical specimens are shown.

Lingual Aspect (Fig. 6–3)

The lingual outline of the maxillary central incisor is the reverse of that found on the labial aspect. The lingual aspect of the crown is different, however, when we compare the surface of the lingual aspect with that of the labial aspect. From the labial aspect, the surface of the crown is smooth generally. The lingual aspect has convexities and a concavity. The outline of the cervical line is similar, but immediately below the cervical line a smooth convexity is to be found; this is called the *cingulum* (Fig. 6–1).

Mesially and distally confluent with the cingulum are the *marginal ridges*. Between the marginal ridges, below the cingulum, a shallow concavity is present called the *lingual fossa*. Outlining the lingual fossa, the linguoincisal edge is raised somewhat, being on a level with the marginal ridges mesially and distally, completing the lingual portion of the incisal ridge of the central incisor.

From the foregoing description, we note that the lingual fossa is bordered mesially by the mesial marginal ridge, incisally by the lingual portion of the incisal ridge, distally by the distal marginal ridge, and cervically by the cingulum. Usually there are developmental grooves extending from the cingulum into the lingual fossa.

The crown and root taper lingually, making the crown calibration at the two labial line

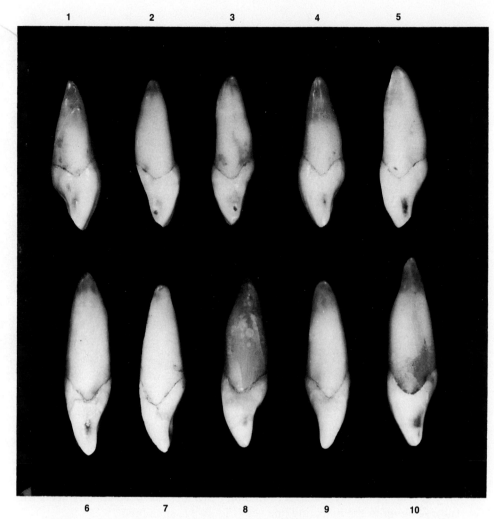

Figure 6-10. Maxillary central incisor, mesial aspect. Ten typical specimens are shown.

angles greater than the calibration at the two lingual line angles and making the lingual portion of the root narrower than the labial portion. A cross section of the root at the cervix shows the root to be generally triangular with rounded angles. One side of the triangle is labial, with the mesial and distal sides pointing lingually. The mesial side of this triangle is a trifle longer than the distal side (see Fig. 13–8, specimens *C 3, 4, 5, 6*).

Mesial Aspect (Figs. 6–4 and 6–10)

The mesial aspect of this tooth has the fundamental form of an incisor: The crown is wedge-shaped, or triangular, with the base of the triangle at the cervix and the apex at the incisal ridge (Fig. 4–21, *A*).

Usually a line drawn through the crown and the root form the mesial aspect through the center of the tooth will bisect the apex of the root and also the incisal ridge of the crown. The incisal ridge of the crown is therefore on a line with the center of the root. This

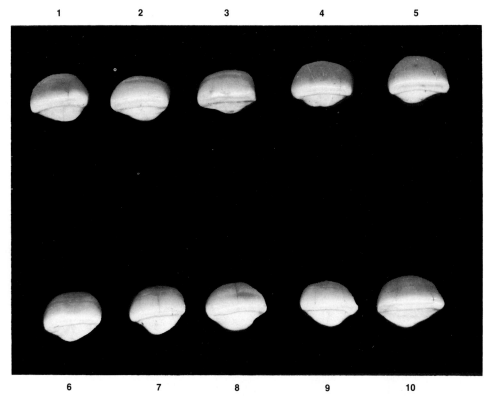

1   2   3   4   5

6   7   8   9   10

Figure 6–11. Maxillary central incisor, incisal aspect. Ten typical specimens are shown.

alignment is characteristic of maxillary central and lateral incisors. A straight line drawn through the center of the crown and root from the mesial or distal aspects will rarely if ever pass lingual to the incisal edge. Maxillary incisors are occasionally seen with the incisal ridges *lingual* to the bisecting line see (Fig. 6–12, specimen *1*).

Labially and lingually, immediately coronal to the cervical line are the crests of curvature of these surfaces. These crests of contour give the crown its greatest labiolingual measurement.

Normally, the curvature labially and lingually is approximately 0.5 mm in extent (Fig. 6–4) before continuing the outlines to the incisal ridge.

The labial outline of the crown from the crest of curvature to the incisal ridge is very slightly convex. The lingual outline is convex at the point where it joins the crest of curvature at the cingulum; it then becomes concave at the mesial marginal ridge, and it becomes slightly convex again at the linguoincisal ridge and the incisal edge.

The cervical line outlining the cementoenamel junction mesially on the maxillary central incisor curves incisally to a noticeable degree. This cervical curvature is greater on the mesial surface of this tooth than on any surface of any other tooth in the mouth. The curvature varies in extent, depending on the length of the crown and the measurement of the crown labiolingually. On an average central incisor of 10.5 to 11 mm in crown length, the curvature will be 3 to 4 mm. (See "Curvatures of the Cervical Lines," Chapter 5.)

The root of this tooth from the mesial aspect is cone-shaped, and the apex of the root is usually bluntly rounded.

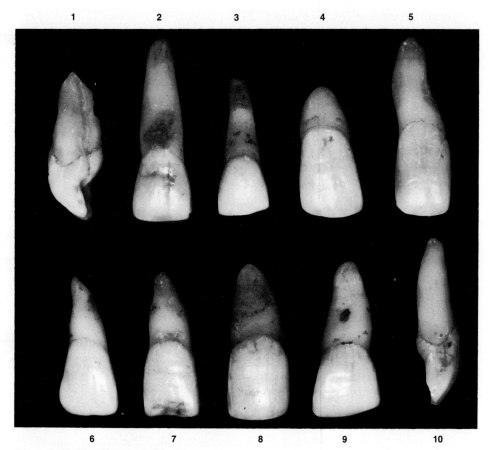

Figure 6–12. Maxillary central incisor.
Ten specimens with uncommon variations are shown.
1, Extralingual inclination of incisal portion of crown. Note developmental groove traversing root and part of crown.
2, Root extremely long.
3, Specimen small in all dimensions.
4, Crown extremely long, root very short.
5, Specimen malformed; crown unusually long; cervix very wide.
6, Root short and tapering.
7, Same as specimen *6.*
8, Crown nearly as wide at the cervix as at contact areas, crown long, root short.
9, Root with unusual curvature.
10, Crown and root narrow labiolingually; root comparable with specimen *2.*

Distal Aspect (Fig. 6–5)

There is little difference between the distal and mesial outlines of this tooth. When looking at the central incisor from the distal aspect, we may note that the crown gives the impression of being somewhat thicker toward the incisal third. Because of the slope of the labial surface distolingually, more of that surface is seen from the distal aspect; this creates the illusion of greater thickness. Actually, most teeth are turned a little on their root bases, in order to adapt to the dental arch curvature. The maxillary central incisor is no exception.

The curvature of the cervical line outlining the cementoenamel junction is less in extent on the distal than on the mesial surfaces. Most teeth show this characteristic.

Incisal Aspect (Figs. 6–6 and 6–11)

The specimen of this tooth is posed in the illustrations so that the incisal edge is centered over the root. A view of the crown from this aspect superposes it over the root entirely so that the latter is not visible.

From this aspect, the labial face of the crown is relatively broad and flat in comparison with the lingual surface, especially toward the incisal third. Nevertheless, the cervical portion of the crown labially is convex, although the arc described is broad.

The incisal ridge may be seen clearly, and a differentiation between the incisal edge and the remainder of the incisal ridge, with its slope toward the lingual, is easily distinguished.

The outline of the lingual portion tapers lingually toward the cingulum. The cingulum of the crown makes up the cervical portion of the lingual surface.

The mesiolabial and distolabial line angles are prominent from the incisal aspect. The relative positions of these line angles should be compared with the mesiolingual and distolingual line angles—which are represented by the borders of the mesial and distal marginal ridges. The mesiodistal calibration of the crown at the labial line angles is greater than the same calibration at the lingual line angles.

The crown of this tooth shows more bulk from the incisal aspect than one would expect from viewing it from the mesial or distal aspect. There are relatively broad surfaces at the site of contact areas mesially and distally. Comparison should also be made between the dimensions of the crown labiolingually and mesiodistally. The labiolingual calibration of the crown is more than two-thirds as great as the mesiodistal calibration. A cursory examination would not indicate this comparison.

Bilaterally, the outline of the incisal aspect is rather uniform. The lingual portion shows some variation, however, in that a line drawn from the mesioincisal angle to the center of the cingulum lingually will be a longer line than one drawn from the same point on the cingulum to the distoincisal angle. The crown conforms to a triangular outline reflected by the outline of the root cross section at the cervix mentioned formerly.

Maxillary Lateral Incisor

Because the maxillary lateral incisor supplements the central incisor in function, the crowns bear a close resemblance. The lateral incisor is smaller in all dimensions except root length (Table 6–2). Since it resembles the maxillary central incisor in form, direct comparisons will be made with the central incisor in its description.

This tooth differs from the central incisor in this—its development may vary considerably. Maxillary lateral incisors vary in form more than any other tooth in the mouth except the third molar. If the variation is too great, it is considered a developmental anomaly. A not uncommon situation is to find maxillary lateral incisors with a nondescript, pointed form; such teeth are called "peg-shaped" laterals (see Fig. 6–21, specimens 7 and 8). In some individuals, the lateral incisors are missing entirely; in these cases, the maxillary central incisor may be in contact distally with the canine.

One type of malformed maxillary lateral incisor will have a large pointed tubercle as part of the cingulum; some will have deep developmental grooves which extend down on the root lingually with a deep fold in the cingulum; and some will show twisted roots, distorted crowns, and so forth (Fig. 6–21).

Table 6–2. Maxillary Lateral Incisor

First evidence of calcification 1 year
Enamel completed 4 to 5 years
Eruption 8 to 9 years
Root completed 11 years

Measurement Table

	Cervico-incisal Length of Crown	Length of Root	Mesiodistal Diameter of Crown	Mesiodistal Diameter of Crown at Cervix	Labio-or Bucco-lingual Diameter of Crown	Labio-or Bucco-lingual Diameter at Cervix	Curvature of Cervical Line—Mesial	Curvature of Cervical Line—Distal
Dimensions suggested for carving technique	9.0*	13.0	6.5	5.0	6.0	5.0	3.0	2.0

* In millimeters.

141

Detailed Description of the Maxillary Lateral Incisor from All Aspects

Figures 6–13 through 6–21 present the maxillary lateral incisors in various aspects.

Labial Aspects (Figs. 6–13 and 6–19)

Although the labial aspect of the maxillary lateral incisor may appear to favor that of the central incisor, usually it has more curvature, with a rounded incisal ridge and rounded incisal angles mesially and distally. Although the crown is smaller in all dimensions, its proportions usually correspond to those of the central incisor.

The mesial outline of the crown from the labial aspect resembles that of the central incisor, with a more rounded mesioincisal angle. The crest of contour mesially is usually at the point of junction of the middle and incisal thirds; occasionally, in the so-called square forms, the mesioincisal angle is almost as sharp as that found on most maxillary central incisors (Fig. 6–19, specimens *4* and *5*). However, a more rounded mesioincisal angle is seen more frequently.

The distal outline of the crown from the labial aspect differs somewhat from that of the central incisor. The distal outline is always more rounded, and the crest of contour is more cervical, usually in the center of the middle third. Some forms describe a semicircular outline distally from the cervix to the center of the incisal ridge (Fig. 6–19, specimens *3* and *7*).

The labial surface of the crown is more convex than that of the central incisor except in some square and flat-faced forms.

This tooth is relatively narrow mesiodistally, usually about 2 mm narrower than the central incisor. The crown on the average will measure from 2 to 3 mm shorter cervicoin-

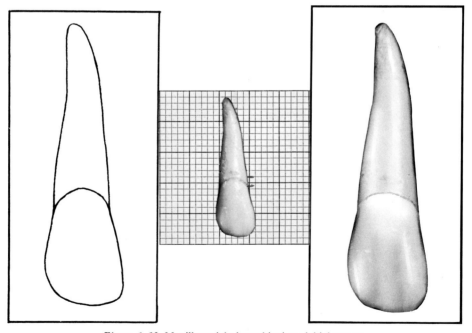

Figure 6–13. Maxillary right lateral incisor, labial aspect.

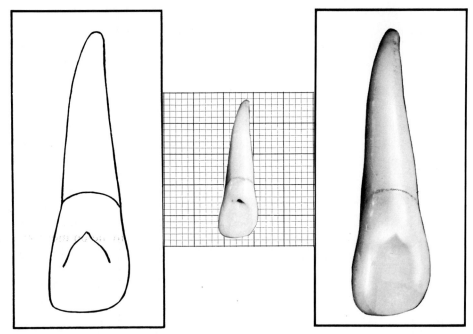

Figure 6–14. Maxillary right lateral incisor, lingual aspect.

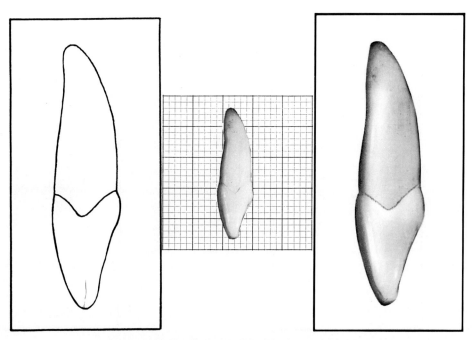

Figure 6–15. Maxillary right lateral incisor, mesial aspect.

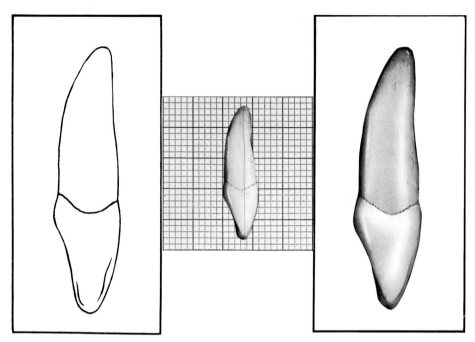

Figure 6–16. Maxillary right lateral incisor, distal aspect.

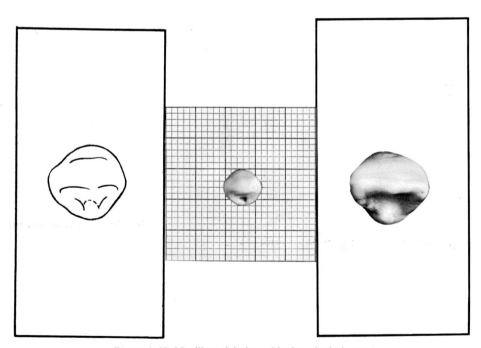

Figure 6–17. Maxillary right lateral incisor, incisal aspect.

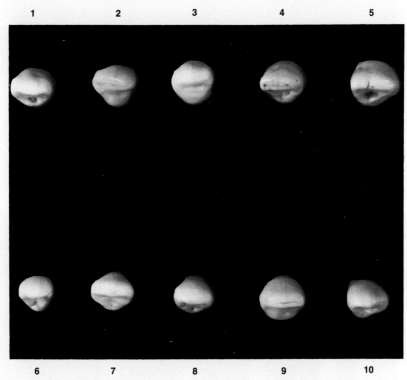

Figure 6–18. Maxillary lateral incisor, incisal aspect. Ten typical specimens are shown.

cisally than that of the central incisor, although the root is usually as long if not somewhat longer than that of the central incisor.

As a rule, its root length is greater in proportion to its crown length than that of the central incisor. The root is often about 1½ times the length of the crown.

The root tapers evenly from the cervical line to a point approximately two-thirds of its length apically. In most cases, it curves sharply from this location in a distal direction and ends in a pointed apex. Although the curvature distally is typical, some roots are straight (Fig. 6–19, specimens *4, 7,* and *9*), and some may be found curving mesially. As mentioned previously, this tooth may show considerable variance in its crown form; the root form may be more characteristic.

Lingual Aspect (Fig. 6–14)

Mesial and distal marginal ridges are marked, and the cingulum is usually prominent, with a tendency toward deep developmental grooves within the lingual fossa, where it joins the cingulum. The linguoincisal ridge is well developed, and the lingual fossa is more concave and circumscribed than that found on the central incisor. The tooth tapers toward the lingual, resembling a central incisor in this respect. It is not uncommon to find a deep developmental groove at the side of the cingulum, usually on the distal side, which may extend up on the root for part or all of its length. Faults in the enamel of the crown are often found in the deep portions of these developmental grooves (Fig. 6–21, specimens *3* and *4*).

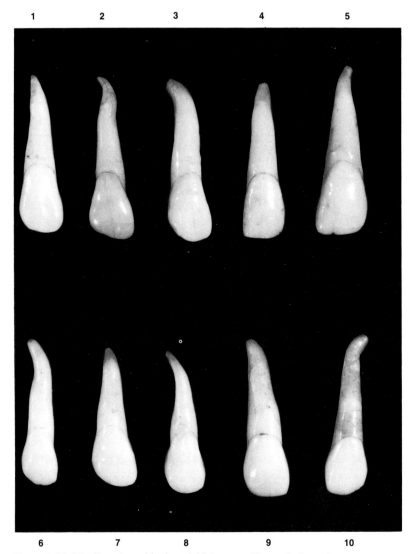

Figure 6–19. Maxillary lateral incisor, labial aspect. Ten typical specimens are shown.

Mesial Aspect (Figs 6–15 and 6–20)

The mesial aspect of the maxillary lateral incisor is similar to that of a small central incisor except that the root appears longer. The crown is shorter, the root is relatively longer, and the labiolingual measurement of the crown and root is a millimeter or so less than the maxillary central incisor of the same mouth.

The curvature of the cervical line is marked in the direction of the incisal ridge, although because of the small size of the crown the actual extent of curvature is less than that found on the central incisor. The heavy development of the incisal ridge accordingly makes the incisal portion appear somewhat thicker than that of the central incisor.

The root appears as a tapered cone from this aspect, with a bluntly rounded, apical end. This varies in individuals, sometimes being quite blunt, while at other times it is

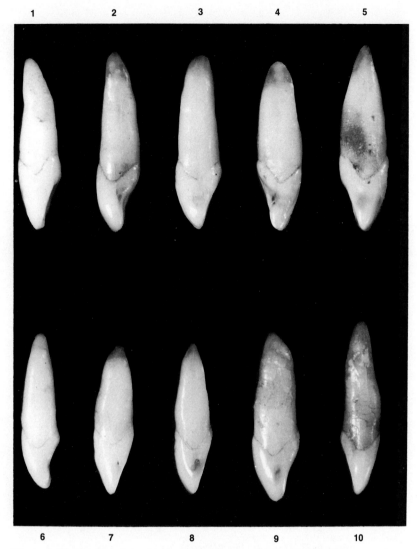

Figure 6–20. Maxillary lateral incisor, mesial aspect. Ten typical specimens are shown.

pointed. In a good many cases, the labial outline of the root from this aspect is straight. As in the central incisor, a line drawn through the center of the root tends to bisect the incisal ridge of the crown.

Distal Aspect (Fig. 6–16)

Because of the placement of the crown on the root, the width of the crown distally appears thicker than it does on the mesial aspect from marginal ridge to labial face. The curvature of the cervical line is usually a millimeter or so less in depth than on the mesial side. It is not uncommon to find a developmental groove distally on this crown extending on the root for part or all of its length.

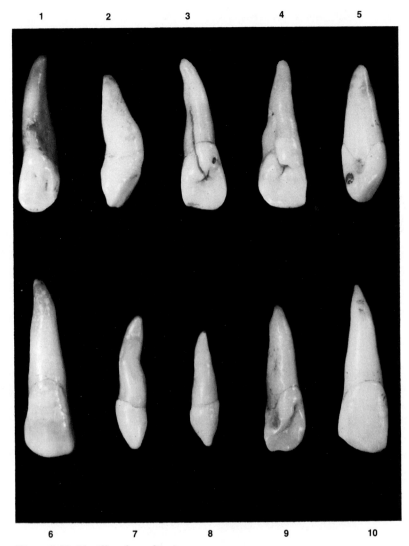

Figure 6–21. Maxillary lateral incisor.
Ten specimens with uncommon variations are shown.
 1, Odd twist to crown and root.
 2, Malformed generally.
 3, Deep developmental groove distally; note pit in lingual fossa.
 4, Same as specimen *3* with pit and groove connected.
 5, Deep concavity above contact area of the crown.
 6, Abnormally large but well formed.
 7, Single-cusp development and malformed root, so called "peg lateral incisor."
 8, Same as specimen *7,* except root is straight.
 9, Same as specimen *5,* with deep lingual pit in addition.
 10, Resemblance to a small maxillary central incisor more marked than the average.

Incisal Aspect (Figs. 6–17 and 6–18)

The incisal aspect of this tooth sometimes resembles that of the central incisor, or it may resemble that of a small canine. If the tooth conforms in development to its central incisor neighbor in other respects, it will, from the incisal aspect, resemble a central incisor except in size (Fig. 6–18, specimens 5 and 9). The cingulum, however, may be large; the incisal ridge also; the labiolingual dimension may be greater than usual in comparison with the mesiodistal dimension. If these variations are present, the tooth has a marked resemblance to a small canine (Fig. 6–18, specimens *3* and *10*).

All maxillary lateral incisors exhibit more convexity labially and lingually from the incisal aspect than maxillary central incisors.

References

Black, G. V. (1897). *Descriptive Anatomy of the Human Teeth,* 4th ed. Philadelphia: S. S. White Dental Manufacturing.

Carbonell, V. M. (1963). Variations in frequency of shovel-shaped incisors in different populations. In Brothwell, D. R. (ed.), *Dental Anthropology.* New York: Macmillan.

Dahlberg, A. A., and Mikkelson, O. (1947). The shovel-shaped character in the teeth of the Pima Indians. Proceedings of the 16th Annual Meeting. Am. J. Phys. Anthropol. 5:234.

Dewey, M. (1916). *Dental Anatomy.* St. Louis, Mo.: Mosby.

Hrdlicka, A. (1920). Shovel-shaped teeth. Am. J. Phys. Anthropol. 3:429.

7 The Permanent Mandibular Incisors

The mandibular incisors are *four* in number. The mandibular *central* incisors are centered in the mandible, one on either side of the median line, with the mesial surface of each one in contact with the mesial surface of the other. The right and left mandibular *lateral* or *second* incisors are distal to the central incisors. They are in contact with the central incisors mesially and with the canines distally.

The mandibular incisors have smaller mesiodistal dimensions than any of the other teeth. The central incisor is somewhat smaller than the lateral incisor, which is the reverse of the situation in the maxilla.

These teeth are similar in form and have smooth crown surfaces that show few traces of developmental lines. Mamelons on the incisal ridges are worn off soon after eruption, if the occlusion is normal, leaving the incisal ridges smooth and straight (compare specimens 7 and 8, Fig. 7–9). The contact areas are near the incisal ridges mesially and distally, and lines drawn through the contact areas are near the same level on both central and lateral incisors; here also the situation is unlike the maxillary incisors. The mandibular incisors show uniform development, with few instances of malformations or anomalies.

The anatomic form of these teeth differs entirely from that of the maxillary incisors. The inclination of the crowns differs from the mesial and distal aspects; the labial faces are inclined lingually so that the incisal ridges are lingual to a line bisecting the root. After normal wear has taken place, obliterating the mamelons, the incisal surfaces thus created show a *labial inclination* when the occlusion has been normal. It will be remembered that the incisal surfaces of maxillary incisors have a *lingual* inclination. With this arrangement, the incisal planes of the mandibular and maxillary incisors are parallel with each other, fitting together during incising action.

Mandibular Central Incisor

Normally, the mandibular central incisor is the smallest tooth in the dental arches (Table 7–1). The crown has little more than half the mesiodistal diameter of the maxillary central incisor; however, the labiolingual diameter is only about 1 mm less. The lines of greatest masticatory stress are brought to bear on the mandibular incisors in a labiolingual direction, making this reinforcement necessary.

Table 7–1. Mandibular Central Incisor

First evidence of calcification	3 to 4 months
Enamel completed	4 to 5 years
Eruption	6 to 7 years
Root completed	9 years

Measurement Table

	Cervico-incisal Length of Crown	Length of Root	Mesiodistal Diameter of Crown	Mesiodistal Diameter of Crown at Cervix	Labio- or Bucco-lingual Diameter of Crown	Labio- or Bucco-lingual Diameter of Crown at Cervix	Curvature of Cervical Line—Mesial	Curvature of Cervical Line—Distal
Dimensions suggested for carving technique	9.0*	12.5	5.0	3.5	6.0	5.3	3.0	2.0

* In millimeters.

151

The single root is very narrow mesiodistally and corresponds to the narrowness of the crown, although the root and crown are wide labiolingually. The length of the root is as great, if not greater, than that of the maxillary central incisor.

Detailed Description of the Mandibular Central Incisor from All Aspects

Figures 7–1 through 7–12 show the mandibular central incisor in various aspects.

Labial Aspect (Figs. 7–2, 7–7 through 7–9)

The labial aspect of the mandibular central incisor is regular, tapering evenly from the relatively sharp mesial and distal incisal angles to the apical portion of the root. The incisal ridge of the crown is straight and is at approximately a right angle to the long axis of the tooth. Usually, the mesial and distal outlines of the crown make a straight drop downward from the incisal angles to the contact areas, which are incisal to the junction of incisal and middle thirds of the crown. The mesial and distal sides of the crown taper evenly from the contact areas to the narrow cervix.

The mesial and distal root outlines are straight with the mesial and distal outlines of the crown down to the apical portion. The apical third of the root terminates in a small pointed taper, in most cases curving distally. Sometimes the roots are straight (Fig. 7–9, specimens *2* and *10*).

The labial face of the mandibular central incisor crown is ordinarily smooth, with a flattened surface at the incisal third; the middle third is more convex, narrowing down to the convexity of the root at the cervical portion.

Except in newly erupted teeth, central incisors show few traces of developmental lines.

The labial surface of the root of the mandibular central incisor is regular and convex.

Lingual Aspect (Figs. 7–1, 7–3, 7–7, and 7–8)

The *lingual* surface of the crown is smooth, with very slight concavity at the incisal third between the inconspicuous marginal ridges. In some instances, the marginal ridges are more prominent near the incisal edges (Fig. 7–11, specimens *2* and *8*). In these cases, the concavity between the marginal ridges is more distinct.

The lingual surface becomes flat and then convex as progression is made from the incisal third to the cervical third.

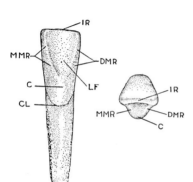

Figure 7–1. Mandibular right central incisor, lingual and incisal aspects. *IR,* incisal ridge; *DMR,* distal marginal ridge; *LF,* lingual fossa; *CL,* cervical line; *C,* cingulum; *MMR,* mesial marginal ridge.

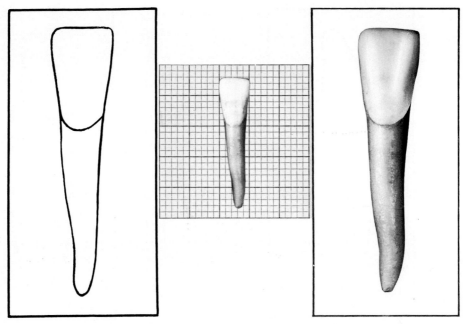

Figure 7–2. Mandibular right central incisor, labial aspect.

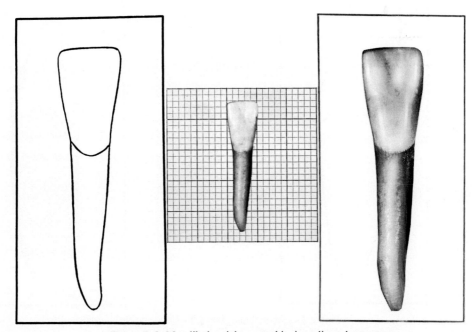

Figure 7–3. Mandibular right central incisor, lingual aspect.

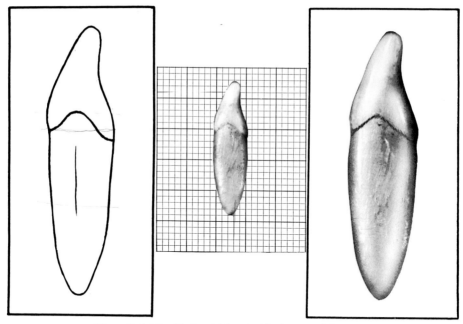

Figure 7–4. Mandibular right central incisor, mesial aspect.

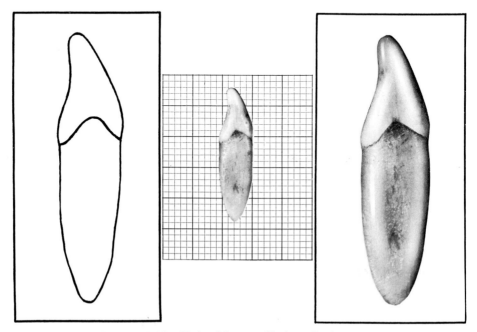

Figure 7–5. Mandibular right central incisor, distal aspect.

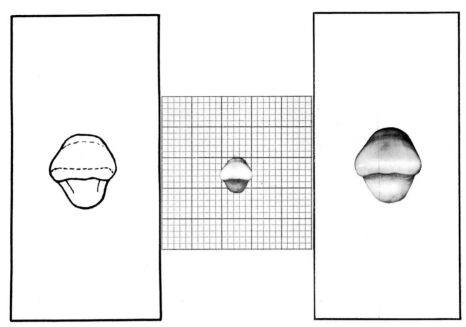

Figure 7–6. Mandibular right central incisor, incisal aspect.

No developmental lines mark the cingulum development on this tooth at the cervical third. No other tooth in the mouth, except the mandibular lateral incisor, shows so few developmental lines and grooves. The outlines and surfaces of the mandibular incisors are regular and symmetrical.

Mesial Aspect (Figs. 7–4, 7–7, 7–8, and 7–10)

The curvature labially and lingually above the cervical line is less than that found on maxillary incisors.

The outline of the labial face of the crown is straight above the cervical curvature, sloping rapidly from the crest of curvature to the incisal ridge. The lingual outline of the crown is a straight line inclined labially for a short distance above the smooth convexity of the cingulum; the straight outline joins a concave line at the middle third of the crown, which extends upward to join the rounded outline of a narrow incisal ridge. The incisal ridge is rounded or worn flat, and its center is usually lingual to the center of the root.

The curvature of the cervical line representing the cementoenamel junction on the mesial surface is marked, curving incisally approximately one-third the length of the crown.

The root outlines from the mesial aspect are straight with the crown outline from the cervical line, keeping the root diameter uniform through the cervical third and part of the middle third; the outline of the root begins to taper in the middle third area, tapering rapidly in the apical third to either a bluntly rounded or a pointed root end.

The mesial surface of the crown is convex and smooth at the incisal third and becomes broader and flatter at the middle third cervical to the contact area; it then becomes quite flat, with a tendency toward concavity immediately below the middle third of the crown and above the cervical line (Fig. 7–10, specimens *5, 8,* and *10*).

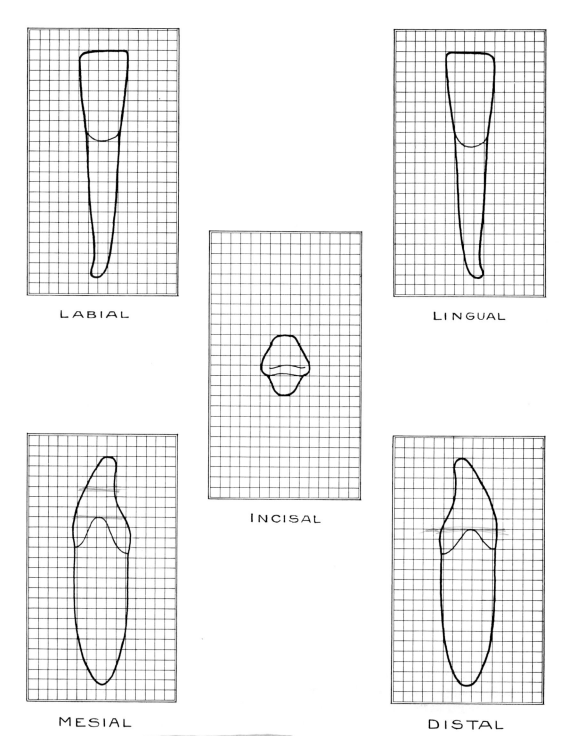

LABIAL

LINGUAL

INCISAL

MESIAL

DISTAL

Figure 7-7. Mandibular right central incisor. Graph outlines of five aspects are shown.

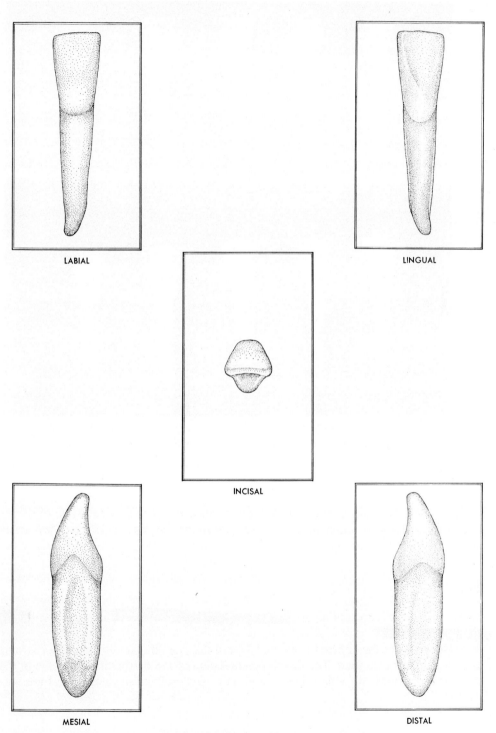

LABIAL

LINGUAL

INCISAL

MESIAL

DISTAL

Figure 7–8. Mandibular right central incisor.

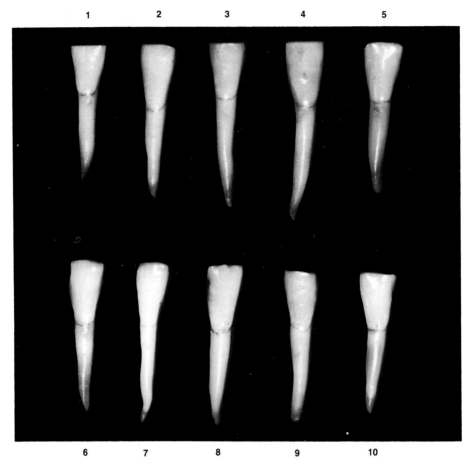

Figure 7–9. Mandibular central incisor, labial aspect. Ten typical specimens are shown.

The mesial surface of the root is flat just below the cervical line. Most of these roots have a broad developmental depression for most of the root length. The depressions usually are deeper at the junction of the middle and apical thirds (Fig. 7–10, specimens *3* and *9*).

Distal Aspect (Figs. 7–5, 7–7, and 7–8)

The cervical line representing the cementoenamel junction curves incisally about 1 mm less than on the mesial.

The distal surface of the crown and root of the mandibular central incisor is similar to that of the mesial surface. The developmental depression on the distal surface of the root may be more marked, with a deeper and more well-defined developmental groove at its center.

Incisal Aspect (Figs. 7–1, 7–6 through 7–8, and 7–11)

This aspect illustrates the bilateral symmetry of the mandibular central incisor. The mesial half of the crown is almost identical with the distal half.

1   2   3   4   5

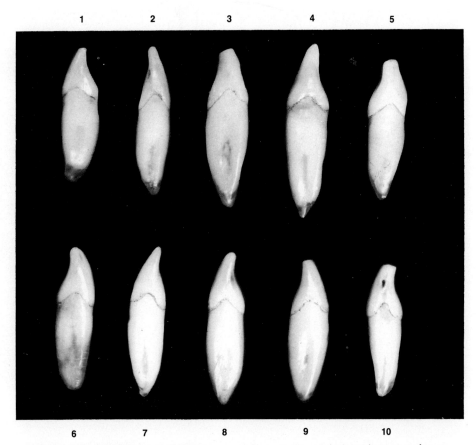

6   7   8   9   10

Figure 7–10. Mandibular central incisor, mesial aspect. Ten typical specimens are shown.

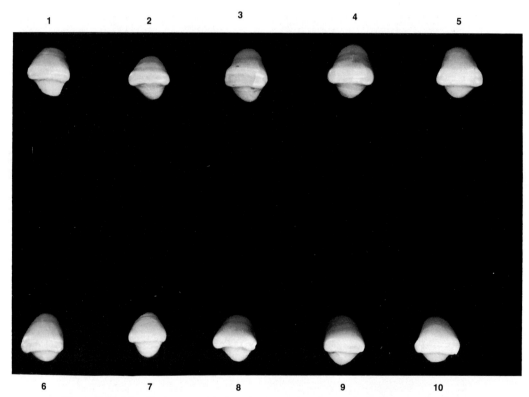

Figure 7–11. Mandibular central incisor, incisal aspect. Ten typical specimens are shown.

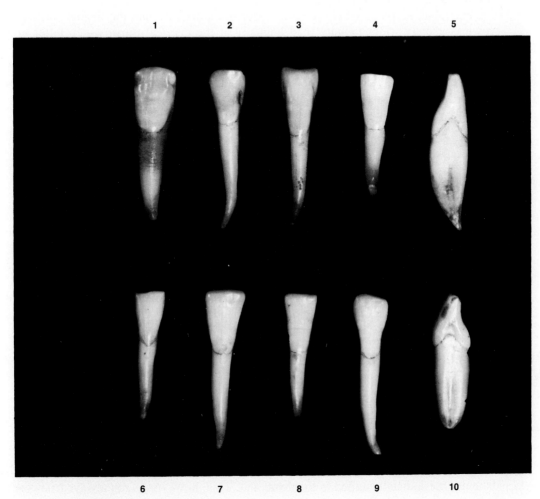

Figure 7–12. Mandibular central incisor.
    Ten specimens with uncommon variations are shown.
    1, Crown and root very broad mesiodistally; malformed enamel at incisal third of crown.
    2, Crown wide at incisal third, with short crown. Root length extreme.
    3, Unusual contours at middle third of crown; cervix narrow.
    4, Well-formed crown; short root.
    5, No curvature labially at cervical third; extreme labial curvature at root end.
    6, Specimen well formed but undersized.
    7, Contact areas pointed at incisal edge; crown and root very long.
    8, Crown long and narrow; root short.
    9, Crown measurement at cervical third same as root; crown and root of extreme length.
    10, Crown and root very wide labiolingually; greater curvature than average above cervical line at the cervical third of the crown.

The incisal edge is almost at right angles to a line bisecting the crown labiolingually. This feature is characteristic of the tooth and serves as a mark of identification in differentiation between mandibular central and lateral incisors (see ''Mandibular Lateral Incisor''). Note the comparison between the diameter of these crowns labiolingually and their diameters mesiodistally. The labiolingual diameter is always *greater.*

The labial surface of the crown is wider mesiodistally than the lingual surface. The crown is usually wider labially than lingually at the cervical third, which latter area is represented by a smooth cingulum.

The labial surface of the crown at the incisal third, although rather broad and flat in comparison with the cervical third, has a tendency toward *convexity,* whereas the lingual surface of the crown at the incisal third has an inclination toward *concavity.*

When this tooth is posed from the incisal aspect so that the line of vision is on a line with the long axis of the tooth, more of the labial surface may be seen than of the lingual surface.

Mandibular Lateral Incisor

The mandibular lateral incisor is the second mandibular tooth from the median line, right or left. It resembles the mandibular central incisor so closely that only a brief description of each aspect of the lateral incisor will be necessary. Direct comparison will be made with the mandibular central incisor, and the variations will be mentioned. The two incisors operate in the dental arch as a team; therefore, their functional form is related.

The mandibular lateral incisor is somewhat larger (compare measurements), but generally speaking, its form closely resembles the mandibular central incisor (Table 7–2).

Brief Description of the Mandibular Lateral Incisor from All Aspects

Figures 7–13 through 7–21 show the mandibular lateral incisor from various aspects.

Labial and Lingual Aspects

The labial and lingual aspects show the added fraction of approximately 1 mm of crown diameter mesiodistally added to the distal half. This, however, is not always true (see Fig. 7–19, specimens *3* and *6*).

Mesial and Distal Aspects

The mesial side of the crown is often longer than the distal side, causing the incisal ridge, which is straight, to slope downward in a distal direction (Fig. 7–19, specimen *1*). The distal contact area is more toward the cervical than the mesial contact area to contact properly the mesial contact area of the mandibular canine.

Except for size, there is no marked difference between the mesial and distal surfaces of central and lateral incisors. Even the curvatures of the cervical line mesially and distally are similar in extent. There is a tendency toward a deeper concavity immediately above the cervical line on the distal surface of the mandibular lateral incisor.

Although the crown of the mandibular lateral incisor is somewhat longer than that of the central incisor (usually a fraction of a millimeter), the root may be considerably longer. The tooth is, therefore, in most instances, a little larger in all dimensions. The root form is similar to that of the central incisor, including the developmental depressions mesially and distally.   *Text continued on page 169*

Table 7–2. Mandibular Lateral Incisor

First evidence of calcification   3 to 4 months
Enamel completed   4 to 5 years
Eruption   7 to 8 years
Root completed   10 years

Measurement Table

	Cervico-incisal Length of Crown	Length of Root	Mesiodistal Diameter of Crown	Mesiodistal Diameter of Crown at Cervix	Labio-or Bucco-lingual Diameter of Crown	Labio-or Bucco-lingual Diameter of Crown at Cervix	Curvature of Cervical Line— Mesial	Curvature of Cervical Line— Distal
Dimensions suggested for carving technique	9.5*	14.0	5.5	4.0	6.5	5.8	3.0	2.0

* In millimeters.

163

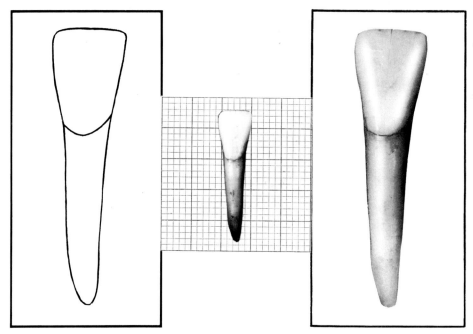

Figure 7–13. Mandibular right lateral incisor, labial aspect.

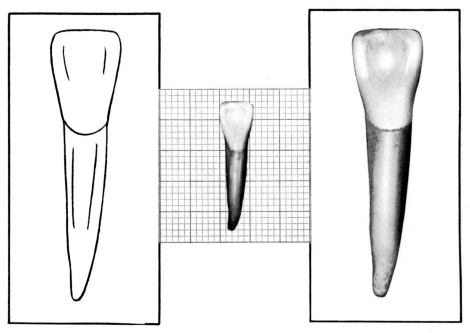

Figure 7–14. Mandibular right lateral incisor, lingual aspect.

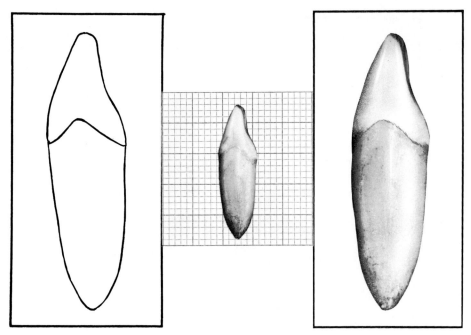

Figure 7–15. Mandibular right lateral incisor, mesial aspect.

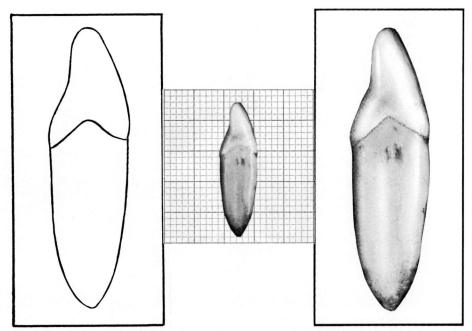

Figure 7–16. Mandibular right lateral incisor, distal aspect.

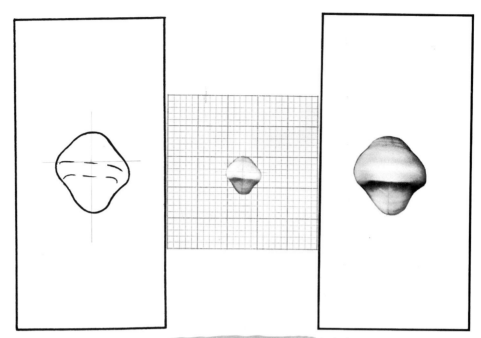

Figure 7–17. Mandibular right lateral incisor, incisal aspect.

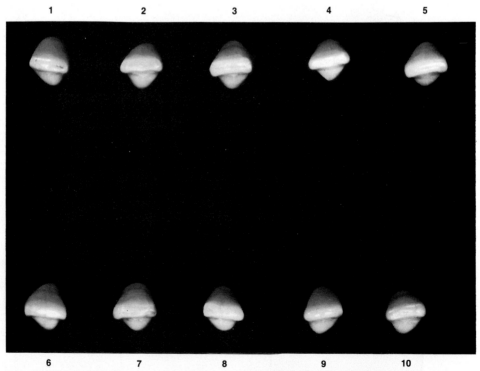

Figure 7–18. Mandibular lateral incisor, incisal aspect. Ten typical specimens are shown.

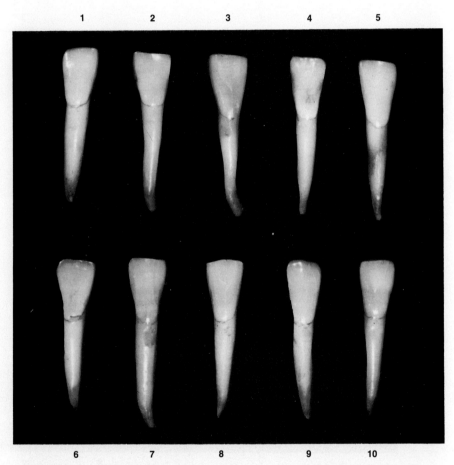

Figure 7–19. Mandibular lateral incisor, labial aspect. Ten typical specimens are shown.

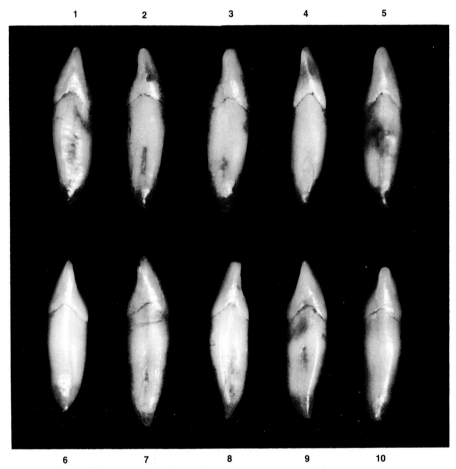

Figure 7–20. Mandibular lateral incisor, mesial aspect. Ten typical specimens are shown.

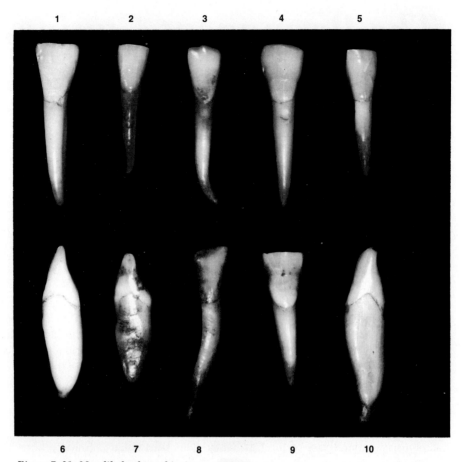

Figure 7–21. Mandibular lateral incisor.
Ten specimens with uncommon variations are shown.

1, Tooth very large; cervix, constricted in comparison with crown width.

2, Specimen well formed, smaller than average.

3, Root extra long; extreme curvature at apical third; mesial and middle mamelons intact on incisal ridge.

4, Extreme mesiodistal measurement for crown length; contact areas very broad cervicoincisally.

5, Specimen undersized.

6, Incisal ridge thin; little or no curvature at cervical third of crown.

7, Incisal edge labial to center of root; root rounded; cingulum with more curvature above root than average.

8, Malformed crown and root; root with extreme length.

9, Crown very wide; root short.

10, Very slight curvature at cervical third of crown; entire tooth oversize, malformation at root end.

Incisal Aspect

The incisal aspect of the mandibular lateral incisor provides a feature that can usually serve to identify this tooth. The incisal edge is not at approximate right angles to a line bisecting the crown and root labiolingually, as was found when observing the central incisor: The edge follows the curvature of the mandibular dental arch, giving the crown of the mandibular lateral incisor the appearance of being twisted slightly on its root base. It is interesting to note that the labiolingual root axes of mandibular central and lateral incisors remain almost parallel in the alveolar process, even though the incisal ridges are not directly in line.

8 The Permanent Canines, Maxillary and Mandibular

The maxillary and mandibular canines bear a close resemblance to each other, and their functions are closely related. The four canines are placed at the "corners" of the mouth, each one the third tooth from the median line, right and left, in the maxilla and mandible. They are the longest teeth in the mouth; the crowns are usually as long as those of the maxillary central incisors, and the single roots are longer than those of any of the other teeth. The middle labial lobes have been highly developed incisally into strong well-formed cusps. Crowns and roots are markedly convex on most surfaces.

The shape of the crowns, with their single pointed cusps, their locations in the mouth, and the extra anchorage furnished by the long, strongly developed roots, makes these canines resemble those of the Carnivora. This resemblance to the prehensile teeth of the Carnivora gives rise to the term *canine*.

Because of the labiolingual thickness of crown and root and the anchorage in the alveolar process of the jaws, these teeth are perhaps the most stable in the mouth. The crown portions of the canines are shaped in a manner that promotes cleanliness. This self-cleansing quality, along with the efficient anchorage in the jaws, tends to preserve these teeth throughout life. When teeth are lost, the canines are usually the last ones to go. They are very valuable teeth, when considered either as units of the natural dental arches or as possible assistants in stabilizing replacements of lost teeth in prosthetic procedures.

Both maxillary and mandibular canines have another quality that must not be overlooked: The positions and forms of these teeth and their anchorage in the bone, along with the bone ridge over the labial portions of the roots, called the *canine eminence,* have a cosmetic value. They help to form a foundation that ensures normal facial expression at the "corners" of the mouth. Loss of all of these teeth makes it extremely difficult, if not impossible, to make replacements that will restore that natural appearance of the face for any length of time. It would therefore be difficult to place a value on the canines, their importance being made manifest by their efficiency in function, their stability, and their help in maintaining natural facial expression.

In *function,* the canines support the incisors and premolars, since they are located between these groups. The canine crowns have some characteristics of functional form which will bear a resemblance to incisor form, and some which resemble the premolar form.

Maxillary Canine

The outline of the labial or lingual aspect of the maxillary canine is a series of curves or arcs except for the angle made by the tip of the cusp. This cusp has a mesial incisal ridge and a distoincisal ridge.

The mesial half of the crown makes contact with the lateral incisor, and the distal half contacts the first premolar. Therefore, the contact areas of the maxillary canine are at different levels cervicoincisally.

From a labial view, the mesial half of the crown resembles a portion of an incisor, whereas the distal half resembles a portion of a premolar. This tooth seems to be a compromise in the change from anterior to posterior teeth in the dental arch.

It is apparent that the construction of this tooth has reinforcement, labiolingually, to offset directional lines of the force brought against it when in use. The incisional portion is thicker labiolingually than that of either the maxillary central or the lateral incisor.

The labiolingual measurement of the crown is about 1 mm greater than that of the maxillary central incisor (Table 8–1). The mesiodistal measurement is approximately 1 mm less.

The cingulum shows greater development than that of the central incisor.

The root of the maxillary canine is usually the longest of any root with the possible exception of that of the mandibular canine, which may be as long at times. The root is thick labiolingually, with developmental depressions mesially and distally that help to furnish the secure anchorage this tooth has in the maxilla.

Detailed Description of the Maxillary Canine from All Aspects

Figures 8–1 through 8–12 present the maxillary canine in various aspects.

Labial Aspect (Figs. 8–2, 8–7 through 8–9)

The crown and root are narrower mesiodistally than those of the maxillary central incisor. The difference is about 1 mm in most mouths. The cervical line labially is convex, with the convexity toward the root portion.

Mesially, the outline of the crown may be convex from the cervix to the center of the mesial contact area, or the crown may exhibit a slight concavity above the contact area from the labial aspect. The center of the contact area mesially is approximately at the junction of middle and incisal thirds of the crown.

Distally, the outline of the crown is usually concave between the cervical line and the distal contact area. The distal contact area is usually at the center of the middle third of the crown. The two levels of contact areas mesially and distally should be noted (see Fig. 5–12, *B* and *C*).

Unless the crown has been worn unevenly, the cusp tip is on a line with the center of the root. The cusp has a mesial slope and a distal slope, the mesial slope being the shorter of the two. Both slopes show a tendency toward concavity before wear has taken place (Fig. 8–9, specimens *5* and *6*). These depressions are developmental in character.

The labial surface of the crown is smooth, with no developmental lines of note except shallow depressions mesially and distally, dividing the three labial lobes. The middle labial lobe shows much greater development than the other lobes. This produces a ridge on the labial surface of the crown. A line drawn over the crest of this ridge, from the cervical line to the tip of the cusp, is a curved one inclined mesially at its center. All areas mesial to the contrast of this ridge exhibit convexity except for insignificant developmental lines in the

Table 8–1. Maxillary Canine

	First evidence of calcification	4 to 5 months
	Enamel completed	6 to 7 years
	Eruption	11 to 12 years
	Root completed	13 to 15 years

Measurement Table

	Cervico-incisal Length of Crown	Length of Root	Mesiodistal Diameter of Crown	Mesiodistal Diameter of Crown at Cervix	Labio- or Bucco-lingual Diameter of Crown	Labio- or Bucco-lingual Diameter at Cervix	Curvature of Cervical Line— Mesial	Curvature of Cervical Line— Distal
Dimensions suggested for carving technique	10.0*	17.0	7.5	5.5	8.0	7.0	2.5	1.5

* In millimeters.

172

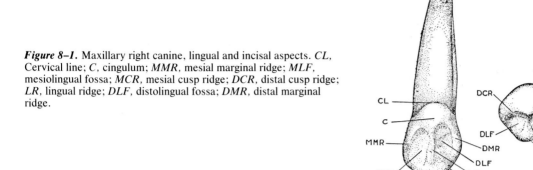

Figure 8–1. Maxillary right canine, lingual and incisal aspects. *CL,* Cervical line; *C,* cingulum; *MMR,* mesial marginal ridge; *MLF,* mesiolingual fossa; *MCR,* mesial cusp ridge; *DCR,* distal cusp ridge; *LR,* lingual ridge; *DLF,* distolingual fossa; *DMR,* distal marginal ridge.

enamel. Distally to the labial ridge (see incisal aspect), there is a tendency toward concavity at the cervical third of the crown, although convexity is noted elsewhere in all areas approaching the labial ridge (Fig. 8–11, specimens *7, 8,* and *9*).

The root of the maxillary canine appears slender from the labial aspect when compared with the bulk of the crown; it is conical in form with a bluntly pointed apex. It is not uncommon for this root to have a sharp curve in the vicinity of the apical third. This curvature may be in a mesial or distal direction—in most instances, the latter (Fig. 8–9, compare specimens *1* and *6*). The labial surface of the root is smooth and convex at all points.

Text continued on page 178

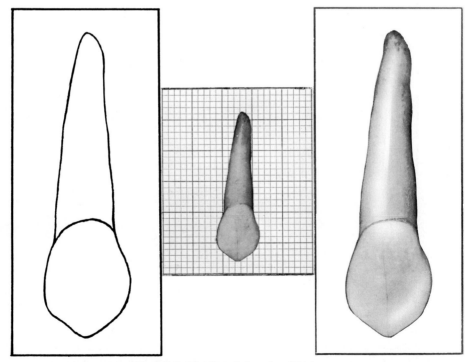

Figure 8–2. Maxillary left canine, labial aspect.

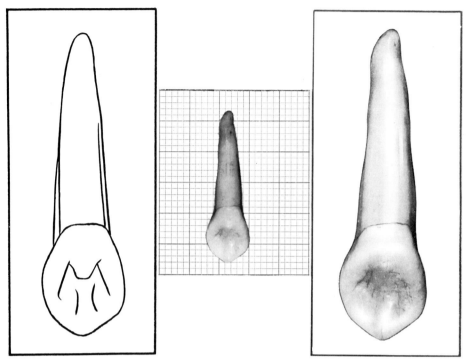

Figure 8–3. Maxillary left canine, lingual aspect.

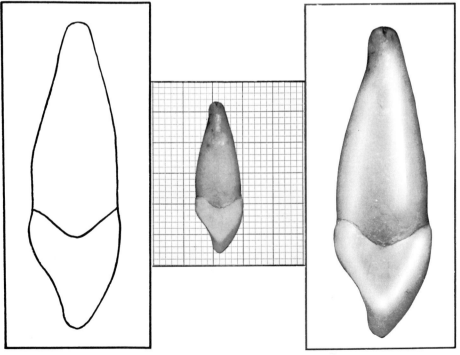

Figure 8–4. Maxillary left canine, mesial aspect.

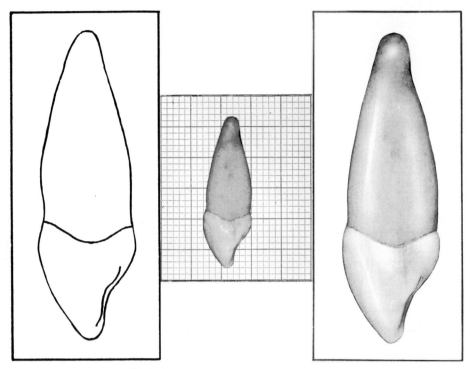

Figure 8–5. Maxillary left canine, distal aspect.

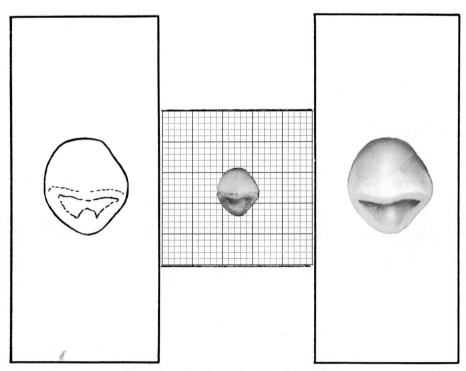

Figure 8–6. Maxillary left canine, incisal aspect.

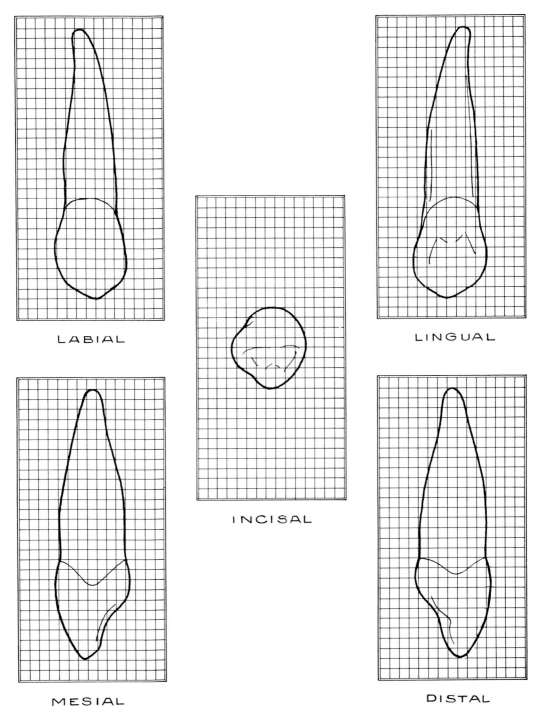

LABIAL

INCISAL

LINGUAL

MESIAL

DISTAL

Figure 8–7. Maxillary right canine. Graph outlines of five aspects are shown.

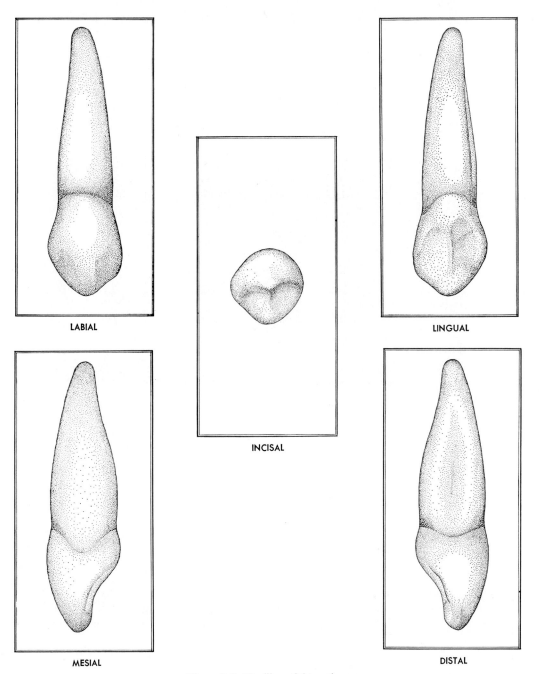

Figure 8–8. Maxillary right canine.

LABIAL

LINGUAL

INCISAL

MESIAL

DISTAL

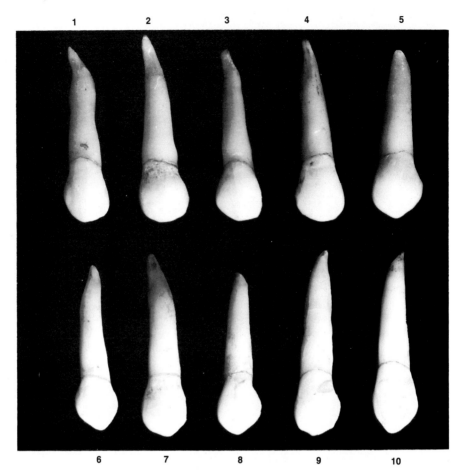

Figure 8–9. Maxillary canine, labial aspect. Ten typical specimens are shown.

Lingual Aspect (Figs. 8–3, 8–7, and 8–8)

The crown and root are narrower lingually than labially.

The cervical line from this aspect differs somewhat from the curvature found labially. The cervical line shows a more even curvature. The line may be straight for a short interval at this point.

The cingulum is large, and in some instances is pointed like a small cusp (Fig. 8–10, specimen 7). In the latter types, definite ridges are found on the lingual surface of the crown below the cingulum and between strongly developed marginal ridges. Although depressions are to be found between these ridge forms, there are seldom any deep developmental grooves.

Occasionally, a well-developed lingual ridge is seen which is confluent with the cusp tip; this extends to a point near the cingulum. There may be shallow concavities between this ridge and the marginal ridges. When these concavities are present, they are called mesial and distal lingual fossae (Figs. 8–1 and 8–8).

Sometimes the lingual surface of the canine crown is so smooth that fossae or minor ridges are difficult to distinguish. There is a tendency toward concavities, however, where the fossae are usually found, and heavy marginal ridges with a well-formed cingulum are to

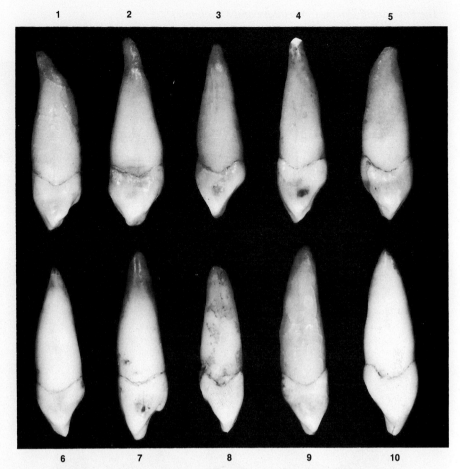

Figure 8–10. Maxillary canine, mesial aspect. Ten typical specimens are shown.

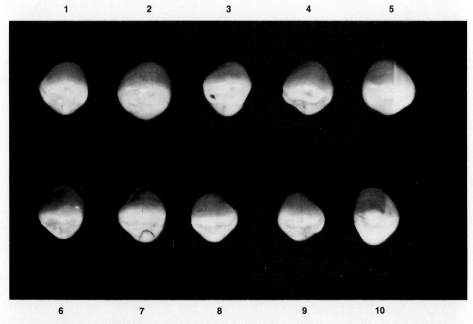

Figure 8–11. Maxillary canine, incisal aspect. Ten typical specimens are shown.

179

1   2   3   4   5

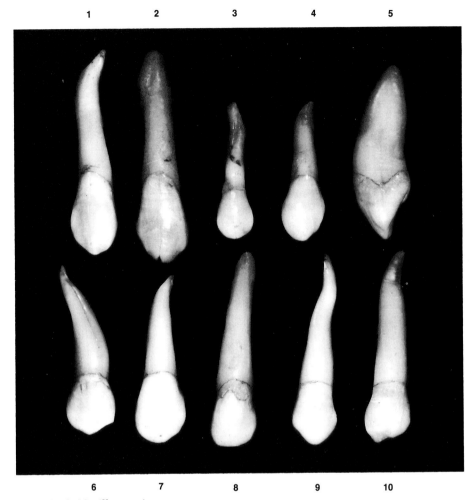

6   7   8   9   10

Figure 8–12. Maxillary canine.

Ten specimens with uncommon variations are shown.

1, Crown very long, with extreme curvature at apical third of the root.

2, Entire tooth unusually long. Note hypercementosis at root end.

3, Very short crown; root small and malformed.

4, Mesiodistal dimension of crown at contact area extreme; calibration at cervix narrow in comparison; root short for crown of this size.

5, Extreme labiolingual calibration; root with unusual curvature.

6, Tooth malformed generally.

7, Large crown; short root.

8, Root overdeveloped and very blunt at apex.

9, Odd curvature of root; extra length.

10, Crown poorly formed; root extra long.

be expected. The smooth cingulum, marginal ridges, and lingual portion of the incisal ridges are usually confluent, with little evidence of developmental grooves.

The lingual portion of the root of the maxillary canine is narrower than the labial portion. Because of this formation, much of the mesial and distal surface of the root is visible from the lingual aspect. Developmental depressions mesially and distally may be seen on most of these roots, extending most of the root length. The lingual ridge of the root is rather narrow, but it is smooth and convex at all points from the cervical line to the apical end (Fig. 8–3).

Mesial Aspect (Figs. 8–4, 8–7, 8–8, and 8–10)

The mesial aspect of the maxillary canine presents the outline of the functional form of an anterior tooth. It shows greater bulk generally, however, and greater labiolingual measurement than any of the other anterior teeth.

The outline of the crown is wedge-shaped, the greatest measurement being at the cervical third and the wedge point being represented by the tip of the cusp.

The curvature of the crown below the cervical line labially and lingually corresponds in extent to the curvature of maxillary central and lateral incisors. Nevertheless, the crest of that curvature is found at a level more incisal, since the middle labial and the lingual lobes are more highly developed (Fig. 8–10, specimens 5 and 10). Many canines show a flattened area labially at the cervical third of the crown, which appears as a straight outline from the mesial aspect. It is questionable just how much wear has to do with this effect (Fig. 8–10, specimens 1 and 2).

Below the cervical third of the crown, the labial face may be presented by a line only slightly convex from the crest of curvature at the cervical third to the tip of the cusp. The line usually becomes straighter as it approaches the cusp.

The entire labial outline from the mesial aspect exhibits more convexity from the cervical line to the cusp tip than the maxillary central incisor does from cervix to incisal edge.

The lingual outline of the crown from the mesial aspect may be represented by a convex line describing the cingulum, which convexity straightens out as the middle third is reached, becoming convex again in the incisal third (Fig. 8–10, specimen 10).

The cervical line which outlines the base of the crown from this aspect curves toward the cusp, on the average, approximately 2.5 mm (cementoenamel junction).

The outline of the root from this aspect is conical, with a tapered or bluntly pointed apex. The root may curve labially toward the apical third. The labial outline of the root may be almost perpendicular, with most of the taper appearing on the lingual side (Fig. 8–10, specimen 4 and 9).

The position of the tip of the cusp in relation to the long axis of the root is different from that of maxillary central and lateral incisors. Although the specimen illustrations in Figures 8–4 and 8–5 do not show this difference, most specimens shown in Figure 8–10 show it conclusively. A line bisecting the cusp is labial to a line bisecting the root. Lines bisecting the roots of central and lateral incisors also bisect the incisal ridges.

The mesial surface of the canine crown presents convexities at all points except for a small circumscribed area above the contact area, where the surface is concave and flat between that area and the cervical line.

The mesial surface of the root appears broad, with a shallow developmental depression for part of the root length. Developmental depressions on the heavy roots help to anchor the teeth in the alveoli and help to prevent rotation and displacement.

Distal Aspect (Figs. 8–5, 8–7, and 8–8)

The distal aspect of the maxillary canine shows somewhat the same form as the mesial aspect, with the following variations: The cervical line exhibits less curvature toward the cusp ridge; the distal marginal ridge is heavier and more irregular in outline; the surface displays more concavity usually above the contact area, and the developmental depression on the distal side of the root is more pronounced.

Incisal Aspect (Figs. 8–6, 8–7, 8–8, and 8–11)

The incisal aspect of the maxillary canine emphasizes the proportions of this tooth mesiodistally and labiolingually. In general, the labiolingual dimension is greater than the mesiodistal. Occasionally, the two measurements are about equal (Fig. 8–11, specimen *8*). Other instances appear with the crown larger than usual in a *labiolingual* direction (Fig. 8–11, specimen *10*).

From the incisal aspect, if the tooth is correctly posed so that the long axis of the root is directly in the line of vision, the tip of the cusp is *labial* to the *center* of the *crown labiolingually* and *mesial* to the *center mesiodistally*.

If the tooth were to be sectioned labiolingually beginning at the center of the cusp of the crown, the two sections would show the root rather evenly bisected, with the mesial portion carrying a narrower portion of the crown mesiodistally than that carried by the distal section of the tooth. (Note the proportions demonstrated by the fracture line in the enamel of specimen *9*, Fig. 8–11). Nevertheless, the mesial section shows a crown portion with greater labiolingual bulk. The crown of this tooth gives the impression of having all of the *distal portion stretched* to make *contact* with the first premolar.

The ridge of the middle labial lobe is very noticeable labially from the incisal aspect. It attains its greatest convexity at the cervical third of the crown, becoming broader and flatter at the middle and incisal thirds.

The cingulum development makes up the cervical third of the crown lingually. The outline of the cingulum may be described by a shorter arc than the one labially from this aspect. This comparison coincides with the relative mesiodistal dimensions of the root lingually and labially.

A line bisecting the cusp and cusp ridges drawn in the mesiodistal direction is almost always straight and bisects the short arcs representative of the mesial and distal contact areas. This fact emphasizes the close relation between maxillary canines and some lateral incisors, since they resemble each other in this characteristic (compare specimen *7*, Fig. 8–11, with specimen *1*, Fig. 6–18). As was mentioned in Chapter 6, there are two types of maxillary lateral incisors, some resembling canines from the incisal aspect and some resembling central incisors. The latter are supposed to be in the majority. Naturally, the lateral incisors that resemble canines are relatively wide labiolingually and those resembling central incisors are narrow in that direction.

The incisal aspect of most canines, maxillary or mandibular, may be outlined in many cases by a series of arcs. Specimen *6*, Fig. 8–11, for example, could be drawn almost perfectly with the aid of a "French curve," a drawing instrument used in drafting to draw arcs of varying degrees.

Mandibular Canine

Because maxillary and mandibular canines bear a close resemblance to each other, direct comparisons will be made with the maxillary canine in describing the mandibular canine.

The mandibular canine crown is narrower mesiodistally than that of the maxillary canine, although it is just as long in most instances and in many instances is longer by 0.5 to 1 mm (Table 8–2). The root may be as long as the maxillary canine, but usually it is somewhat shorter. The labiolingual diameter of crown and root is usually a fraction of a millimeter less, adapting this measurement to the other anteriors.

The lingual surface of the crown is smoother, with less cingulum development and less bulk to the marginal ridges. The lingual portion of this crown resembles the form of the lingual surfaces of mandibular lateral incisors.

Table 8–2. Mandibular Canine

First evidence of calcification 4 to 5 years
Enamel completed 6 to 7 years
Eruption 9 to 10 years
Root completed 12 to 14 years

Measurement Table

	Cervico-incisal Length of Crown	Length of Root	Mesiodistal Diameter of Crown	Mesiodistal Diameter of Crown at Cervix	Labio- or Bucco-lingual Diameter of Crown	Labio- or Bucco-lingual Diameter at Cervix	Curvature of Cervical Line— Mesial	Curvature of Cervical Line— Distal
Dimensions suggested for carving technique	11.0*	16.0	7.0	5.5	7.5	7.0	2.5	1.0

* In millimeters.

183

The cusp of the mandibular canine is not as well developed as that of the maxillary canine, and the cusp ridges are thinner labiolingually. Usually the cusp tip is on a line with the center of the root, from the mesial or distal aspect, but sometimes it lies lingual to the line, comparable with mandibular incisors.

A variation in the form of the mandibular canine is *bifurcated* roots. This variation is not rare (Fig. 8–24, specimens *1, 2, 5,* and *6*).

Detailed Description of the Mandibular Canine from All Aspects

Figures 8–13 through 8–24 present the mandibular canine in various aspects.

Labial Aspect (Figs. 8–14, 8–19 through 8–21)

The mesiodistal dimensions of the mandibular canine are less than those of the maxillary canine. The difference is usually about 1 mm. The mandibular canine is broader mesiodistally than either of the mandibular incisors, for example, about 1 mm wider than the mandibular lateral incisor.

The essential differences between mandibular and maxillary canines viewed from the labial aspect may be described as follows:

The crowns of the mandibular canines *appear* longer. Sometimes they are longer, but the effect of greater length is emphasized by the narrowness of the crown mesiodistally and the height of the contact areas above the cervix.

The mesial outline of the crown of the mandibular canine is nearly straight with the mesial outline of the root, the mesial contact area being near the mesioincisal angle.

When the cusp ridges have not been affected by wear, the cusp angle is on a line with the center of the root, as on the maxillary canine. The mesial cusp ridge is the shorter.

The distal contact area of the mandibular canine is more toward the incisal than that of the maxillary canine, but not up to the level of the mesial area.

The cervical line labially has a semicircular curvature apically.

Many mandibular canines give the impression from this aspect of being bent distally on the root base. The maxillary canine crowns are more likely to be in line with the root.

The mandibular canine root is shorter by 1 or 2 mm on the average than that of the maxillary canine, and its apical end is more sharply pointed. Root curvatures are infre-

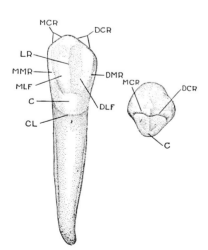

Figure 8–13. Mandibular right canine, lingual and incisal aspects. *DCR,* Distal cusp ridge; *DMR,* distal marginal ridge; *DLF,* distolingual fossa; *CL,* cervical line; *C,* cingulum; *MLF,* mesiolingual fossa; *MMR,* mesial marginal ridge; *LR,* lingual ridge; *MCR,* mesial cusp ridge.

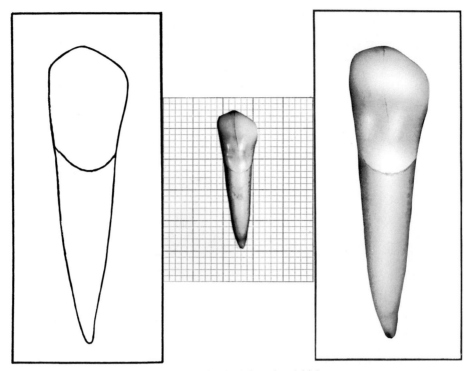

Figure 8–14. Mandibular left canine, labial aspect.

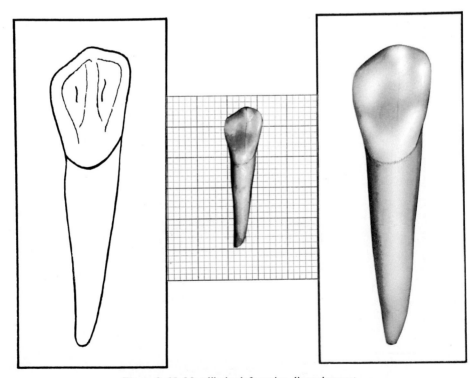

Figure 8–15. Mandibular left canine, lingual aspect.

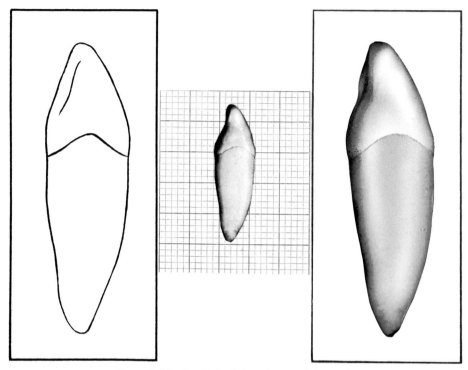

Figure 8–16. Mandibular left canine, mesial aspect.

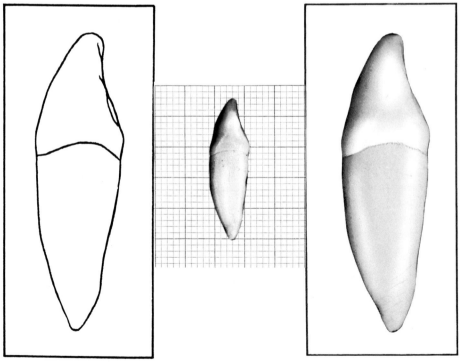

Figure 8–17. Mandibular left canine, distal aspect.

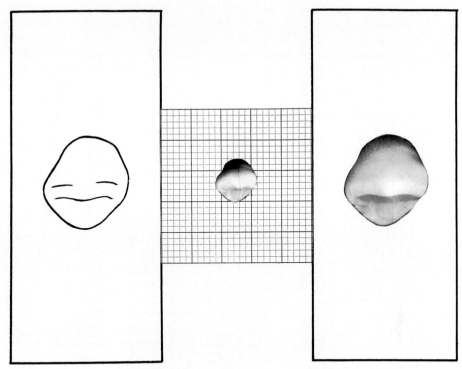

Figure 8–18. Mandibular left canine, incisal aspect.

quent. When curvature of root ends is present, it is often in a mesial direction (Fig. 8–21, specimens *1, 2, 3, 4*).

Lingual Aspect (Figs. 8–15, 8–19, and 8–20)

In comparing the lingual aspect of the mandibular canine with the maxillary canine the following differences are noted.

The lingual surface of the crown of the mandibular canine is flatter, simulating the lingual surfaces of mandibular incisors. The cingulum is smooth and poorly developed. The marginal ridges are less distinct. This is true of the lingual ridge except toward the cusp tip, where it is raised. Generally speaking, the lingual surface of the crown is smooth and regular.

The lingual portion of the root is narrower relatively than that of the maxillary canine. It narrows down to little more than half the width of the labial portion.

Mesial Aspect (Figs. 8–16, 8–19, 8–20, and 8–22)

From the mesial aspect, there are characteristic differences between the two teeth in question. The mandibular canine has less curvature labially on the crown, with very little curvature directly above the cervical line. The curvature at the cervical portion, as a rule, is less than 0.5 mm. The lingual outline of the crown is curved in the same manner as that of the maxillary canine, but it differs in degree.

Text continued on page 192

188   *The Permanent Canines, Maxillary and Mandibular*

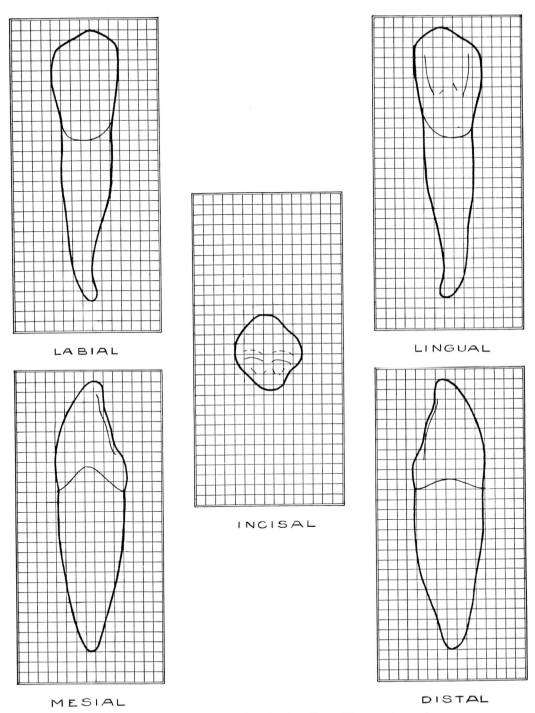

LABIAL

LINGUAL

INCISAL

MESIAL

DISTAL

Figure 8–19. Mandibular right canine. Graph outlines of five aspects are shown.

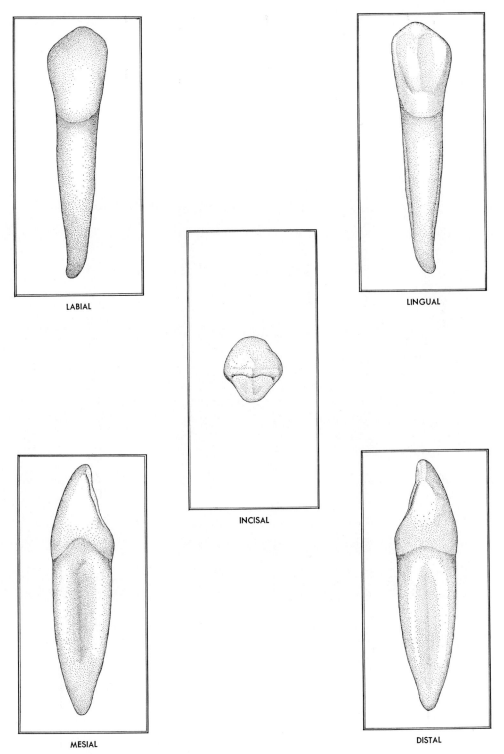

LABIAL

LINGUAL

INCISAL

MESIAL

DISTAL

Figure 8–20. Mandibular right canine.

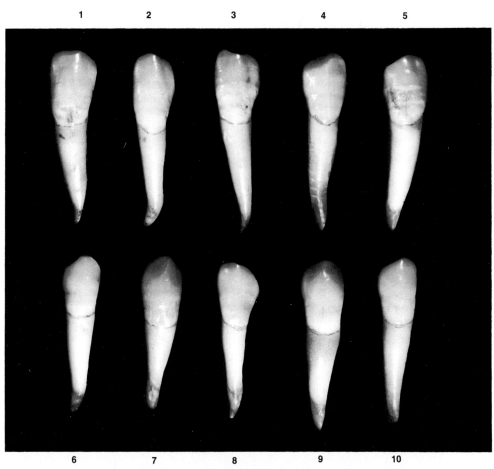

Figure 8–21. Mandibular canine, labial aspect. Ten typical specimens are shown.

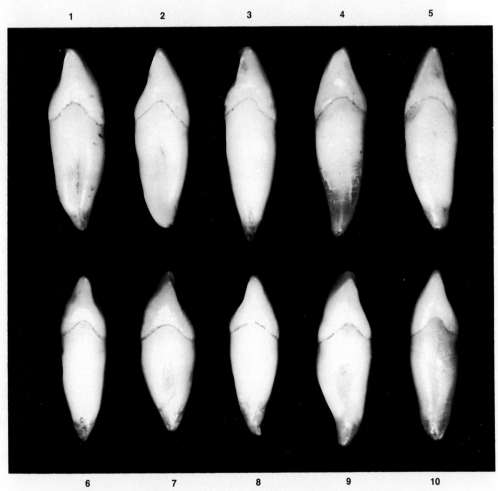

Figure 8–22. Mandibular canine, mesial aspect. Ten typical specimens are shown.

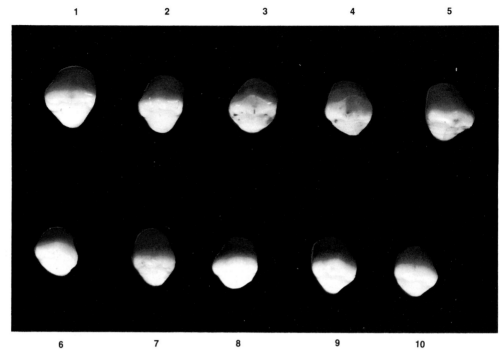

Figure 8–23. Mandibular canine, incisal aspect. Ten typical specimens are shown.

The cingulum is not as pronounced, and the incisal portion of the crown is thinner labiolingually, which allows the cusp to appear more pointed and the cusp ridge more slender. The tip of the cusp is more nearly centered over the root, with a lingual placement in some cases comparable to the placement of incisal ridges on mandibular incisors.

The cervical line curves more toward the incisal portion than does the cervical line on the maxillary canine.

The roots of the two teeth are quite similar from the mesial aspect, with the possible exception of a more pointed root tip. The developmental depression mesially on the root of the mandibular canine is more pronounced and sometimes quite deep.

Distal Aspect (Figs. 8–17, 8–19, and 8–20)

There is little difference from the distal aspect between mandibular and maxillary canines except those features mentioned under *mesial aspect,* which are common to both.

Incisal Aspect (Figs. 8–18, 8–19, 8–20, and 8–23)

The outlines of the crowns of mandibular and maxillary canines from the incisal aspect are often similar. The main differences to be noted are these.

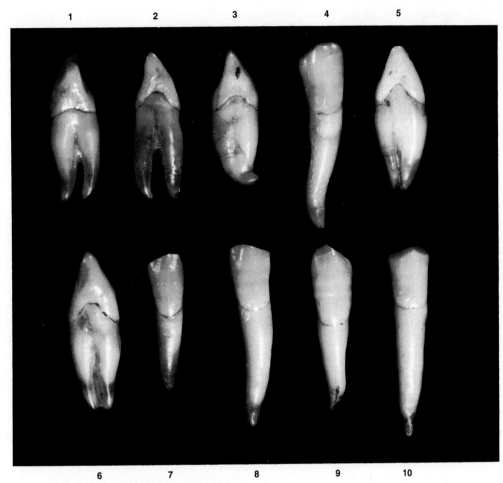

Figure 8–24. Mandibular canine.

    1, Well-formed crown; two roots, one lingual and one labial.
    2, Same as specimen *1*, with longer roots.
    3, Well-formed crown portion; poorly formed root.
    4, Root longer than average, with extreme curvature.
    5, Deep developmental groove dividing the root.
    6, Same as specimen *5*.
    7, Crown resembling mandibular lateral incisor; root short.
    8, Root extra long, with odd mesial curvature starting at cervical third.
    9, Crown extra long and irregular in outline. Root short and poorly formed at apex.
    10, Crown with straight mesial and distal sides, wide at cervix, with a root of extreme length.

    The mesiodistal dimension of the mandibular canine is less than the labiolingual dimension. In this there is a similarity, but the outlines of the mesial surface are less curved. The cusp tip and mesial cusp ridge are more likely to be inclined in a lingual direction, in the mandibular canine with the distal cusp ridge and the contact area extension distinctly so. It will be remembered that the cusp ridges of the maxillary canine with the contact area extensions were more nearly in a straight line mesiodistally from the incisal aspect.

9 *The Permanent Maxillary Premolars*

The maxillary premolars are four in number: two in the right maxilla and two in the left maxilla. They are posterior to the canines and immediately anterior to the molars.

The premolars are so named because they are anterior to the molars in the permanent dentition. In zoology, the premolars are those teeth that succeed the deciduous molars regardless of the number to be succeeded. The term *bicuspid,* which is widely used when we describe human teeth, presupposes two cusps, a supposition that makes the term misleading, since mandibular premolars in the human subject may show a variation in the number of cusps from one to three. Among Carnivora, in the study of comparative dental anatomy, premolar forms differ so greatly that a more desriptive single term than premolar is out of the question. Since the term *premolar* is the one most widely used by all sciences interested in dental anatomy, human and comparative, it is the one that will be given preference here.

The maxillary premolars are developed from the same number of lobes as anterior teeth, which is four. The primary difference in development is the well-formed lingual cusp, developed from the lingual lobe, which is represented by the cingulum development on incisors and canines. The middle buccal lobe on the premolars, corresponding to the middle labial lobe of the canines, remains highly developed, the maxillary premolars resembling the canines when viewed from the buccal aspect. The buccal cusp of the maxillary first premolar, especially, is long and sharp, assisting the canine as a prehensile or tearing tooth. The mandibular first premolar assists the mandibular canine in the same manner.

The *second* premolars, both maxillary and mandibular, have cusps less sharp than the others, and their cusps intercusp with opposing teeth when the jaws are brought together; this makes them more efficient as grinding teeth and they function much like the molars, to a lesser degree.

The maxillary premolar crowns are shorter than those of the maxillary canines, and the roots are shorter also. The root lengths equal those of the molars. The crowns are a little longer than those of the molars.

Because of the cusp development buccally and lingually, the marginal ridges are in a more horizontal plane and are considered part of the occlusal surface of the crown rather than of the lingual surface, as in the case of incisors and canines.

When premolars have two roots, one is placed buccally and one lingually.

Maxillary First Premolar

The maxillary first premolar has two cusps, a buccal and a lingual, each being sharply defined. The buccal cusp is usually about 1 mm longer than the lingual cusp. The crown is angular and the buccal line angles prominent (Table 9–1).

The crown is shorter than the canine by 1.5 to 2 mm on the average. Although this tooth resembles the canine from the buccal aspect, it differs in that the contact areas mesially and distally are at about the same level. The root is shorter. If the buccal cusp form has not been changed by wear, the mesial slope of the cusp is longer than the distal slope. The opposite arrangement is true of the maxillary canine. Generally, the first premolar is not as wide in a mesiodistal direction as the canine.

Most maxillary first premolars have two roots (Fig. 9–10) and two pulp canals. When only one root is present, two pulp canals are usually found anyway.

The maxillary first premolar has some characteristics commmon to all posterior teeth. Briefly, these characteristics as differentiated from those of anterior teeth are as follows:

1. Greater relative faciolingual measurement as compared with the mesiodistal measurement
2. Broader contact areas
3. Contact areas more nearly at the same level
4. Less curvature of the cervical line mesially and distally
5. Shorter crown, cervico-occlusally when compared with anterior teeth

Detailed Description of the Maxillary First Premolar from All Aspects

Figures 9–1 through 9–15 present the maxillary first premolar in various aspects.

Buccal Aspect (Figs. 9–2, 9–7 through 9–9)

From this aspect, the crown is roughtly trapezoidal (see Fig. 4–23, *c*). The crown exhibits little curvature at the cervical line. The crest of curvature of the cervical line buccally is near the center of the root buccally.

The mesial outline of the crown is slightly concave from the cervical line to the mesial contact area. The contact area is represented by a relatively broad curvature, the crest of which lies immediately occlusal to the halfway point from the cervical line to the tip of the buccal cusp.

The mesial slope of the buccal cusp is rather straight and longer than the distal slope, which is shorter and more curved. This arrangement places the tip of the buccal cusp distal to a line bisecting the buccal surface of the crown. The mesial slope of the buccal cusp is sometimes notched; in other instances, a concave outline is noted at this point (Fig. 9–9, specimens *7, 9,* and *10*).

The distal outline of the crown below the cervical line is straighter than that of the mesial, although it may be somewhat concave also. The distal contact area is represented by a broader curvature than is found mesially, and the crest of curvature of the contact area tends to be a little more occlusal when the tooth is posed with its long axis vertical. Even so, the contact areas are more nearly level with each other than those found on anterior teeth.

The width of the crown of the maxillary first premolar mesiodistally is about 2 mm less at the cervix than at its width at the points of its greatest mesiodistal measurement.

Table 9–1. Maxillary First Premolar

First evidence of calcification	1½ to 1¾ years
Enamel completed	5 to 6 years
Eruption	10 to 11 years
Root completed	12 to 13 years

Measurement Table

	Cervico-occlusal Length of Crown	Length of Root	Mesiodistal Diameter of Crown	Mesiodistal Diameter of Crown at Cervix	Labio- or Bucco-lingual Diameter of Crown	Labio- or Bucco-lingual Diameter at Cervix	Curvature of Cervical Line— Mesial	Curvature of Cervical Line— Distal
Dimensions suggested for carving technique	8.5*	14.0	7.0	5.0	9.0	8.0	1.0	0.0

* In millimeters.

Figure 9–1. Maxillary right first premolar, mesial and occlusal aspects. *LR*, Lingual root; *CL*, cervical line; *MMDG*, mesial marginal developmental groove; *LC*, lingual cusp; *BC*, buccal cusp; *MCA*, mesial contact area; *BCR*, buccal cervical ridge; *MDD*, mesial developmental depression; *BR*, buccal root; *MBCR*, mesiobuccal cusp ridge; *MMR*, mesial marginal ridge; *MTF*, mesial triangular fossa (shaded area); *CDG*, central developmental groove; *MLCR*, mesiolingual cusp ridge; *DLCR*, distolingual cusp ridge; *DTF*, distal triangular fossa; *DMR*, distal marginal ridge; *DBCR*, distobuccal cusp ridge.

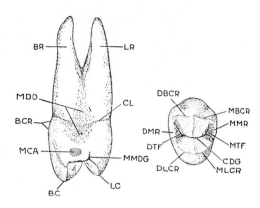

The buccal cusp is long, coming to a pointed tip and resembling the canine in this respect, although contact areas in this tooth are near the same level.

The buccal surface of the crown is convex, showing strong development of the middle buccal lobe. The continuous ridge from cusp tip to cervical margin on the buccal surface of the crown is called the *buccal ridge*.

Mesial and distal to the buccal ridge, at or occlusal to the middle third, developmental depressions are usually seen which serve as demarcations between the middle buccal lobe and the mesio- and distobuccal lobes. Although the latter lobes show less development, they are nevertheless prominent and serve to emphasize strong mesiobuccal and distobuccal line angles on the crown (Fig. 4–23, *c*).

The roots are 3 or 4 mm shorter than those of the maxillary canine, although the outline of the buccal portion of the root form bears a close resemblance.

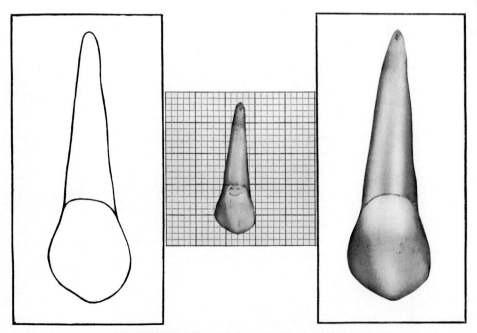

Figure 9–2. Maxillary left first premolar, buccal aspect.

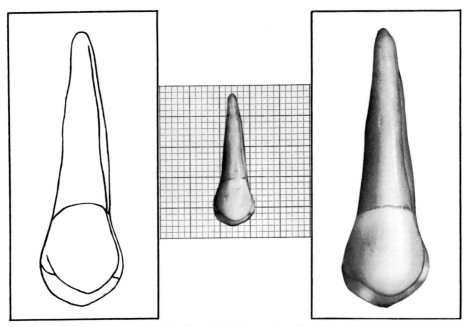

Figure 9–3. Maxillary left first premolar, lingual aspect.

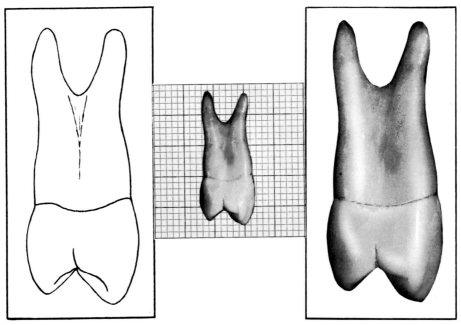

Figure 9–4. Maxillary left first premolar, mesial aspect.

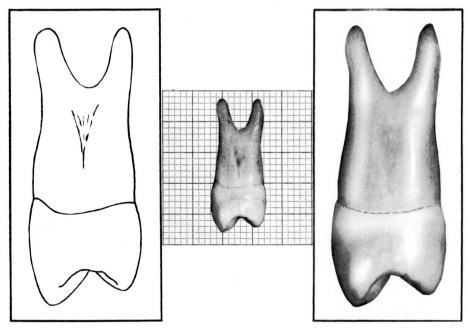

Figure 9–5. Maxillary left first premolar, distal aspect.

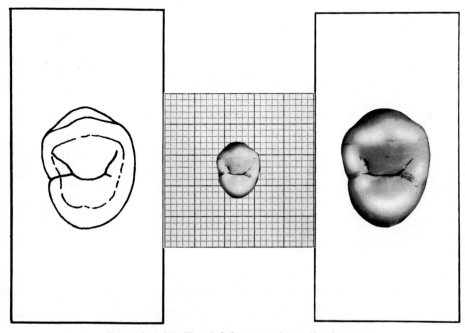

Figure 9–6. Maxillary left first premolar, occlusal aspect.

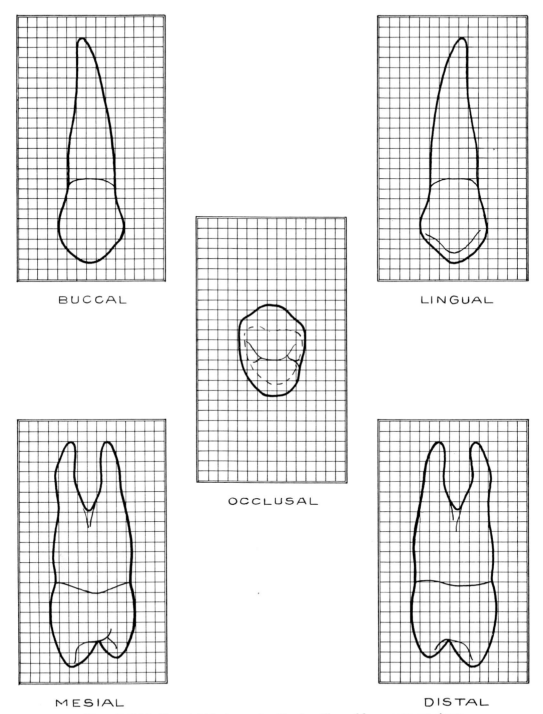

BUCCAL

LINGUAL

OCCLUSAL

MESIAL

DISTAL

Figure 9–7. Maxillary right first premolar. Graph outlines of five aspects are shown.

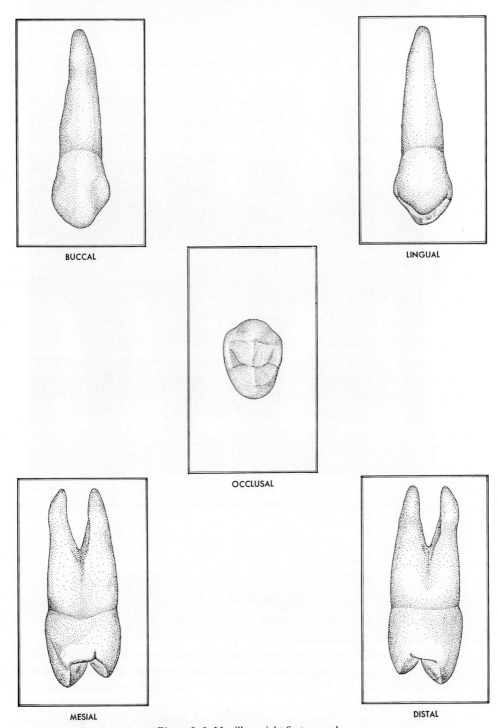

BUCCAL

LINGUAL

OCCLUSAL

MESIAL

DISTAL

Figure 9–8. Maxillary right first premolar.

1   2   3   4   5

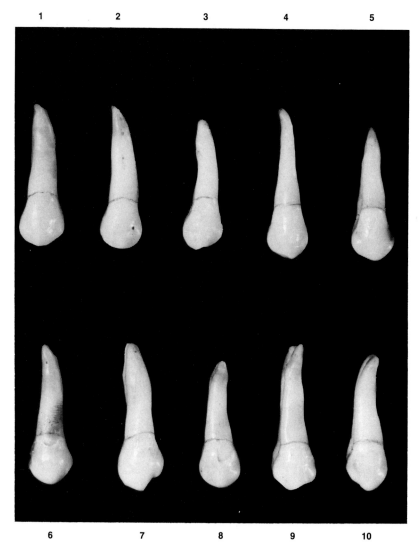

6   7   8   9   10

Figure 9–9. Maxillary first premolars, buccal aspect. Ten typical specimens are shown.

Lingual Aspect (Fig. 9–3, 9–7, and 9–8)

From the lingual aspect, the gross outline of the maxillary first premolar is the reverse of the gross outline of the buccal aspect.

The crown tapers toward the lingual, since the lingual cusp is narrower mesiodistally than the buccal cusp. The lingual cusp is smooth and spheroidal from the cervical portion to the area near the cusp tip. The cusp tip is pointed, with mesial and distal slopes meeting at an angle of about 90 degrees.

Naturally, the spheroidal form of the lingual portion of the crown is convex at all points. Sometimes the crest of the smooth lingual portion that terminates at the point of the lingual cusp is called the *lingual ridge*.

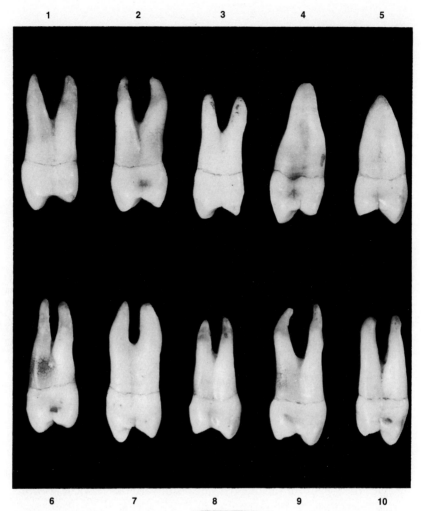

Figure 9–10. Maxillary first premolars, mesial aspect. Ten typical specimens are shown.

The mesial and distal outlines of the lingual portion of the crown are convex, these outlines being continuous with the mesial and distal slopes of the lingual cusp, straightening out as they join the mesial and distal sides of the lingual root at the cervical line.

The cervical line lingually is regular, with slight curvature toward the root and the crest of curvature centered on the root. Since the lingual portion of the crown is narrower than the buccal portion, it is possible to see part of the mesial and distal surfaces of crown and root from the lingual aspect, depending upon the posing of the tooth and the line of vision.

Since the lingual cusp is not so long as the buccal cusp, the tips of both cusps, with their mesial and distal slopes, may be seen from the lingual aspect.

The lingual portion of the root—or the lingual portion of the lingual root if two roots are present—is smooth and convex at all points. The apex of the lingual root of a two-root specimen tends to be more blunt than the buccal root apex.

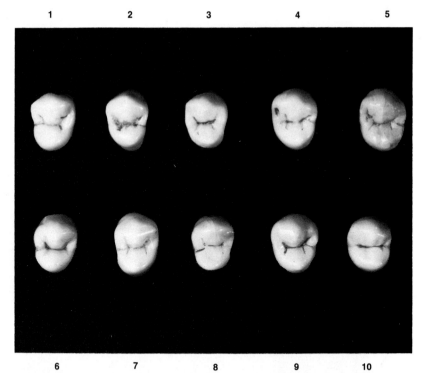

1   **2**   **3**   **4**   **5**

6   **7**   **8**   **9**   **10**

Figure 9–11. Maxillary first premolars, occlusal aspect. Ten typical specimens are shown.

Mesial Aspect (Figs. 9–1, 9–4, 9–7, 9–8, and 9–10)

The mesial aspect of the crown of the maxillary first premolar is also roughly trapezoidal. However, the longest of the uneven sides is toward the cervical portion and the shortest is toward the occlusal portion (see Fig. 4–23, *e*).

Another characteristic that is representative of all posterior maxillary teeth is that the tips of the cusps are well within the confines of the root trunk. (For a definition of root trunk, see Figures 11–3 and 11–8.) That is, the measurement from the tip of the buccal cusp to the tip of the lingual cusp is less than the buccolingual measurement of the root at its cervical portion.

Most maxillary first premolars have two roots, one buccal and one lingual; these are clearly outlined from the mesial aspect.

The cervical line may be regular in outline (Fig. 9–10, specimen *1*) or irregular (Fig. 9–10, specimen *4*). In either case, the curvature occlusally is less (about 1 mm on the average) than the cervical curvature on the mesial of any of the anterior teeth. The extent of the curvature of the cervical line mesially on these teeth is constant within a fraction of a millimeter and is similar to the average curvature to the mesial of all posterior teeth.

From the mesial aspect, the buccal outline of the crown curves outward below the cervical line; the crest of curvature is often located approximately at the junction of cervical and middle thirds. Or the crest of curvature may be located within the cervical third (Fig. 9–10, specimens *1* and *10*). From the crest of curvature, the buccal outline continues as a line of less convexity to the tip of the buccal cusp, which is directly below the center of the buccal root (when two roots are present).

1 2 3 4 5

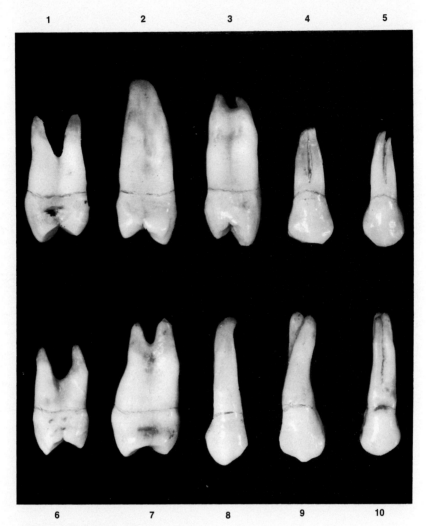

6 7 8 9 10

Figure 9–12. Maxillary first premolars.
Ten specimens with uncommon variations are shown.
  1, Constricted occlusal surface; short roots.
  2, Single root of extreme length.
  3, Constricted occlusal surface; mesial developmental groove indistinct on mesial surface of root.
  4, Short root form, with two buccal roots fused.
  5, Short root form, with two buccal roots showing bifurcation.
  6, Short roots, with considerable separation.
  7, Buccolingual calibration greater than usual.
  8, Root extremely long; distal contact area high.
  9, Twisted buccal root.
  10, Three roots fused; roots are also uncommonly long.

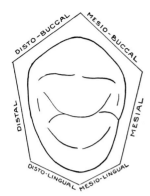

Figure 9–13. Maxillary first premolar, occlusal aspect. This aspect resembles a hexagonal figure.

Figure 9–14. Maxillary first premolar, occlusal aspect. *A*, Crest of buccal ridge; *B*, crest of lingual ridge; *C*, crest of mesial contact area; *D*, crest of distal contact area.

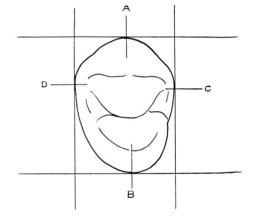

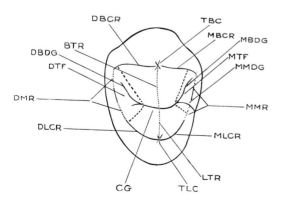

Figure 9–15. Maxillary first premolar, occlusal aspect. *TBC*, Tip of buccal cusp; *MBCR*, mesiobuccal cusp ridge; *MBDG*, mesiobuccal developmental groove; *MTF*, mesial triangular fossa; *MMDG*, mesial marginal developmental groove; *MMR*, mesial marginal ridge; *MLCR*, mesiolingual cusp ridge; *LTR*, lingual triangular ridge; *TLC*, tip of lingual cusp; *CG*, central groove; *DLCR*, distolingual cusp ridge; *DMR*, distal marginal ridge; *DTF*, distal triangular fossa; *DBDG*, distobuccal developmental groove; *BTR*, buccal triangular ridge; *DBCR*, distobuccal cusp ridge. (Compare with Figure 9–1.)

The lingual outline of the crown may be described as a smoothly curved line starting at the cervical line and ending at the tip of the lingual cusp. The crest of this curvature is most often near the center of the middle third. Some specimens show a more abrupt curvature at the cervical third (Fig. 9–10, specimens *2* and *9*).

The tip of the lingual cusp is on a line, in most cases, with the lingual border of the lingual root. The lingual cusp is always shorter than the buccal cusp, the average difference being about 1 mm. This difference, however, may be greater (Fig. 9–10, specimens *1, 4,* and *10*). From this aspect, it is noted that the cusps of the maxillary first premolar are long and sharp, with the mesial marginal ridge at about the level of the junction of the middle and occlusal thirds.

A distinguishing feature of this tooth is found on the mesial surface of the crown. Immediately cervical to the mesial contact area, centered on the mesial surface and bordered buccally and lingually by the mesiobuccal and mesiolingual line angles, is a marked depression called the *mesial developmental depression* (Fig. 9–1). This mesial concavity continues apically beyond the cervical line, joins a deep developmental depression between the roots, and ends at the root bifurcation. On single-root specimens, the concavity on the crown and root is plainly seen also, although it may not be so deeply marked: Maxillary second premolars do not have this feature.

Another distinguishing feature of the maxillary first premolar is a well-defined developmental groove in the enamel of the mesial marginal ridge. This groove is in alignment with the developmental depression on the mesial surface of the root but is not usually connected with it. This marginal groove is continuous with the central groove of the occlusal surface of the crown, crossing the marginal ridge immediately lingual to the mesial contact area and terminating a short distance cervical to the mesial marginal ridge on the mesial surface (Fig. 9–10, specimen *10*).

The buccal outline of the buccal root, above the cervical line, is straight, with a tendency toward a lingual inclination. On those buccal roots having a buccal inclination above the root bifurcation, the outline may be relatively straight up to the apical portion of the buccal root or it may curve bucally at the middle third. Buccal roots may take a buccal or lingual inclination, apical to middle thirds.

The lingual outline of the lingual root is rather straight above the cervical line. It may not exhibit much curvature between the cervix and the apex. Many cases, however, show considerable curvature to lingual roots apical to the middle thirds. It may take a buccal or lingual inclination (Fig. 9–10, specimens *1, 2,* and *9*).

The root trunk is long on this tooth, making up about half of the root length. The bifurcation on those teeth with two roots begins at a more occlusal point mesially than distally. Generally speaking, when bifurcated, the root is bifurcated for half its total length.

Except for the deep developmental groove and depression at or below the bifurcation, the mesial surface of the root portion of this tooth is smoothly convex buccally and lingually. Even when one root only is present, the developmental depression is very noticeable for most of the root length. The latter instances show roots with buccal and lingual outlines ending in a blunt apex above the center of the crown (Fig. 9–10, specimens *4* and *5*).

Distal Aspect (Figs. 9–5, 9–7, and 9–8)

From the distal aspect, the anatomy of crown and root of the maxillary first premolar differs from that of the mesial aspect as follows.

The crown surface is convex at all points except for a small flattened area just cervical to the contact area and buccal to the center of the distal surface.

The curvature of the cervical line is less on the distal than on the mesial surface, often showing a line straight across from buccal to lingual.

There is no evidence of a deep developmental groove crossing the distal marginal ridge of the crown. If a developmental groove should be noticeable, it is shallow and insignificant.

The root trunk is flattened on the distal surface above the cervical line with no outstanding developmental signs.

The bifurcation of the roots is abrupt near the apical third, with no developmental groove leading to it such as one finds mesially.

Occlusal Aspects (Figs. 9–6, 9–7, 9–8, 9–11, 9–13, 9–14, and 9–15)

The occlusal aspect of the maxillary first premolar resembles roughly a six-sided or hexagonal figure (Fig. 9–13). The six sides are made up of the mesiobuccal (which is mesial to the buccal ridge), mesial, mesiolingual (which is mesial to the lingual ridge), distolingual, distal, and distobuccal. This hexagonal figure, however, is not equilateral. The two buccal sides are nearly equal, the mesial side is shorter than the distal side and the mesiolingual side is shorter than the distolingual side (Fig. 9–13).

The relation and position of various anatomic points are to be considered from the occlusal aspect. A drawing of the outline of this occlusal aspect, when placed within a rectangle the dimensions of which represent the mesiodistal and buccolingual width of the crown, demonstrates the relative positions of the mesial and distal contact areas and also those of the buccal and lingual ridges (Fig. 9–14; see also Fig. 9–6).

The crest of the distal contact area is somewhat buccal to that of the mesial contact area, and the crest of the buccal ridge is somewhat distal to that of the lingual ridge. The crests of curvature represent the highest points on the buccal and lingual ridges and the mesial and distal contact areas.

Close observation of the crown from this aspect reveals the following characteristics (Fig. 9–14).

1. The distance from the buccal crest (*A*) to the mesial crest (*C*) is slightly longer than the distance from the buccal crest to the distal crest (*D*).
2. The distance from the mesial crest to the lingual crest is much shorter than the distance from the distal crest to the lingual crest.
3. The crown is wider on the buccal than on the lingual.
4. The buccolingual dimension of the crown is much greater than the mesiodistal dimension.

The occlusal surface of the maxillary first premolar is circumscribed by the cusp ridges and marginal ridges. The mesiobuccal and distobuccal cusp ridges are in line with each other, and their alignment is in a distobuccal direction. In other words, even though they are in the same alignment, the distobuccal cusp ridge is buccal to the mesiobuccal cusp ridge (Fig. 9–15).

The angle formed by the convergence of the mesiobuccal cusp ridge and the mesial marginal ridge approaches a right angle. The angle formed by the convergence of the distobuccal cusp ridge and the distal marginal ridge is acute. The mesiolingual and distolingual cusp ridges are confluent with the mesial and distal marginal ridges; these cusp ridges are curved, following a seimcircular outline from the marginal ridges to their convergence at the tip of the lingual cusp.

When looking at the occlusal aspect of the maxillary first premolar, posing the tooth so that the line of vision is in line with the long axis, we see more of the buccal surface of the crown than of the lingual surface. It should be remembered that when we look at the tooth from the mesial aspect, the tip of the buccal cusp is nearer the center of the root trunk than is the lingual cusp.

The occlusal surface of this tooth has no supplemental grooves in most cases, a fact that makes the surface relatively smooth. A well-defined *central developmental groove* divides the surface evenly buccolingually. It is located at the bottom of the central sulcus of the occlusal surface, extending from a point just mesial to the distal marginal ridge to the mesial marginal ridge, where it joins the *mesial marginal development groove;* this latter groove crosses the mesial marginal ridge and ends on the mesial surface of the crown (Figs. 9–1 and 9–4).

Two collateral developmental grooves join the central groove just inside the mesial and distal marginal ridges. These grooves are called the *mesiobuccal developmental groove* and the *distobuccal developmental groove.* The junctions of the grooves are deeply pointed and are named the *mesial* and *distal developmental pits.*

Just distal to the mesial marginal ridge, the triangular depression that harbors the mesiobuccal developmental groove is called the *mesial triangular fossa.* The depression in the occlusal surface, just mesial to the distal marginal ridge, is called the *distal triangular fossa.*

Although no supplemental grooves are present in most instances, smooth developmental depressions may be visible radiating from the central groove and giving the occlusal surface an uneven appearance.

The *buccal traingular ridge* of the buccal cusp is prominent, arising near the center of the central groove and converging with the tip of the buccal cusp. The *lingual triangular ridge* is less prominent; it also arises near the center of the central groove and converges with the tip of the lingual cusp.

The lingual cusp is pointed more sharply than the buccal cusp.

Maxillary Second Premolar

The maxillary second premolar supplements the maxillary first premolar in function. The two teeth resemble each other so closely that only a brief description of each aspect of the second premolar will be necessary. Direct comparison will be made between it and the first premolar, variations being mentioned.

The maxillary second premolar is less angular, giving a more rounded effect to the crown from all aspects. It has a single root.

Considerable variations in the relative sizes of the two teeth may be seen, since the second premolar does not appear true to form as often as does the first premolar (Table 9–2). The maxillary second premolar may have a crown that is noticeably smaller cervico-occlusally and also mesiodistally. On the other hand, it may be larger in those dimensions. Usually the root length of the second premolar is as great, if not a millimeter or so greater, than that of the first premolar. The two teeth have about the same dimensions *on the average,* except for the tendency toward greater length of the second premolar root.

Brief Description of the Maxillary Second Premolar from All Aspects

Figures 9–16 through 9–24 show the maxillary second premolar in various aspects.

Table 9–2. Maxillary Second Premolar

First evidence of calcification   2 to 2¼ years
Enamel completed   6 to 7 years
Eruption   10 to 12 years
Root completed   12 to 14 years

Measurement Table

	Cervico-occlusal Length of Crown	Length of Root	Mesiodistal Diameter of Crown	Mesiodistal Diameter of Crown at Cervix	Labio- or Bucco-lingual Diameter of Crown	Labio- or Bucco-lingual Diameter at Cervix	Curvature of Cervical Line—Mesial	Curvature of Cervical Line—Distal
Dimensions suggested for carving technique	8.5*	14.0	7.0	5.0	9.0	8.0	1.0	0.0

* In millimeters.

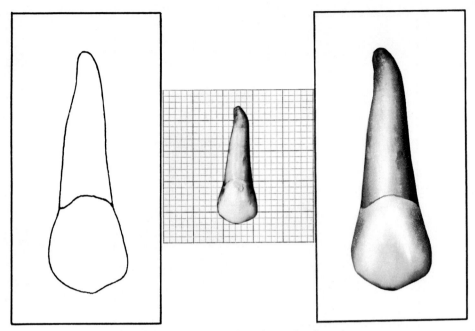

Figure 9–16. Maxillary left second premolar, buccal aspect.

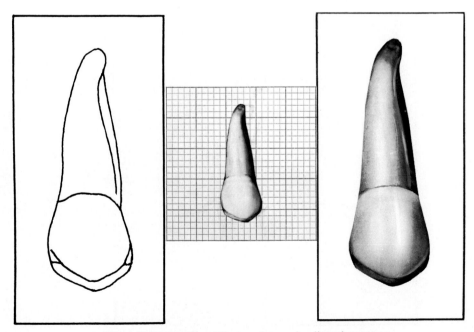

Figure 9–17. Maxillary left second premolar, lingual aspect.

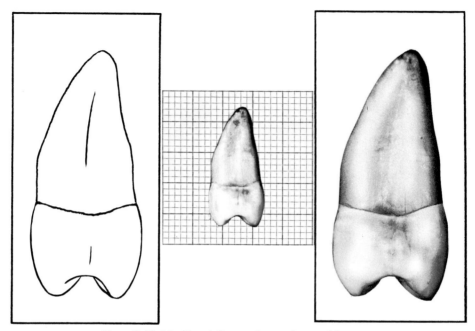

Figure 9–18. Maxillary left second premolar, mesial aspect.

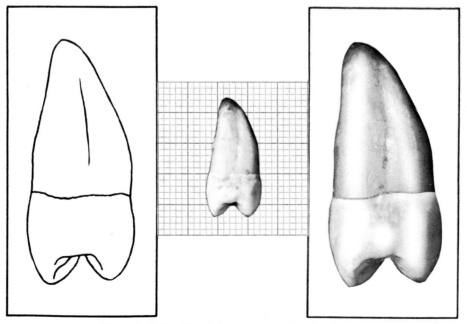

Figure 9–19. Maxillary left second premolar, distal aspect.

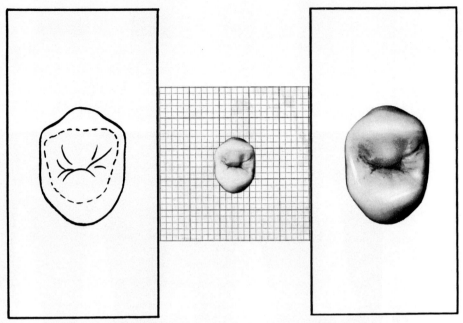

Figure 9–20. Maxillary left second premolar, occlusal aspect.

Buccal Aspect

From the buccal aspect, it may be noticed that the buccal cusp of the second premolar is not as long as that of the first premolar and it appears less pointed. Also, the mesial slope of the buccal cusp ridge is usually shorter than the distal slope. The oppostie is true of the first premolar.

In a good many instances, the crown and root of the second premolar are thicker at their cervical portions. This is not the rule, however (Fig. 9–21, specimens 5, 6, 7, and 9). The buccal ridge of the crown may not be so prominent when compared with the first premolar.

Lingual Aspect

From the lingual aspect, little variation may be seen except that the lingual cusp is longer, making the crown longer on the lingual side.

Mesial Aspect

The mesial aspect shows the difference in cusp length between the two teeth. The cusps of the second premolar are shorter, with the buccal and lingual cusps more nearly the same length. There may be greater distance between cusp tips—a condition that widens the occlusal surface buccolingually.

There is no developmental depression on the mesial surface of the crown as on the first premolar; the crown surface is convex instead. A shallow developmental groove appears on the single tapered root.

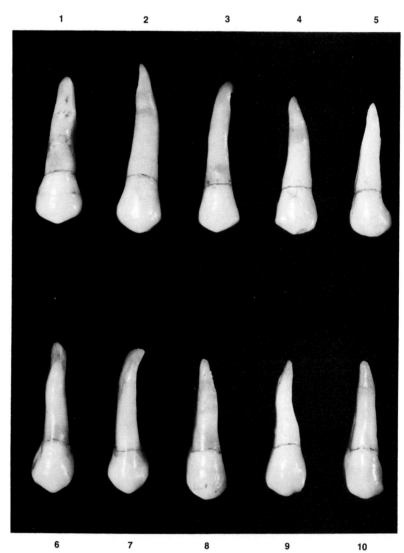

Figure 9–21. Maxillary second premolars, buccal aspect. Ten typical specimens are shown.

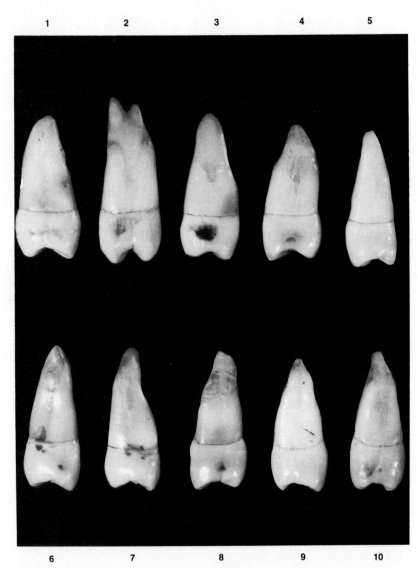

Figure 9–22. Maxillary second premolars, mesial aspect. Ten typical specimens are shown.

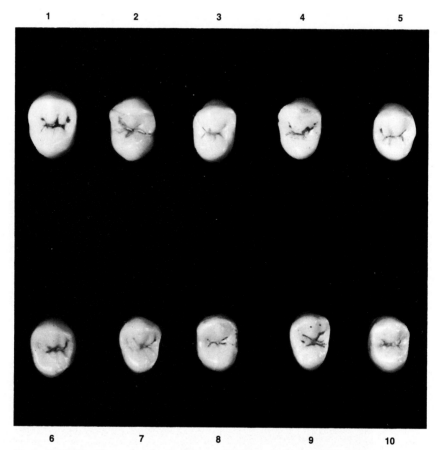

Figure 9–23. Maxillary second premolars, occlusal aspect. Ten typical specimens are shown.

There is no deep developmental groove crossing the mesial marginal ridge, and except for the variation in root form, there is no outstanding variation to be noted when we view the distal aspect.

Occlusal Aspect

From the occlusal aspect, some differences are to be noted between the two premolars. The outline of the crown is more rounded or oval, rather than angular. There are, of course, exceptions. The central developmental groove is shorter and more irregular, and there is a

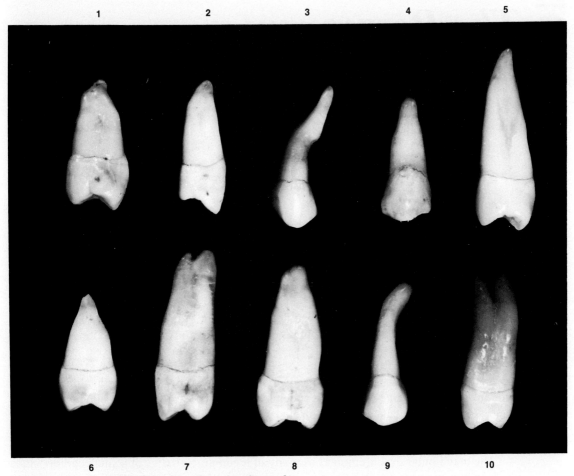

Figure 9-24. Maxillary second premolars.
Ten specimens with uncommon variations are shown.
   1, Root dwarfed and malformed.
   2, Broad occlusal surface; lingual outline of crown straight.
   3, Malformed root.
   4, Crown very broad mesiodistally; root dwarfed.
   5, Root extremely long.
   6, Root dwarfed and very pointed at apex.
   7, Root extremely long; bifurcation at root end.
   8, Crown wider than usual buccolingually, curvature at cervical third extreme.
   9, Root malformed, thick at apical third.
  10, Root unusually long, bifurcated at apical third.

tendency toward multiple supplementary grooves radiating from the central groove. These supplementary grooves terminate in shallow depressions in the enamel that may extend out to the cusp ridges.

   This arrangement makes for an irregular occlusal surface and gives the surface a very wrinkled appearance.

10 *The Permanent Mandibular Premolars*

The mandibular premolars are four in number: Two are situated in the right side of the mandible and two in the left side. They are immediately posterior to the mandibular canines and anterior to the molars.

The mandibular first premolars are developed from four *lobes* as were the maxillary premolars. The mandibular second premolars are, in most instances, developed from five lobes, three buccal and two lingual lobes.

The first premolar has a large buccal *cusp,* which is long and well formed, with a small nonfunctioning lingual cusp that in some specimens is no longer than the cingulum found on some maxillary canines (Fig. 10–10, specimens *3* and *8;* Fig. 10–12, specimens *4* and *7*). The second premolar has three well-formed cusps in most cases, one large buccal cusp and two smaller lingual cusps. The form of both mandibular premolars fails to conform to the implications of the term "bicuspid," the term implying two functioning cusps.

The mandibular first premolar has many of the characteristics of a small canine, since its sharp buccal cusp is the only part of it occluding with maxillary teeth. It functions along with the mandibular canine. The mandibular second premolar has more of the characteristics of a small molar because its lingual cusps are well developed, a fact that places both marginal ridges high and produces a more efficient occlusion with antagonists in the opposite jaw. The mandibular second molar functions by being supplementary to the mandibular first molar.

The first premolar is always the smaller of the two *mandibular* premolars, whereas the opposite is true, in many cases, of the *maxillary* premolars.

Mandibular First Premolar

The mandibular first premolar is the fourth tooth from the median line and the first posterior tooth in the mandible. This tooth is situated between the canine and second premolar and has some characteristics common to each of them.

The characteristics that resemble those of the *mandibular canine* are as follows:

1. The buccal cusp is long and sharp and is the only occluding cusp.
2. The buccolingual measurement is similar to that of the canine.
3. The occlusal surface slopes sharply lingually in a cervical direction.

218

4. The mesiobuccal cusp ridge is shorter than the distobuccal cusp ridge.
5. The outline form of the occlusal aspect resembles the outline form of the incisal aspect of the canine (compare Figs. 10–6 and 8–18).

The characteristics that resemble those of the *second mandibular premolar* are as follows:

1. Except for the longer cusp, the outline of crown and root from the buccal aspect resembles the second premolar.
2. The contact areas, mesially and distally, are near the same level.
3. The curvatures of the cervical line mesially and distally are similar.
4. The tooth has more than one cusp.

Although the root of the mandibular first premolar is shorter as a rule than that of the mandibular second premolar, it is closer to the length of the second premolar root than it is to that of the mandibular canine (Table 10–1).

Detailed Description of the Mandibular First Premolar from All Aspects

Figures 10–1 through 10–12 show the mandibular first premolar in various aspects.

Buccal Aspect (Figs. 10–2, 10–7, 10–8, and 10–9)

From the buccal aspect, the form of the mandibular first premolar crown is nearly symmetrical bilaterally. The middle buccal lobe is well developed, resulting in a large, pointed buccal cusp. The mesial cusp ridge is shorter than the distal cusp ridge. The contact areas are broad from this aspect; they are almost at the same level mesially and distally, this level being a little more than half the distance from cervical line to cusp tip. The measurement mesiodistally at the cervical line is small when it is compared with the measurement at the contact areas.

From the buccal aspect, the crown is roughly trapezoidal (see Fig. 4–23, *c*). The cervical margin is represented by the shortest of the uneven sides.

The crown exhibits little curvature at the cervical line buccally, caused by the slight curvature of the cervical line on the mesial and distal surfaces of the tooth. The crest of curvature of the cervical line buccally approaches the center of the root buccally.

The mesial outline of the crown is straight or slightly concave above the cervical line to a point where it joins the curvature of the mesial contact area. The center of the contact area mesially is occlusal to the cervical line, a distance equal to a little more than half the crown length. The outline of the mesial slope of the buccal cusp usually shows some concavity unless wear has obliterated the original form.

The tip of the buccal cusp is pointed and is, in most cases, located a little mesial to the center of the crown buccally (Fig. 10–9, specimens *3, 7, 8,* and *9*). The mandibular canine has the same characteristic to a greater degree.

The distal outline of the crown is slightly concave above the cervical line to a point where it is confluent with the curvature describing the distal contact area. This curvature is broader than that describing the curvature of the mesial contact area. The distal slope of the buccal cusp usually exhibits some concavity.

The cervix of the mandibular first premolar crown is narrow mesiodistally when compared with the crown width at the contact areas.

Table 10–1. Mandibular First Premolar

First evidence of calcification   1¾ to 2 years
Enamel completed   5 to 6 years
Eruption   10 to 12 years
Root completed   12 to 13 years

Measurement Table

	Cervico-occlusal Length of Crown	Length of Root	Mesiodistal Diameter of Crown	Mesiodistal Diameter of Crown at Cervix	Labio- or Bucco-lingual Diameter of Crown	Labio- or Bucco-lingual Diameter of Crown at Cervix	Curvature of Cervical Line—Mesial	Curvature of Cervical Line—Distal
Dimensions suggested for carving technique	8.5*	14.0	7.0	5.0	7.5	6.5	1.0	0.0

* In millimeters.

220

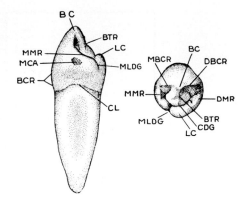

Figure 10–1. Mandibular right first premolar, mesial and occlusal aspects. *BC*, Buccal cusp; *BTR*, buccal triangular ridge; *LC*, lingual cusp; *MLDG*, mesiolingual developmental groove; *CL*, cervical line; *BCR*, buccal cervical ridge; *MCA*, mesial contact area; *MMR*, mesial marginal ridge; *MBCR*, mesiobuccal cusp ridge; *DBCR*, distobuccal cusp ridge; *CDG*, central developmental groove; *DMR*, distal marginal ridge.

The root of this tooth is 3 or 4 mm shorter than that of the mandibular canine, although the outline of the buccal portion of the root bears a close resemblance to the canine.

The buccal surface of the crown is more convex than in the maxillary premolars, especially at the cervical and middle thirds.

The development of the middle buccal lobe is outstanding, ending in a pointed buccal cusp. Developmental depressions are often seen between the three lobes (Fig. 10–9, specimens *2, 3, 8,* and *10*).

The continuous ridge from the cervical margin to the cusp tip is called the *buccal ridge*.

In general, the enamel of the buccal surface of the crown is smooth and shows no developmental grooves and few developmental lines. If the latter are present, they are seen as very fine horizontal cross lines at the cervical portion.

Text continued on page 226

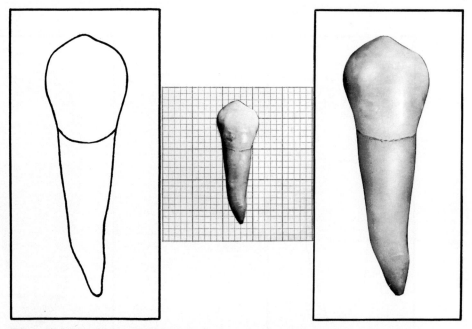

Figure 10–2. Mandibular right first premolar, buccal aspect. The specimen in this photograph shows a mesial inclination of the root. Mandibular premolars and canines have this tendency, although most of the roots of these teeth will curve, if at all, in a distal direction.

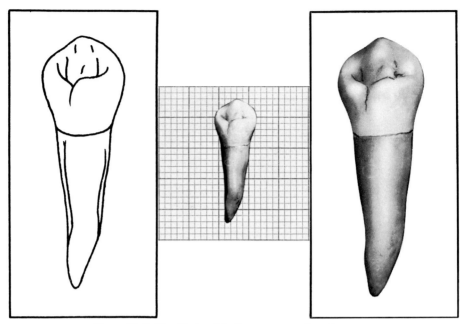

Figure 10–3. Mandibular right first premolar, lingual aspect.

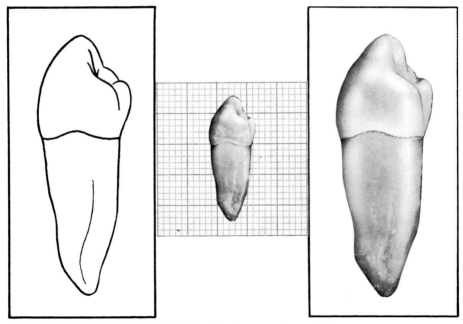

Figure 10–4. Mandibular right first premolar, mesial aspect.

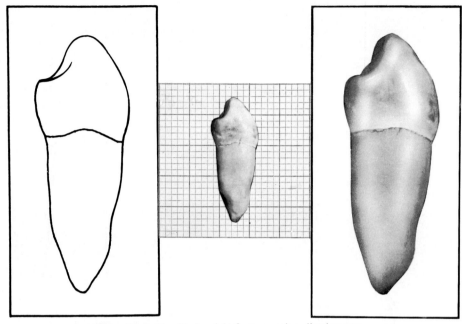

Figure 10–5. Mandibular right first premolar, distal aspect.

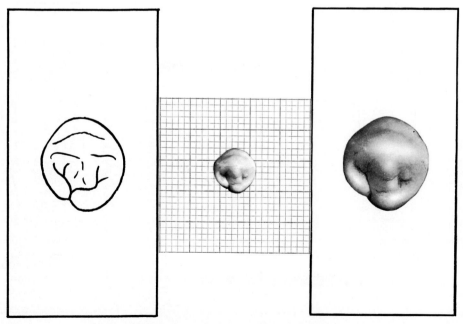

Figure 10–6. Mandibular right first premolar, occlusal aspect.

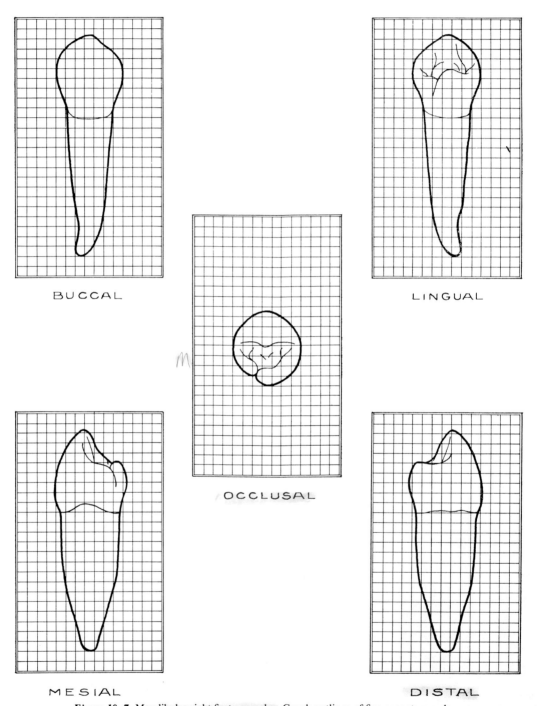

BUCCAL

LINGUAL

OCCLUSAL

MESIAL

DISTAL

Figure 10–7. Mandibular right first premolar. Graph outlines of five aspects are shown.

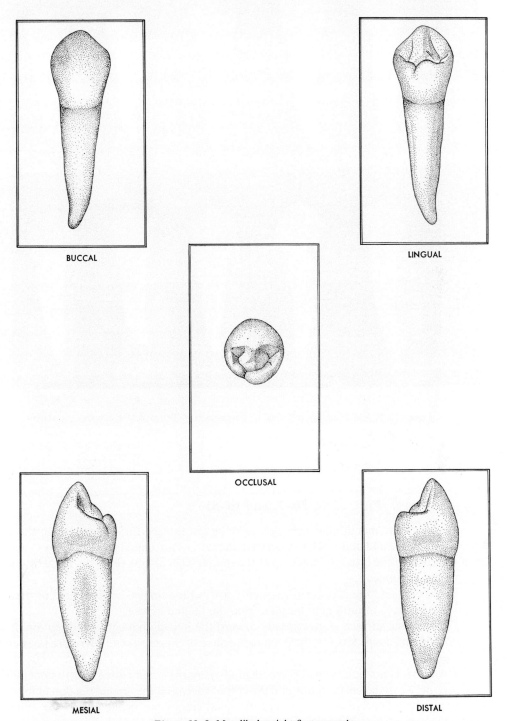

BUCCAL

LINGUAL

OCCLUSAL

MESIAL

DISTAL

Figure 10-8. Mandibular right first premolar.

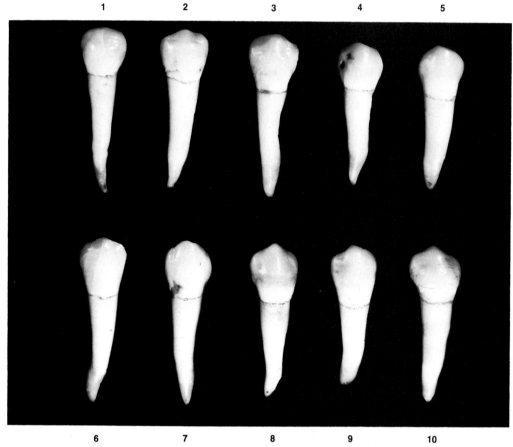

Figure 10–9. Mandibular first premolar, buccal aspect. Ten typical specimens are shown.

Lingual Aspect (Figs. 10–3, 10–7, and 10–8)

The crown of the mandibular first premolar tapers toward the lingual, since the lingual measurement mesiodistally is less than that buccally. The lingual cusp is always small. The major portion of the crown is made up of the middle buccal lobe (Fig. 10–11). This makes it resemble the canine.

The crown and the root taper markedly toward the lingual so that most of the mesial and distal surfaces of both may be seen from the lingual aspect.

The occlusal surface slopes greatly toward the lingual in a cervical direction down to the short lingual cusp. Most of the occlusal surface of this tooth can therefore be seen from this aspect.

The cervical portion of the crown lingually is narrow and convex, with concavities in evidence between the cervical line and the contact areas on the lingual portion of mesial and distal surfaces. The contact areas and marginal ridges are pronounced and extend out above the narrow cervical portion of the crown.

Although the lingual cusp is short and poorly developed (resembling a strongly developed cingulum at times), it usually shows a pointed tip. This cusp tip is in alignment with the buccal triangular ridge of the occlusal surface, which is in plain view. The mesial and distal occlusal fossae are on each side of the triangular ridge (Fig. 10–1).

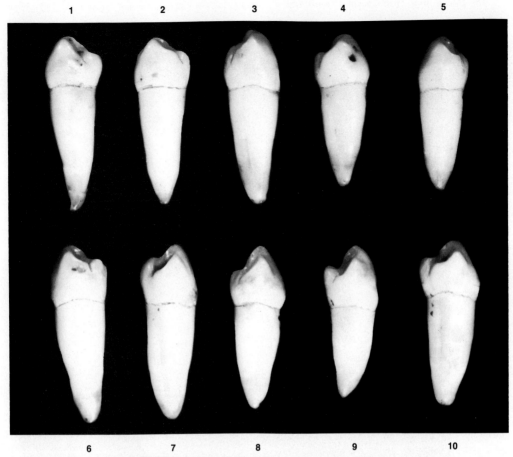

Figure 10–10. Mandibular first premolar, mesial aspect. Ten typical specimens are shown.

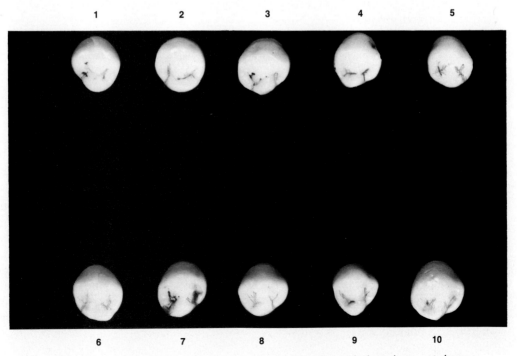

Figure 10–11. Mandibular first premolar, occlusal aspect. Ten typical specimens are shown.

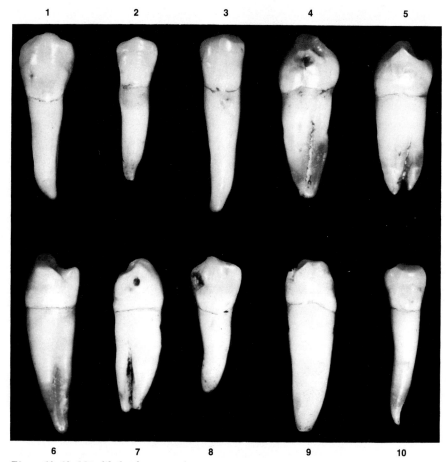

Figure 10–12. Mandibular first premolar.
Ten specimens with uncommon variations are shown.
  1, Crown oversize.
  2, Crown and root diminutive.
  3, Mesial and distal sides of crown straight, cervix wide mesiodistally; root extra long.
  4, Unusual formation of lingual portion of crown; root with deep developmental groove mesially.
  5, Bifurcated root.
  6, Lingual cusp long; little lingual curvature; root of extra length.
  7, No lingual cusp; root bifurcated.
  8, Dwarfed root.
  9, Crown poorly formed; root unusually long.
  10, Very long curved root for crown so small.

A characteristic of the lingual surface of the mandibular first premolar is the *mesiolingual developmental groove*. This groove acts as a line of demarcation between the mesiobuccal lobe and the lingual lobe and extends into the mesial fossa of the occlusal surface.

The root of this tooth is much narrower on the lingual side, and there is a narrow ridge, smooth and convex, the full length of the root. This formation allows most of the mesial and distal surfaces of the root to be seen. Often developmental depressions in the root may be seen with developmental grooves mesially. The root of this tooth tapers evenly from the cervix to a pointed apex.

Mesial Aspect (Figs. 10–4, 10–7, 10–8, and 10–10)

From the mesial aspect, the mandibular first premolar shows an outline that is fundamental and characteristic of all mandibular posterior teeth when viewed from the mesial or distal aspect. The crown outline is roughly rhomboidal (see Fig. 4–23, *e*), and the tip of the buccal cusp is nearly centered over the root. The convexity of the outline of the lingual lobe is lingual to the outline of the root. The surface of the crown presents an overhang above the root trunk in a lingual direction. The tip of the cusp will be on a line approximately with the lingual border of the root. This differs from the condition found in maxillary posterior teeth, where both buccal and lingual cusp tips are well within the confines of the root trunks.

The mandibular first premolar, when viewed from the mesial aspect, often shows the buccal cusp centered over the root (Fig. 10–4). In other instances, the buccal cusp tip is a little buccal to the center, corresponding to the typical placement of buccal cusps on all mandibular posterior teeth.

The buccal outline of the crown from this aspect is prominently curved from the cervical line to the tip of the buccal cusp; the crest of the curvature is near the middle third of the crown. This accented convexity and the location of the crest of contour are characteristic of all mandibular posterior teeth on the buccal surfaces.

The lingual outline of the crown, representative of the lingual outline of the lingual cusp, is a curved outline of less convexity than that of the buccal surface. The crest of curvature lingually approaches the middle third of the crown, the curvature ending at the tip of the lingual cusp, which is in line with the lingual border of the root.

The distance from the cervical line lingually to the tip of the lingual cusp is about two thirds of that from the cervical line buccally to the tip of the buccal cusp.

The mesiobuccal lobe development is prominent from this aspect; it creates by its form the mesial contact area and the mesial marginal ridge, which in turn has a sharp inclination lingually in a cervical direction. The lingual border of the mesial marginal ridge merges with the developmental depression mesiolingually; this harbors the mesiolingual developmental groove.

Some of the occlusal surface of the crown mesially may be seen with the mesial portion of the buccal triangular ridge. The slope of this ridge parallels the mesial marginal ridge, although the crest of the triangular ridge is above it. The sulcus formed by the convergence of buccal and lingual triangular ridges is directly above the mesiolingual groove from this aspect.

The cervical line on the mesial surface is rather regular, curving occlusally. The crest of the curvature is centered buccolingually, the average curvature being about 1 mm in extent. It may, however, be a fraction of a millimeter, or the line may be straight across buccolingually.

The surface of the crown mesially is smooth except for the mesiolingual groove. The surface is plainly convex at the mesial contact area, which is centered on a line with the tip of the buccal cusp. Immediately below the convexity of the contact area, the surface is sharply concave between that area and the cervical line. The distance between the contact area and the cervical line is very short.

The root outline from the mesial aspect is a tapered form from the cervix, ending in a relatively pointed apex in line with the tip of the buccal cusp. The lingual outline may be straight, the buccal outline more curved.

The mesial surface of the root is smooth and flat from the buccal margin to the center. From this point, it too converges sharply toward the root center lingually, often displaying a deep developmental groove in this area. Shallow grooves are nearly always in evidence, and occasionally, a deep developmental groove will end in a bifurcation at the apical third (Fig. 10–12, specimens *5* and *7*).

Distal Aspect (Figs. 10–5, 10–7, and 10–8)

The distal aspect of the mandibular first premolar differs from the mesial aspect in some respects. The distal marginal ridge is higher above the cervix, and it does not have the extreme lingual slope of the mesial marginal ridge, being more nearly at right angles to the axis of crown and root. The marginal ridge is confluent with the lingual cusp ridge; it has no developmental groove on the distal marginal ridge. The major portion of the distal surface of the crown is smoothly convex, the spheroidal form having an unbroken curved surface. Below this curvature and just above the cervical line, a concavity is to be noted which is linear in form and which extends buccolingually. The distal contact area is broader than the mesial, although it is centered in the same relation to the crown outlines. The center of the distal contact area is at a point midway between buccal and lingual crests of curvature and midway between the cervical line and the tip of the buccal cusp.

The curvature of the cervical line distally may be the same as that found mesially, although less curvature distally is the general rule when one is describing all posterior teeth.

The surface of the root distally exhibits more convexity than was found mesially. A shallow developmental depression is centered on the root, but rarely does it contain a deep developmental groove.

The distal surface slopes from the buccal margin toward the center of the root lingually, but the slope is more gradual than that found mesially.

Occlusal Aspects (Figs. 10–6, 10–7, 10–8, and 10–11)

The occlusal aspects of many specimens show considerable variation in the gross outlines of this tooth. Both mandibular premolars exhibit more variations in form occlusally than the maxillary premolars.

The usual outline form of the mandibular first premolar from the occlusal aspect is roughly diamond-shaped and similar to the incisal aspect of mandibular canines (Fig. 10–11, specimens *1, 3, 4,* and *7* through *10*). Some of these teeth have a circular form similar to that of some mandibular second premolars (specimen *2*); others conform to the gross outlines of the more common second premolars (specimens *5* and *6*).

The characteristics common to all mandibular first premolars, regardless of type, when viewed from the occlusal aspect are these:

1. The middle buccal lobe makes up the major bulk of the tooth crown.
2. The buccal ridge is prominent.
3. The mesiobuccal and distobuccal line angles are prominent even though rounded.
4. The curvatures representing the contact areas, immediately lingual to the buccal line angles, are relatively broad, the distal area being the broader of the two.
5. The crown converges sharply to the center of the lingual surface, starting from points approximating the mesial and distal contact areas. This formation makes that part of the crown represented by buccal cusp ridges, marginal ridges, and lingual lobe triangular in form, with the base of the triangle at the buccal cusp ridges and the point of the triangle at the lingual cusp.
6. The marginal ridges are well developed.
7. The lingual cusp is small.
8. The occlusal surface shows a heavy buccal triangular ridge and a small lingual triangular ridge.
9. The occlusal surface harbors two depressions. These are called the *mesial* and *distal fossae* because of their irregularity of form, although they correspond in location to the mesial and distal triangular fossae of other posterior teeth.

The most common type of mandibular first premolars shows a mesiolingual developmental depression and groove. These constrict the mesial surface of the crown and create a smaller mesial contact area which is in contact with the mandibular canine. The distal portion of the crown is described by a larger arc that creates a broader contact area in contact with the second mandibular premolar, which has a broader proximal surface than the canine (see Figs. 5–5, *A*, and 5–13).

The mesial fossa is more linear in form, being more sulcate and containing the *mesial developmental groove,* which extends buccolingually. This groove is confluent with its extension, which becomes the *mesiolingual developmental groove* as it passes over the mesiolingual surface. The distal fossa is more circular in most cases and is circumscribed by the distobuccal cusp ridge, the distal marginal ridge, the buccal triangular ridge, and the distolingual cusp ridge.

The distal fossa may contain a distal developmental groove that is crescent-shaped (Fig. 10–11, specimen *2*). It may harbor a distal developmental pit with accessory supplemental grooves radiating from it (specimen *10*), or it may contain a linear groove running mesiodistally with an arrangement resembling the typical triangular fossa (specimens *4, 5,* and *6*).

Because of the position of this crown over the root, most of the buccal surface may be seen from the occlusal aspect, whereas very little of the lingual surface is in view.

Mandibular Second Premolar

The mandibular second premolar resembles the mandibular first premolar from the buccal aspect only. Although the buccal cusp is not as pronounced, the mesiodistal measurement of the crown and its general outline are similar (Table 10–2). The tooth is larger and has better development in other respects. This tooth assumes two common forms. The first form, which probably occurs most often, is the *three-cusp* type, which appears more angular from the occlusal aspect (Fig. 10–17). The second form is the *two-cusp* type, which appears more rounded from the occlusal aspect (Fig. 10–20, specimens *1, 2, 7,* and *10*).

The two types differ mainly in the occlusal design. The outlines and general appearance from all other aspects are similar.

The single root of the second premolar is larger and longer than that of the first premolar. The root is seldom if ever bifurcated, although some specimens show a deep developmental groove buccally (Fig. 10–18, specimens *3* and *6*). Often a flattened area appears in this location.

Detailed Description of the Mandibular Second Premolar from All Aspects

To describe the separate aspects of this tooth, direct comparisons are made with the mandibular first premolar except for the occlusal aspect. Figures 10–13 through 10–21 present the mandibular second premolar in various aspects.

Buccal Aspect (Figs. 10–13 and 10–18)

From the buccal aspect, the mandibular second premolar presents a shorter buccal cusp than the first premolar, with mesiobuccal and distobuccal cusp ridges presenting angulation of less degree. The contact areas, both mesial and distal, are broad. The contact areas appear to be higher because of the short buccal cusp.

Table 10–2. Mandibular Second Premolar

First evidence of calcification	2¼ to 2½ years
Enamel completed	6 to 7 years
Eruption	11 to 12 years
Root completed	13 to 14 years

Measurement Table

	Cervico-occlusal Length of Crown	Length of Root	Mesiodistal Diameter of Crown	Mesiodistal Diameter of Crown at Cervix	Labio- or Bucco-lingual Diameter of Crown	Labio- or Bucco-lingual Diameter at Cervix	Curvature of Cervical Line—Mesial	Curvature of Cervical Line—Distal
Dimensions suggested for carving technique	8.0*	14.5	7.0	5.0	8.0	7.0	1.0	0.0

* In millimeters.

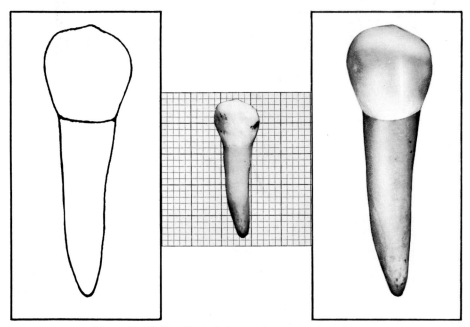

Figure 10–13. Mandibular left second premolar, buccal aspect.

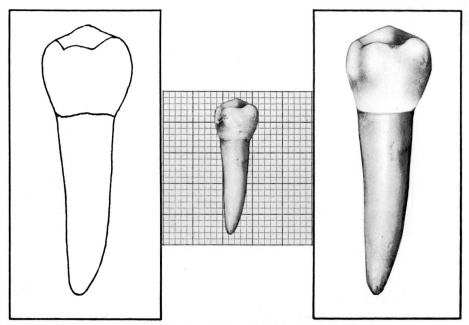

Figure 10–14. Mandibular left second premolar, lingual aspect.

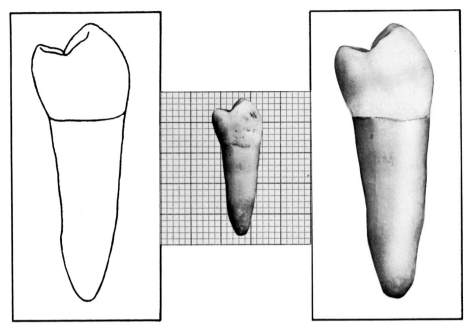

Figure 10–15. Mandibular left second premolar, mesial aspect.

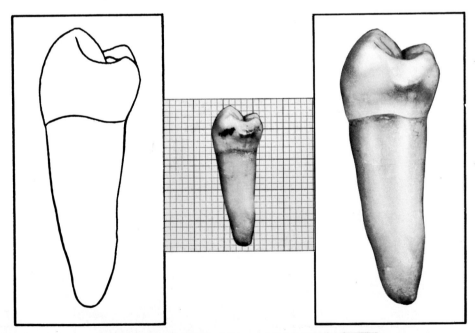

Figure 10–16. Mandibular left second premolar, distal aspect.

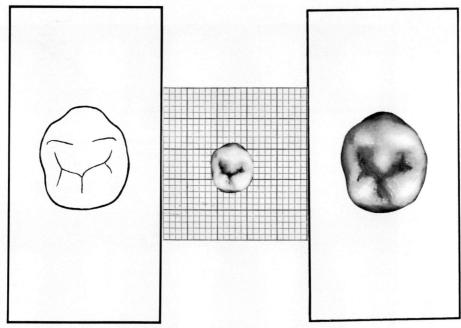

Figure 10–17. Mandibular left second premolar, occlusal aspect.

The root is broader mesiodistally than that of the first premolar, the extra breadth appearing for most of its length, and the root ends in an apex that is more blunt. In other respects, the two teeth are quite similar from this aspect.

Lingual Aspect (Fig. 10–14)

From the lingual aspect, the second premolar crown shows considerable variation from the crown portion of the first premolar. The variations are as follows:

1. The lingual lobes are developed to a greater degree, making the cusp or cusps (depending on the type) longer.
2. Less of the occlusal surface may be seen from this aspect. Nevertheless, since the lingual cusps are not as long as the buccal cusp, part of the buccal portion of the occlusal surface may be seen.
3. In the three-cusp type, the lingual development brings about the greatest variation between the two teeth. There are a mesiolingual and a distolingual cusp, the former being the larger and the longer one in most cases. There is a groove between them, extending a very short distance on the lingual surface and usually centered over the root (Fig. 10–20, specimen 8).

In the two-cusp type, the single lingual cusp development attains equal height with the three-cusp. The two-cusp type has no groove, but it shows a developmental depression distolingually where the lingual cusp ridge joins the distal marginal ridge (Fig. 10–20, specimens 2 and 3).

The lingual surface of the crown of all mandibular second premolars is smooth and spheroidal, having a bulbous form above the constricted cervical portion.

1   2   3   4   5

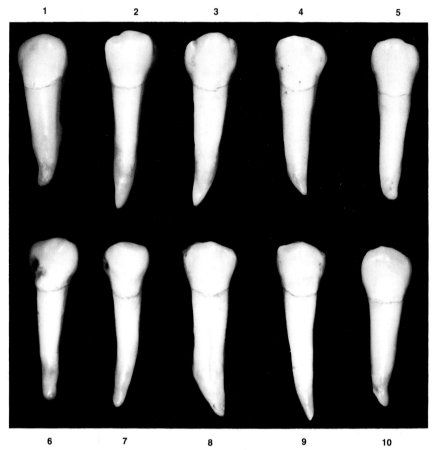

6   7   8   9   10

Figure 10–18. Mandibular second premolar, buccal aspect. Ten typical specimens are shown.

The root is wide lingually, although not quite so wide as the buccal portion. There is less difference in dimension than was found on the first premolar, a fact that creates much less convergence toward the lingual.

Since in most instances the lingual portion of the crown converges little from the buccal portion, less of the mesial and distal sides of this tooth may be seen from this aspect than are seen from the lingual aspect of the first premolar.

The lingual portion of the root is smoothly convex for most of its length.

Considered overall, the second premolar is the larger of the two mandibular premolars.

Mesial Aspect (Figs. 10–15 and 10–19)

From the mesial aspect, the second premolar differs from the first premolar as follows:

1. The crown and root are wider buccolingually.
2. The buccal cusp is not so nearly centered over the root trunk, and it is shorter.
3. The lingual lobe development is greater.
4. The marginal ridge is at right angles to the long axis of the tooth.
5. Less of the occlusal surface may be seen.
6. There is no mesiolingual developmental groove on the crown portion.

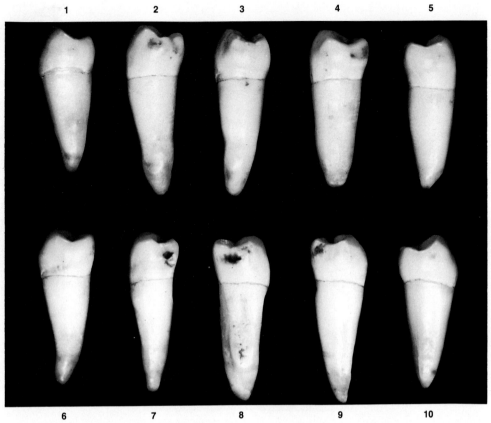

Figure 10–19. Mandibular second premolar, mesial aspect. Ten typical specimens are shown.

7. The root is longer and in most cases slightly convex on the mesial surface; however, this convexity is not always present (Fig. 10–19, specimens *6, 7,* and *8*).
8. The apex of the root is usually more blunt on the second premolar.

Distal Aspect (Fig. 10–16)

This aspect of the mandibular second premolar is similar to the mesial aspect, except that more of the occlusal surface may be seen. This is possible, since the distal marginal ridge is at a lower level than the mesial marginal ridge when we pose the tooth vertically. The crowns of all posterior teeth are tipped distally to the long axes of the roots so that when the specimen tooth is held vertically, more of the occlusal surface may be seen from the distal aspect than from the mesial aspect. This is a characteristic possessed by all posterior teeth, mandibular and maxillary. The angulation of occlusal surfaces to long axes of all posterior teeth is an important observation to remember, not only in the study of individual tooth forms but also later, in the study of alignment and occlusion.

Occlusal Aspect (Figs. 10–17 and 10–20)

As mentioned before, there are two common forms of this tooth. The outline form of each type shows some variation from the occlusal aspect. The two types are similar in that portion which is buccal to the mesiobuccal and distobuccal cusp ridges.

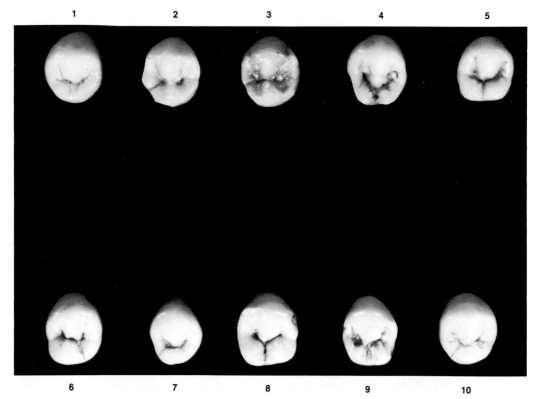

Figure 10–20. Mandibular second premolar, occlusal aspect. Ten typical specimens are shown.

The three-cusp type appears square lingual to the buccal cusp ridges when highly developed (Fig. 10–20, specimen *8*). The round, or two-cusp, type appears round lingual to the buccal cusp ridges (Fig. 10–20, specimen *3*).

The square type (specimen *8*) has three cusps that are distinct; the buccal cusp is the largest, the mesiolingual cusp is next, and the distolingual cusp is the smallest.

Each cusp has well-formed triangular ridges separated by deep developmental grooves. These grooves converge in a *central pit* and form a Y on the occlusal surface. The central pit is located midway between the buccal cusp ridge and the lingual margin of the occlusal surface and slightly distal to the central point between mesial and distal marginal ridges.

Starting at the central pit, the *mesial developmental groove* travels in a mesiobuccal direction and ends in the *mesial triangular fossa* just distal to the mesial marginal ridge. The *distal developmental groove* travels in a distobuccal direction, is somewhat shorter than the mesial groove, and ends in the *distal triangular fossa* mesial to the distal marginal side. The lingual developmental groove extends lingually between the two lingual cusps and ends on the lingual surface of the crown just below the convergence of the lingual cusp ridges. The mesiolingual cusp is wider mesiodistally than the distolingual cusp. This arrangement places the lingual developmental groove distal to center on the crown.

Supplemental grooves and depressions are often seen, radiating from the developmental grooves. Occasionally, a groove crosses one or both of the marginal ridges. On a tooth of this type, the point angles are distinct. Developmental grooves are often deep.

Specimen *8* (Fig. 10–20) is representative. Variations of this development may be seen in specimens *4, 5, 6,* and *9*.

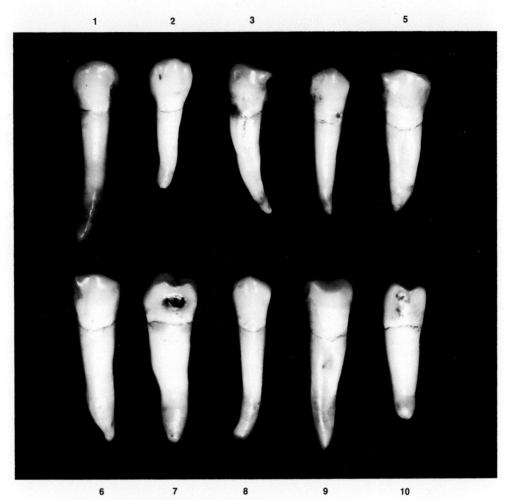

Figure 10–21. Mandibular second premolar.
Ten specimens with uncommon variations are shown.
1, Root extremely long.
2, Root dwarfed.
3, Malformed root; developmental groove on buccal surface.
4, Contact areas on crown high and constricted.
5, Crown oversize; developmental groove buccally on root.
6, Root oversize.
7, Root malformed and of extra length.
8, Root very long with blunt apex; extreme curvature at apical third.
9, Crown and root oversize; developmental groove buccally on root.
10, Crown narrow buccolingually; very little curvature buccally and lingually.

The round, or two-cusp type (specimen *3*) differs considerably from the three-cusp type when viewed from the occlusal aspect. Specimen *3* is a true typal form of the two-cusp type. Variations may be seen in specimens *1, 2, 7,* and *10.*

The *occlusal* characteristics of the two-cusp type are as follows:

1. The outline of the crown is rounded lingual to the buccal cusp ridges.
2. There is some lingual convergence of mesial and distal sides, although no more than is found in some variations of the square type.

3. The mesiolingual and distolingual line angles are rounded.
4. There is one well-developed lingual cusp directly opposite the buccal cusp in a lingual direction.

A *central developmental groove* on the occlusal surface travels in a mesiodistal direction. This groove may be straight (Fig. 10–20, specimen *3*), but it is most often crescent-shaped (specimens *1*, *7*, and *10*). The central groove has its terminals centered in *mesial* and *distal fossae*, which are roughly circular depressions having supplemental grooves and depressions radiating from the central groove and its terminals. The enamel surface inside these fossae and around their peripheries is very irregular, acting as a contrast to the smoothness of cusp ridges, marginal ridges, and the transverse ridge from buccal cusp to lingual cusp.

Some of these teeth show *mesial* and *distal developmental pits* centered in the mesial and distal fossae instead of an unbroken central groove (Fig. 10–20, specimen *2*).

Although photographs do not demonstrate it very well, most of these two-cusp specimens show a developmental depression crossing the distolingual cusp ridge.

References

Kraus, B. S., and Furr, M. L. (1953). Lower first premolar: A definition of discrete morphologic traits. J. Dent. Res. 32:5554.

Ludwig, F. J. (1957). The mandibular second premolars: Morphologic variation and inheritance. J. Dent. Res. 36:263.

11 ≡ *The Permanent Maxillary Molars*

The maxillary molars differ in design from any of the teeth previously described. These teeth assist the mandibular molars in performing the major portion of the work in the mastication and comminution of food. They are the largest and strongest maxillary teeth, by virtue both of their bulk and of their anchorage in the jaws. Although the crowns on the molars may be somewhat shorter than the premolars, their dimensions are greater in every respect. The root portion may be no longer than that of the premolars, but instead of one root or a root bifurcated, the maxillary molar root is broader at the base in all directions and is trifurcated into three well-developed prongs that are actually three full-sized roots emanating from a common broad base above the crown.

Generally speaking, the maxillary molars have large crowns with four well-formed cusps. They have three roots, two buccal and one lingual. The lingual root is the largest. The crowns have two buccal cusps and two lingual cusps. The outlines and curvatures of all the maxillary molars are similar. Developmental variations will be set forth under descriptions of the separate molars.

Before a detailed description of the maxillary first molar is begun, some statements will be made that are applicable to all first molars, mandibular as well as maxillary.

The permanent first molars usually appear in the oral cavity when the child is 6 years old. The mandibular molars precede the maxillary molars. The first permanent molar (maxillary or mandibular) erupts posterior to the second deciduous molar, taking up a position in contact with it. Therefore, the first molar is not a succedaneous tooth, since it has no predecessor. The deciduous teeth are all still in position and functioning when the first molar takes its place. Because the development of the bones of the face is downward and forward, sufficient space has been created normally at the age of 6 for the accommodation of this tooth.

The normal location of the first permanent molar is at the center of the fully developed adult jaw anteroposteriorly. As a consequence of the significance of their positions and the circumstances surrounding their eruption, the first molars are considered the "cornerstones" of the dental arches. A full realization of the significance of these teeth as units in the arches—their function and their positions relative to the other teeth—will be thoroughly understood when there has been an opportunity to study the arrangement of the teeth with their occlusion and the temporomandibular articulation of the jaws. Subsequent chapters cover those phases. The mandibular first molars will be described in Chapter 12.

Maxillary First Molar

The crown of this tooth is wider buccolingually than mesiodistally. Usually the extra dimension buccolingually is about 1 mm (Table 11–1). This, however, varies in individuals (see Fig. 11–17, specimens *1, 5, 7,* and *9*). From the occlusal aspect, the inequality of the measurements in the two directions appears slight. Although the crown is relatively short, it is broad both mesiodistally and buccolingually, which gives the occlusal surface its generous dimensions.

The maxillary first molar is normally the largest tooth in the maxillary arch. It has four well-developed functioning cusps and one supplemental cusp of little practical use. The four large cusps of most physiologic significance are the mesiobuccal, the distobuccal, the mesiolingual, and the distolingual. A supplemental cusp is called the *cusp* or *tubercle of Carabelli*. This morphological trait can take the form of a well-developed fifth cusp, or it can grade down to a series of grooves, depressions, or pits on the mesial portion of the lingual surface. This trait has been used to distinguish populations.

This cusp is found lingual to the mesiolingual cusp, which is the largest of the well-developed cusps. Usually, a developmental groove is found, leaving a record of cusp development unless it has been erased by frictional wear. The fifth cusp or a developmental trace at its usual site serves to identify the maxillary first molar. A specimen of this tooth showing no trace of its typical characteristic would be rare.

There are three *roots* of generous proportions: the mesiobuccal, distobuccal, and lingual. These roots are well separated and well developed, and their placement gives this tooth maximum anchorage against forces that would tend to unseat it. The roots have their greatest spread parallel to the line of greatest force brought to bear against the crown— diagonally in a buccolingual direction. The lingual root is the longest root. It is tapered and smoothly rounded. The mesiobuccal root is not as long, but it is broader buccolingually and shaped (in cross section) so that its resistance to torsion is greater than that of the lingual root. The distobuccal root is the smallest of the three and smoothly rounded.

The development of maxillary first molars rarely deviates from the accepted normal.

Detailed Description of the Maxillary First Molar from All Aspects

Figures 11–1 through 11–18 present the maxillary first molar in various aspects.

Buccal Aspect (Figs. 11–4, 11–13, 11–14, and 11–15)

The crown is roughly trapezoidal, with cervical and occlusal outlines representing the uneven sides. The cervical line is the shorter of the uneven sides (Fig. 4–23, *d*).

When looking at the buccal aspect of this tooth with the line of vision at right angles to the buccal developmental groove of the crown, we see the distal side of the crown in perspective. This is caused by the obtuse character of the distobuccal line angle (see "Occlusal Aspect"). Parts of four cusps are seen, the mesiobuccal, distobuccal, mesio-lingual, and distolingual.

The mesiobuccal cusp is broader than the distobuccal cusp, and its mesial slope meets its distal slope at an obtuse angle. The mesial slope of the distobuccal cusp meets its distal slope at approximately a right angle. The distobuccal cusp is therefore sharper than the mesiobuccal cusp, and it is at least as long and often longer (Fig. 11–15, specimens *4, 6, 7, 8,* and *9*).

The buccal developmental groove that divides the two buccal cusps is approximately equidistant between the mesiobuccal and distolingual line angles. The groove slants

Table 11-1. Maxillary First Molar

First evidence of calcification   At birth
Enamel completed   3 to 4 years
Eruption   6 years
Root completed   9 to 10 years

Measurement Table

	Cervico-occlusal Length of Crown	Length of Root	Mesiodistal Diameter of Crown	Mesiodistal Diameter of Crown at Cervix	Labio- or Bucco-lingual Diameter of Crown	Labio- or Bucco-lingual Diameter at Cervix	Curvature of Cervical Line— Mesial	Curvature of Cervical Line— Distal
Dimensions suggested for carving technique	7. 5*	b l 12 13	10.0	8.0	11.0	10.0	1.0	0.0

* In millimeters.

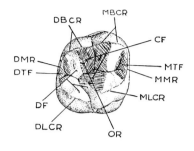

Figure 11–1. Maxillary right first molar, occlusal aspect. *MBCR*, Mesiobuccal cusp ridge; *CF*, central fossa (shaded area); *MTF*, mesial triangular fossa (shaded area); *MMR*, mesial marginal ridge; *MLCR*, mesiolingual cusp ridge; *DF*, distal fossa; *DTF*, distal triangular fossa (shaded area); *DMR*, distal marginal ridge; *DBCR*, distobuccal cusp ridge; *DLCR*, distolingual cusp ridge; *OR*, oblique ridge.

Figure 11–2. Maxillary right first molar, occlusal aspect, developmental grooves. *BG*, Buccal groove; *BGCF*, buccal groove of central fossa; *CGCF*, central groove of central fossa; *FCG*, fifth cusp groove; *LG*, lingual groove; *DOG*, distal oblique groove; *TGOR*, transverse groove of oblique ridge; *CP*, central pit.

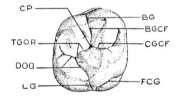

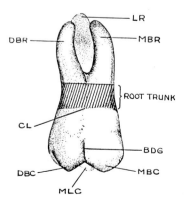

Figure 11–3. Maxillary right first molar, buccal aspect. *DBR*, Distobuccal root; *LR*, lingual root; *MBR*, mesiobuccal root; *CL*, cervical line; *DBC*, distobuccal cusp; *MLC*, mesiolingual cusp; *BDG*, buccal developmental groove; *MBC*, mesiobuccal cusp.

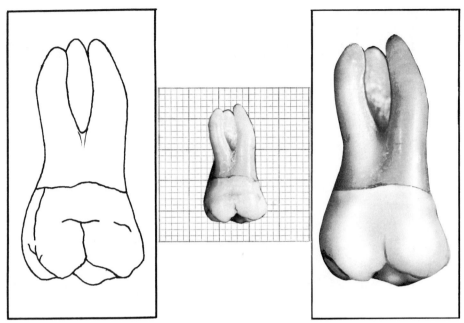

Figure 11–4. Maxillary right first molar, buccal aspect.

occluso-apically in a line of direction parallel to the long axis of the distobuccal root. It terminates at a point approximately half the distance from its origin occlusally to the cervical line of the crown. Although the groove is not deep at any point, it becomes more shallow toward its termination, gradually fading out. Lateral to its terminus, there is a dip in the enamel of the crown that is developmental in character and that extends for some distance mesially and distally.

The cervical line of the crown does not have much curvature from mesial to distal; however, it is not as smooth and regular as that found on some of the other teeth. The line is generally convex with the convexity toward the roots.

The mesial outline of the crown from this aspect follows a nearly straight path downward and mesially, curving occlusally as it reaches the crest of contour of the mesial surface, which is the contact area. This crest is approximately two-thirds the distance from cervical line to tip of mesiobuccal cusp. The mesial outline continues downward and

Figure 11–5. Maxillary right first molar, lingual aspect. *MBR*, Mesiobuccal root; *DBR*, distobuccal root; *CL*, cervical line; *FC*, fifth cusp; *MLC*, mesiolingual cusp; *LDG*, lingual developmental groove; *DLC*, distolingual cusp; *LR*, lingual root.

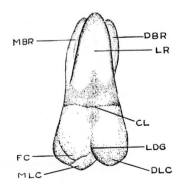

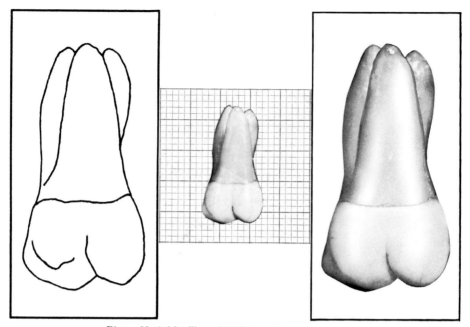

Figure 11-6. Maxillary right first molar, lingual aspect.

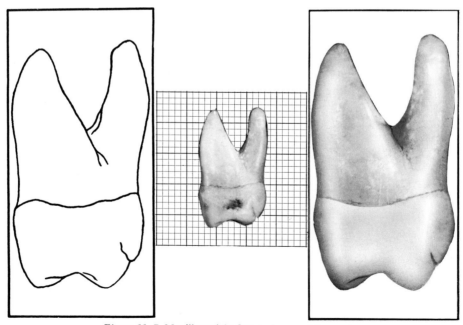

Figure 11-7. Maxillary right first molar, mesial aspect.

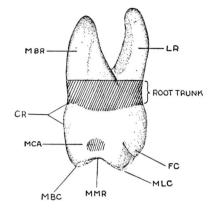

Figure 11-8. Maxillary right first molar, mesial aspect. *LR*, Lingual root; *FC*, fifth cusp; *MLC*, mesiolingual cusp; *MMR*, mesial marginal ridge; *MBC*, mesiobuccal ridge; *MCA*, mesial contact area; *CR*, cervical ridge; *MBR*, mesiobuccal root.

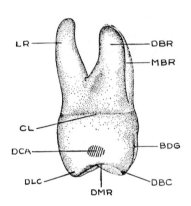

Figure 11-9. Maxillary right first molar, distal aspect. *DBR*, Distobuccal root; *MBR*, mesiobuccal root; *BDG*, buccal developmental groove; *DBC*, distobuccal cusp; *DCA*, distal contact area; *CL*, cervical line; *LR*, lingual root; *DLC*, distolingual cusp; *DMR*, distal marginal ridge.

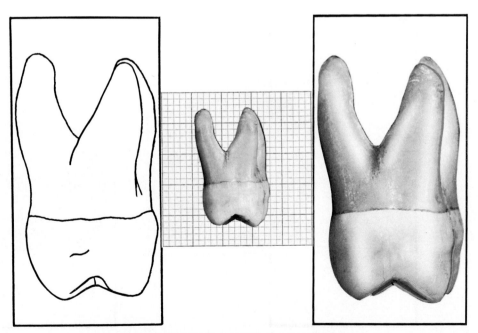

Figure 11-10. Maxillary right first molar, distal aspect.

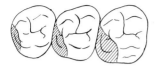

Figure 11–11. Maxillary molar primary cusp triangle. The distolingual lobe, represented by shaded areas, becomes progressively smaller on maxillary molars, starting with the first molar, which presents the greatest development of the lobe. The plain areas, roughly triangular in outline, represent the "maxillary molar primary cusp triangles."

distally and becomes congruent with the outline of the mesial slope of the mesiobuccal cusp.

The distal outline of the crown is convex; the distal surface is spheroidal. The crest of curvature on the distal side of the crown is located at a level approximately half the distance from cervical line to tip of cusp. The distal contact area is in the middle of the middle third.

Often from this aspect, a flattened area or a concave area is seen on the distal surface immediately above the distobuccal cusp at the cervical third of the crown.

All three of the roots may be seen from the buccal aspect. The axes of the roots are inclined distally. The roots are not straight, however, the buccal roots showing an inclination to curvature halfway between the point of bifurcation and the apices. The mesiobuccal root curves distally, starting at the middle third. Its axis usually is at right angles to the cervical line. The distal root is straighter, with its long axis at an acute angle distally with the cervical line. It has a tendency toward curvature mesially at its middle third.

The point of bifurcation of the two buccal roots is located approximately 4 mm above the cervical line. This measurement varies somewhat, of course. Nevertheless, the point is much farther removed from the cervical line than in the deciduous molars. This relation is typical when all permanent molars are compared with all deciduous molars.

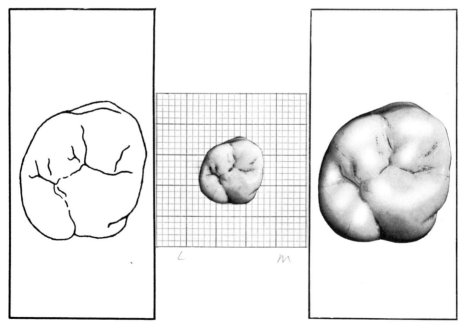

Figure 11–12. Maxillary right first molar, occlusal aspect.

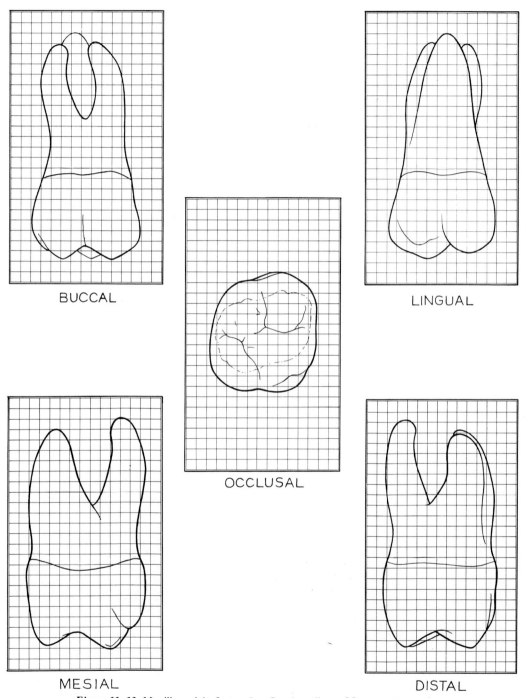

BUCCAL

LINGUAL

OCCLUSAL

MESIAL

DISTAL

Figure 11–13. Maxillary right first molar. Graph outlines of five aspects are shown.

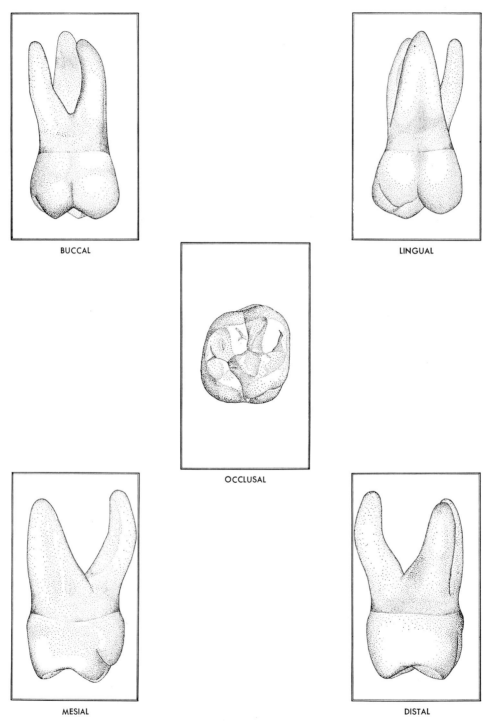

BUCCAL

LINGUAL

OCCLUSAL

MESIAL

DISTAL

Figure 11–14. Maxillary right first molar.

1   3   4   5

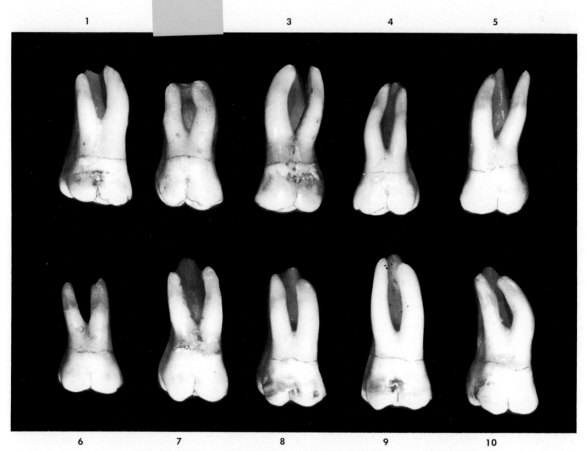

6   7   8   9   10

Figure 11–15. Maxillary first molars, buccal aspect. Ten typical specimens are shown.

There is a deep developmental groove buccally on the root trunk of the maxillary first molar, which starts at the bifurcation and progresses downward, becoming more shallow until it terminates in a shallow depression at the cervical line. Sometimes this depression extends slightly onto the enamel at the cervix.

The reader must keep in mind the fact that molar roots originate as a single root on the base of the crown. They then are divided into three roots, as in the maxillary molars, or into two roots, as in the mandibular molars. The common root base is called the *root trunk* (Figs. 11–3 and 11–8).

In judging the length of the roots and the direction of their axes, we must indicate the part of the root trunk that is congruent with each root as part of it, since it functions as an entity. Usually the lingual root is the longest and the two buccal roots are approximately equal in length. There is considerable variance in this, although the difference is a matter of a millimeter or so only in the average first molars with normal development.

From the buccal aspect, a measurement of the roots inclusively at their greatest extremities mesiodistally is less than a calibration of the diameter of the crown mesiodistally.

There is no invariable rule covering the relative length of crown and root when describing the upper first molar. On the average, the roots are about twice as long as the crown.

1   2   3   4   5

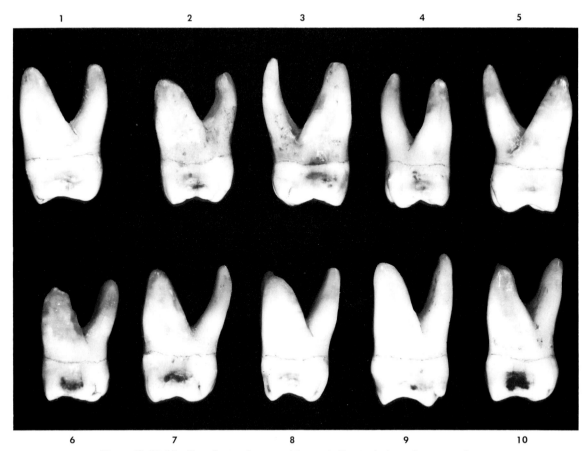

6   7   8   9   10

Figure 11–16. Maxillary first molars, mesial aspect. Ten typical specimens are shown.

Lingual Aspect (Figs. 11–5, 11–6, 11–13, and 11–14)

From the lingual aspect, the gross outline of the maxillary first molar is the reverse of that from the buccal aspect. Photographs or drawings show this only approximately because all teeth have breadth and thickness; consequently, perspective of two dimensions plus the human element (which enters into the technique of posing specimens and the making of drawings and photographs) are bound to result in some error in graphic interpretation.

The variation between the outline of the mesial surface and that of the distal surface is apparent. Because of the roundness of the distolingual cusp, the smooth curvature of the distal outline of the crown becoming confluent with the curvature of the cusp creates an arc that is almost a semicircle. The line that describes the lingual developmental groove is also confluent with the outline of the distolingual cusp, progressing mesially and cervically and ending at a point at the approximate center of the lingual surface of the crown. A shallow depression in the surface extends from the terminus of the lingual groove to the center of the lingual surface of the lingual root at the cervical line and then continues in an apical direction on the lingual root, fading out at the middle third of the root.

The lingual cusps are the only ones to be seen from the lingual aspect. The mesiolingual cusp is much the larger, and before occlusal wear it is always the longest cusp the tooth possesses. Its mesiodistal width is about three fifths of the mesiodistal crown diameter, the distolingual cusp making up the remaining two fifths. The angle formed by the mesial

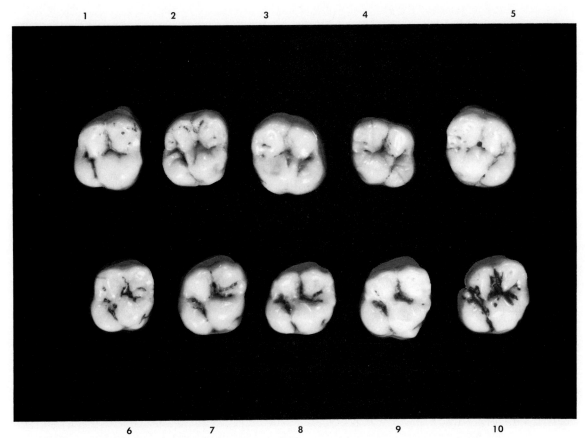

Figure 11–17. Maxillary first molars, occlusal aspect. Ten typical specimens are shown.

outline of the crown and the mesial slope of the mesiolingual cusp is almost 90 degrees. An obtuse angle describes the junction of the mesial and distal slopes of this cusp.

The distolingual cusp is so spheroidal and smooth that it is difficult to describe any angulation on the mesial and distal slopes.

The lingual developmental groove starts approximately in the center of the lingual surface mesiodistally, curves sharply to the distal as it crosses between the cusps, and continues on to the occlusal surface.

The fifth cusp appears attached to the mesiolingual surface of the mesiolingual cusp. It is outlined occlusally by an irregular developmental groove, which may be described as starting in a depression of the mesiolingual line angle of the crown, extending occlusally toward the point of the mesiolingual cusp, then making an obtuse angle turn toward the terminus of the lingual groove and fading out near the lingual groove terminus. If the fifth cusp is well developed, its cusp angle will be sharper and less obtuse than that of the mesiolingual cusp. The cusp ridge of the fifth cusp is approximately 2 mm cervical to the cusp ridge of the mesiolingual cusp (Fig. 11–5).

All three of the roots are visible from the lingual aspect, the large lingual root making up most of the foreground. The lingual portion of the root trunk is continuous with the entire cervical portion of the crown lingually. The lingual root is conical, terminating in a bluntly rounded apex.

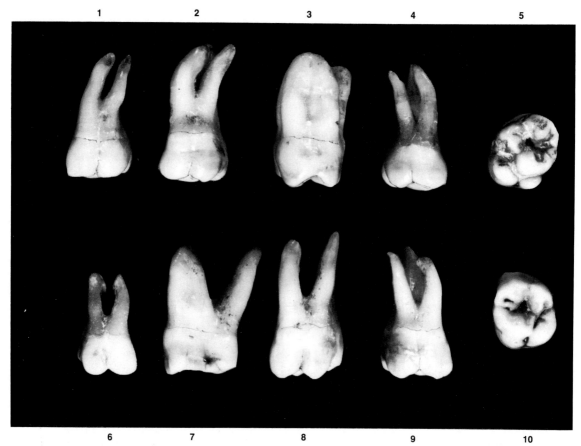

Figure 11–18. Maxillary first molars.
Ten specimens with uncommon variations are shown.
 1, Unusual curvature of buccal roots.
 2, Roots abnormally long with extreme curvature.
 3, Lingual and distobuccal roots fused.
 4, Mesiodistal measurement of root trunk smaller than usual.
 5, Extreme rhomboidal development of crown; fifth cusp with maximum development.
 6, Tooth well developed but much smaller than usual.
 7, Extreme buccolingual measurement.
 8, Extreme length, especially of the distobuccal root; buccal cusps narrow mesiodistally.
 9, Well-developed crown; roots poorly developed.
 10, Extreme development of lingual portion of the crown when compared with the buccal development.

All of the mesial outline of the mesiobuccal root may be seen from this angle and part of its apex.

The distal outline of the distobuccal root is seen above its middle third, including all of its apical outline.

Mesial Aspect (Figs. 11–7, 11–8, 11–13, and 11–14)

From this aspect, the increased buccolingual dimensions may be observed as well as the cervical curvatures of the crown outlines at the cervical third buccally and lingually, and the difference in dimensions between the crown at its greatest measurement and the distance between the cusp tips in a buccolingual direction.

Starting at the cervical line buccally, the outline of the crown makes a short arc buccally to its crest of curvature within the cervical third of the crown. The extent of this curvature is about 0.5 mm (Fig. 11–13). The line of the buccal surface then describes a shallow concavity immediately occlusal to the crest of curvature (see "Buccal Aspect"). The outline then becomes slightly convex as it progresses downward and inward to circumscribe the mesiobuccal cusp, ending at the tip of the cusp well within projected outlines of the root base.

If the tooth is posed so that the line of vision is at right angles to the mesial contact area, the only cusps in sight are the mesiobuccal, the mesiolingual, and the fifth cusps. The distobuccal root is hidden by the mesiobuccal root.

The lingual outline of the crown curves outward and lingually approximately to the same extent as on the buccal side. The level of the crest of curvature is near the middle third of the crown rather than a point within the cervical third, as it is buccally.

If the fifth cusp is well developed, the lingual outline dips inward to illustrate it. If it is undeveloped, the lingual outline continues from the crest of curvature as a smoothly curved arc to the tip of the mesiolingual cusp. The point of the cusp is more clearly centered within projected outlines of the root base than the tip of the mesiobuccal cusp. The mesiolingual cusp is on a line with the long axis of the lingual root.

The mesial marginal ridge, which is confluent with the mesiobuccal and mesiolingual cusp ridges, is irregular, the outline curving cervically about one fifth the crown length and centering its curvature below the center of the crown buccolingually.

The cervical line of the crown is irregular, curving occlusally, but as a rule not more than 1 mm at any one point. If there is definite curvature, it reaches its maximum immediately above the contact area.

The mesial contact area is above the marginal ridge but closer to it than to the cervical line, approximately at the junction of the middle and occlusal thirds of the crown (see Fig. 11–8). It is also somewhat buccal to the center of the crown buccolingually. A shallow concavity is usually found just above the contact area on the mesial surface of the maxillary first molar. This concavity may be continued to the mesial surface of the root trunk at its cervical third.

The mesiobuccal root is broad and flattened on its mesial surface; this flattened surface often exhibits smooth flutings for part of its length. The width of this root near the crown from the buccal surface to the point of bifurcation on the root trunk is approximately two thirds of the crown measurement buccolingually at the cervical line. The buccal outline of the root extends upward and outward from the crown, ending at the blunt apex. The greatest projection on this root is usually buccal to the greatest projection of the crown. The lingual outline of the root is relatively straight from the bluntly rounded apex down to the bifurcation with the lingual root.

The level of the bifurcation is a little closer to the cervical line than is found between the roots buccally. A smooth depression congruent with the bifurcation extends occlusally and lingually almost to the cervical line directly above the mesiolingual line angle of the crown.

The lingual root is longer than the mesial root but is narrower from this aspect. It is banana-shaped, extending lingually with its convex outline to the lingual and its concave outline to the buccal. At its middle and apical thirds, it is outside of the confines of the greatest crown projection. Although its apex is rounded, the root appears more pointed toward the end than the mesiobuccal root.

Distal Aspect (Figs. 11–10, 11–13, and 11–14)

The gross outline of this aspect is similar to that of the mesial aspect. Certain variations must be noted when the tooth is viewed from the distal aspect.

Because of the tendency of the crown to taper distally on the buccal surface, most of the buccal surface of the crown may be seen in perspective from the distal aspect. This is because the buccolingual measurement of the crown mesially is greater than the same measurement distally. All of the decrease in measurement distally is due to the slant of the buccal side of the crown.

The distal marginal ridge dips sharply in a cervical direction, exposing triangular ridges on the distal portion of the occlusal surface of the crown.

The cervical line is almost straight across from buccal to lingual. Occasionally it curves apically 0.5 mm or so.

The distal surface of the crown is generally convex, with a smoothly rounded surface except for a small area near the distobuccal root at the cervical third. This concavity continues on to the distal surface of the distobuccal root, from the cervical line to the area of the root that is on a level with bifurcation separating the distobuccal and lingual roots.

The distobuccal root is narrower at its base than either of the others. An outline of this root, when we view the tooth from the distal aspect, starts buccally at a point immediately above the distobuccal cusp, follows a concave path inward for a short distance, then outward in a buccal direction, completing a graceful convex arc from the concavity to the rounded apex. This line lies entirely within the confines of the outline of the mesiobuccal root. The lingual outline of the root from the apex to the bifurcation is slightly concave. There is no concavity between the bifurcation of the roots and the cervical line. If anything, the surface at this point on the root trunk has a tendency toward convexity.

The bifurcation here is more apical than either of the other two areas on this tooth. The area from cervical line to bifurcation is 5 mm or more in extent.

Occlusal Aspect (Figs. 11–1, 11–2, 11–12, 11–13, 11–14, and 11–17)

From the occlusal aspect, the maxillary first molar is somewhat rhomboidal. An outline following the four major cusp ridges and the marginal ridges is especially so.

A measurement of the crown buccolingually and mesial to the buccal and lingual grooves will be greater than the measurement on that portion of the crown which is distal to these developmental grooves. Also, a measurement of the crown immediately lingual to contact areas mesiodistally is greater than the measurement immediately buccal to the contact areas. Thus it is apparent that the maxillary first molar crown is wider mesially than distally and wider lingually than buccally.

The four major cusps are well developed, with the small minor, or fifth, cusp appearing on the lingual surface of the mesiolingual cusp near the mesiolingual line angle of the crown. The fifth cusp may be indistinct, or all the cusp form may be absent. At this site, however, there will nearly always be traces of developmental lines in the enamel.

The mesiolingual cusp is the largest cusp; it is followed in point of size by the mesiobuccal, distolingual, distobuccal, and fifth cusps.

If reduced to a geometric schematic figure, the occlusal aspect of this molar locates the various angles of the rhomboidal figure as follows: acute angles, mesiobuccal and distolingual; and obtuse angles, mesiolingual and distobuccal.

An analysis of the design of occlusal surfaces of maxillary molars may be summarized as follows: Developmentally, there are only three major cusps to be analyzed as primary, with the mesiolingual cusp (the most primitive), and the two buccal cusps. The distolingual cusp development common to all of the maxillary molars, and any other additional one, such as the cusp of Carabelli on first molars, must be regarded as secondary.

The *maxillary molar primary cusp triangle* supposition follows the Cope-Osborn hypothesis of tooth origins. There was a tritubercular stage in human tooth development when the molar forms with only three cusps explained the background for the triangular arrangement just described.

This primary design is also reflected in the outline of the root trunks of maxillary molars when the teeth are sectioned in those areas (see "Root Sections," Chapter 13).

Another observation that bears out this theory is that the distolingual cusp becomes progressively smaller on second and third maxillary molars, often disappearing as a major cusp (Fig. 11–11).

To repeat, the triangular arrangement of the three important molar cusps is called the maxillary molar primary cusp triangle. The characteristic triangular figure, made by tracing the cusp outlines of these cusps, the mesial marginal ridge, and the oblique ridge of the occlusal surface, is representative of all maxillary molars.

The *occlusal surface* of the maxillary first molar is within the confines of the cusp ridges and marginal ridges. It may be described as follows:

There are two major fossae and two minor fossae. The major fossae are the *central fossa,* which is roughly triangular and mesial to the oblique ridge, and the *distal fossa,* which is roughly linear and distal to the oblique ridge. The two minor fossae are the *mesial triangular fossa,* immediately distal to the mesial marginal ridge, and the *distal triangular fossa,* immediately mesial to the distal marginal ridge (Fig. 11–1).

The *oblique ridge* is a ridge that crosses the occlusal surface obliquely. It is formed by the union of the triangular ridge of the distobuccal cusp and the distal ridge of the mesio-lingual cusp. This ridge is reduced in height in the center of the occlusal surface, being about on a level with the marginal ridges of the occlusal surface. Sometimes it is crossed by a developmental groove that partially joins the two major fossae by means of its shallow sulcate groove.

The *mesial marginal ridge* and the *distal marginal ridge* are irregular ridges confluent with the mesial and distal cusp ridges of the mesial and distal major cusps.

The *central fossa* of the occlusal surface is a concave area bounded by the distal slope of the mesiobuccal cusp, the mesial slope of the distobuccal cusp, the crest of the oblique ridge, and the crests of the two triangular ridges of the mesiobuccal and mesiolingual cusps. The central fossa has connecting sulci within its boundaries, with developmental grooves at the deepest portions of these sulci (sulcate grooves). In addition, it contains supplemental grooves, short grooves that are disconnected, and also the central developmental pit. A worn specimen may show developmental or sulcate grooves only.

In the center of the central fossa, the central developmental pit has sulcate developmental grooves, radiating from it at obtuse angles to each other. This pit is located in the approximate center of that portion of the occlusal surface which is circumscribed by cusp ridges and marginal ridges (Fig. 11–1). From this pit the *buccal developmental groove* radiates buccally at the bottom of the buccal sulcus of the central fossa, continuing on to the buccal surface of the crown between the buccal cusps.

Starting again at the central pit, the *central developmental groove* is seen to progress in a mesial direction at an obtuse angle to the buccal sulcate groove. The central groove at the bottom of the sulcus of the central fossa usually terminates at the apex of the *mesial triangular fossa.* Here it is joined by short supplemental grooves that radiate from its terminus into the triangular fossa. These supplemental grooves often appear as branches of the central groove. Occasionally one or more supplemental grooves cross the mesial marginal ridge of the crown.

The *mesial triangular fossa* is rather indistinct in outline, but it is generally triangular in shape with its base at the mesial marginal ridge and its apex at the point where the supplemental grooves join the central groove.

An additional short developmental groove radiates from the central pit of the central fossa at an obtuse angulation to the buccal and central developmental grooves. Usually it is considered a projection of one of these, since it is very short and usually fades out before reaching the crest of the oblique ridge. When it crosses the oblique ridge transversely, however, as it sometimes does, joining the central and distal fossae with a shallow groove, it is called the *transverse groove of the oblique ridge* (Fig. 11–17, specimens *3, 4,* and *5*).

The *distal fossa* of the maxillary first molar is roughly linear in form and is located immediately distal to the oblique ridge. An irregular developmental groove traverses its deepest portion. This developmental groove is called the *distal oblique groove*. It connects with the *lingual developmental groove* at the junction of the cusp ridges of the mesiolingual and distolingual cusps. These two grooves travel in the same oblique direction to the terminus of the lingual groove, which is centered below the lingual root at the approximate center of the crown lingually (Fig. 11–5, *LDG*). If the fifth cusp development is distinct, a developmental groove outlining it joins the lingual groove near its terminus. Any part of the developmental groove that outlines a fifth cusp is called the *fifth cusp groove*.

The distal oblique groove in most cases shows several supplemental grooves. Two terminal branches usually appear, forming two sides of the triangular depression immediately mesial to the distal marginal ridge. These two sides, in combination with the slope mesial to the distal marginal ridge, form the *distal triangular fossa*. The distal outline of the distal marginal ridge of the crown shows a slight concavity.

The distolingual cusp is smooth and rounded from the occlusal aspect, and an outline of it, from the distal concavity of the distal marginal ridge to the lingual groove of the crown, describes an arch of an ellipse.

The lingual outline of the distolingual cusp is straight with the lingual outline of the fifth cusp, unless the fifth cusp is unusually large. In the latter case the lingual outline of the fifth cusp is more prominent lingually (Fig. 11–7, specimen 9). The cusp ridge of the distolingual cusp usually extends lingually farther than the cusp ridge of the mesiolingual cusp.

Maxillary Second Molar

The maxillary second molar supplements the first molar in function. In describing this tooth, direct comparisons will be made with the first molar both in form and development.

Generally speaking, the roots of this tooth are as long as, if not somewhat longer than, those of the first molar (Table 11–2). The distobuccal cusp is not as large or as well developed, and the distolingual cusp is smaller. No fifth cusp is evident.

The crown of the maxillary second molar is 0.5 mm or so shorter cervico-occlusally than that of the first molar, but the measurement of the crown buccolingually is about the same. Two types of maxillary second molars are found when we are viewing the occlusal aspect: (1) The type that is seen most has an occlusal form which resembles the first molar, although the rhomboidal outline is more extreme. This is accentuated by the lesser measurement lingually. (2) This type bears more resemblance to a typical third molar form. The distolingual cusp is poorly developed and makes the development of the other three cusps predominate. This results in a heart-shaped form from the occlusal aspect that is more typical of the maxillary *third* molar (see Fig. 11–26, specimens *1* and *7*).

Detailed Description of the Maxillary Second Molar from All Aspects

Figures 11–19 through 11–27 present the maxillary second molar in various aspects.

Table 11-2. Maxillary Second Molar

First evidence of calcification   2½ years
Enamel completed   7 to 8 years
Eruption   12 to 13 years
Root completed   14 to 16 years

Measurement Table

	Cervico-occlusal Length of Crown	Length of Root	Mesiodistal Diameter of Crown	Mesiodistal Diameter of Crown at Cervix	Labio- or Bucco-lingual Diameter of Crown	Labio- or Bucco-lingual Diameter at Cervix	Curvature of Cervical Line— Mesial	Curvature of Cervical Line— Distal
Dimensions suggested for carving technique	7.0*	buccal = 11 lingual = 12	9.0	7.0	11.0	10.0	1.0	0.0

* In millimeters.

259

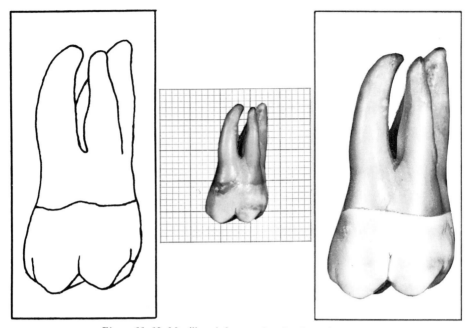

Figure 11–19. Maxillary left second molar, buccal aspect.

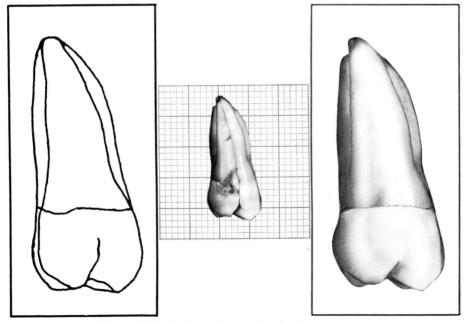

Figure 11–20. Maxillary left second molar, lingual aspect.

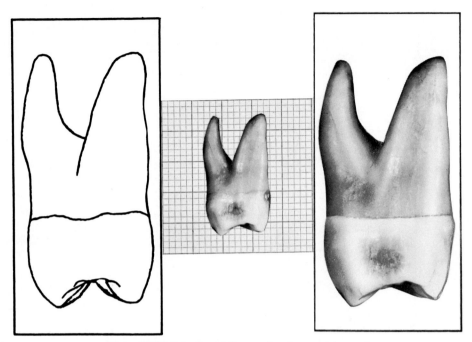

Figure 11–21. Maxillary left second molar, mesial aspect.

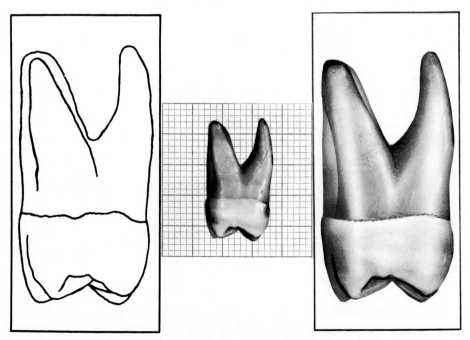

Figure 11–22. Maxillary left second molar, distal aspect.

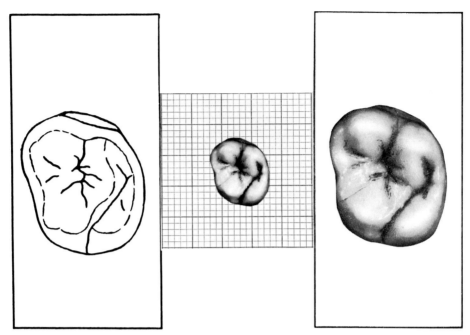

Figure 11–23. Maxillary left second molar, occlusal aspect.

Buccal Aspect (Figs. 11–19 and 11–24)

The crown is a little shorter cervico-occlusally and narrower mesiodistally than the maxillary first molar. The distobuccal cusp is smaller and allows part of the distal marginal ridge and part of the distolingual cusp to be seen.

The buccal roots are about the same length. These roots are more nearly parallel and are inclined distally more than those of the maxillary first molar so that the end of the distobuccal root is slightly distal to the distal extremity of the crown. The apex of the mesiobuccal root is on a line with the buccal groove of the crown instead of the tip of the mesiobuccal cusp, as was found on the first molar.

Lingual Aspect (Fig. 11–20)

Differences between the second and first molars to be noted here in addition to those mentioned before are these:

1. The distolingual cusp of the crown is smaller.
2. The distobuccal cusp may be seen through the sulcus between the mesiolingual and distolingual cusp.
3. No fifth cusp is evident.

The apex of the lingual root is in line with the distolingual cusp tip instead of the lingual groove as was found on the first molar.

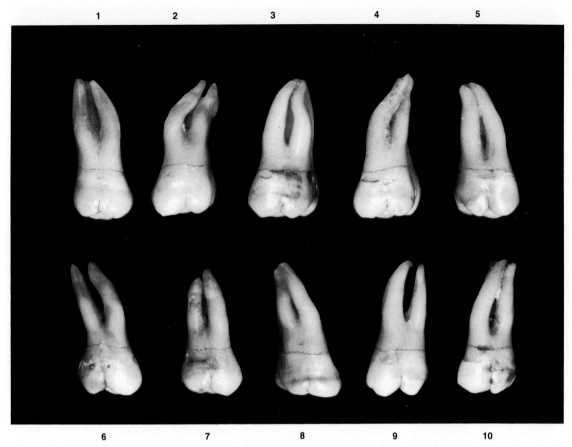

Figure 11–24. Maxillary second molars, buccal aspect. Ten typical specimens are shown.

Mesial Aspect (Figs. 11–21 and 11–25)

The buccolingual dimension is about the same as that of the first molar, but the crown length is less. The roots do not spread as far buccolingually, being within the confines of the buccolingual crown outline.

Distal Aspect (Fig. 11–22)

Because the distobuccal cusp is smaller than in the maxillary first molar, more of the mesiobuccal cusp may be seen from this angle. The mesiolingual cusp cannot be seen. The apex of the lingual root is in line with the distolingual cusp.

Occlusal Aspect (Figs. 11–23 and 11–26)

The rhomboidal type of second maxillary molar is most frequent, although in comparison with the first molar the acute angles of the rhomboid are less and the obtuse angles greater. The buccolingual diameter of the crown is about equal, but the mesiodistal diameter is approximately 1 mm less. The mesiobuccal and mesiolingual cusps are just as large and well developed as in the first molar, but the distobuccal and distolingual cusps are smaller and

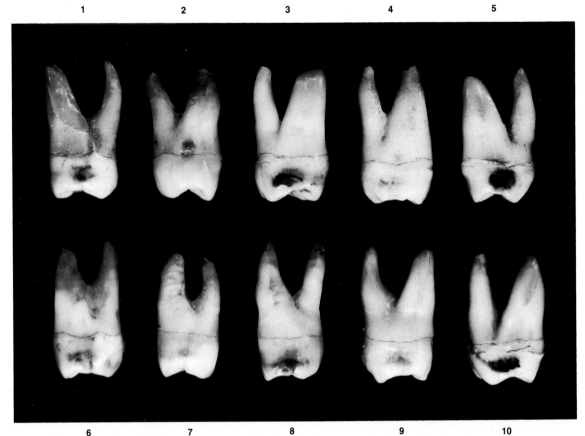

Figure 11–25. Maxillary second molars, mesial aspect. Ten typical specimens are shown.

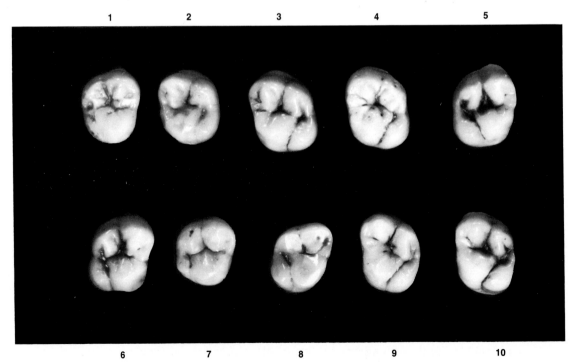

Figure 11–26. Maxillary second molars, occlusal aspect. Ten typical specimens are shown.

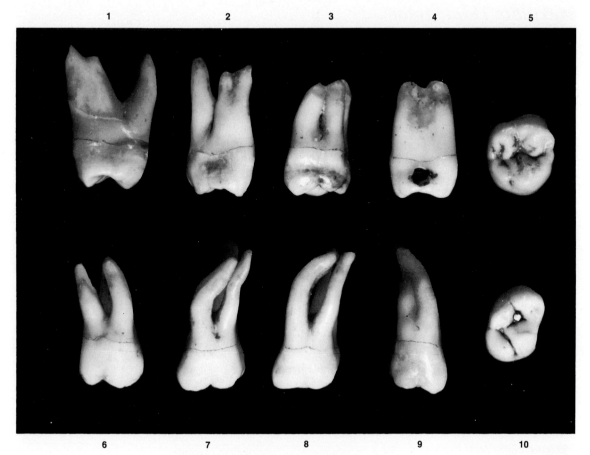

Figure 11–27. Maxillary second molars.
Ten specimens with uncommon variations are shown.
  1, Roots spread similar to first molar.
  2, Bifurcated mesiobuccal root.
  3, Roots very short and fused.
  4, Mesiobuccal and lingual roots with complete fusion.
  5, Crown similar to the typical third molar form.
  6, Short roots with spread similar to first molar.
  7, Roots extra long with abnormal curvatures.
  8, Another variation similar to specimen 7.
  9, Very long roots fused.
  10, Crown with extreme rhomboidal form.

less well developed. Usually, a calibration made of the crown at the greatest diameter buccally and lingually of the distal portion is considerably less than one made at the greatest diameter buccally and lingually of the mesial portion, showing more convergence distally than the maxillary first molar.

It is not uncommon to find more supplemental grooves as well as accidental grooves and pits on the occlusal surface of a maxillary second molar than are usually found on a maxillary first molar.

Maxillary Third Molar

The maxillary third molar often appears as a developmental anomaly. It can vary considerably in size, contour, and relative position to the other teeth (Table 11–3). It is seldom as well developed as the maxillary second molar, to which it often bears resemblance. The third molar supplements the second molar in function, and its fundamental design is similar. The crown is smaller, and the roots are shorter as a rule, with the inclination toward fusion with the resultant anchorage of one tapered root.

The predominating third molar design, when we view the occlusal surface, is that of the heart-shaped type of second molar. The distolingual cusp is very small and poorly developed in most cases, and it may be absent entirely.

All third molars, mandibular and maxillary, show more variation in development than any of the other teeth in the mouth. Occasionally they appear as anomalies bearing little or no resemblance to neighboring teeth. A few of the variations in form are shown in Figure 11–36.

For the purposes at hand, it is necessary to give a short description of the third molar that is considered average in its development and one that would be in good proportion to the other maxillary molars and with an occlusal form considered normal. In describing the normal maxillary third molar, direct comparisons will be made with the maxillary second molar.

Detailed Description of the Maxillary Third Molar from All Aspects

Figures 11–28 through 11–36 present the maxillary third molar in various aspects.

Buccal Aspect (Figs. 11–28 and 11–33)

The crown is shorter cervico-occlusally and narrower mesiodistally than that of the second molar. The roots are usually fused, functioning as one large root, and they are shorter cervicoapically. The fused roots end in a taper at the apex. The roots have a distinct slant to the distal, giving the apices of the fused root a more distal relation to the center of the crown.

Lingual Aspect (Fig. 11–29)

In addition to the differences just mentioned, in comparison with the maxillary second molar, there is usually just one large lingual cusp and therefore no lingual groove. However, in many cases, a third molar with the same essential features has a poorly developed distolingual cusp with a developmental groove lingually (Fig. 11–35, specimen 2).

Mesial Aspect (Figs. 11–30 and 11–34)

Here, aside from the differences in measurement, the main feature is the taper to the fused roots and a bifurcation, usually in the region of the apical third. (Figure 11–30 does not show a bifurcation. See specimens 1, 2, and 3, Fig. 11–34.) The root portion is considerably shorter in relation to the crown length. Both the crown and the root portions are inclined to be poorly developed, with irregular outlines.

Text continued on page 272

Table 11–3. Maxillary Third Molar

First evidence of calcification	7 to 9 years
Enamel completed	12 to 16 years
Eruption	17 to 21 years
Root completed	18 to 25 years

Measurement Table

	Cervico-occlusal Length of Crown	Length of Root	Mesiodistal Diameter of Crown	Mesiodistal Diameter of Crown at Cervix	Labio- or Bucco-lingual Diameter of Crown	Labio- or Bucco-lingual Diameter at Cervix	Curvature of Cervical Line—Mesial	Curvature of Cervical Line—Distal
Dimensions suggested for carving technique	6. 5*	11.0	8.5	6.5	10.0	9.5	1.0	0.0

* In millimeters.

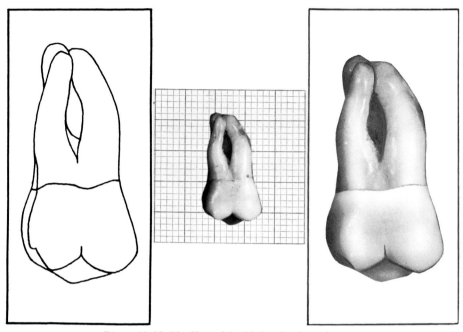

Figure 11–28. Maxillary right third molar, buccal aspect.

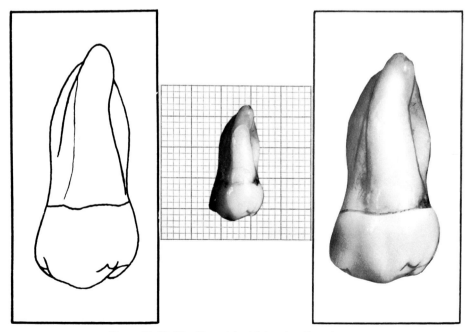

Figure 11–29. Maxillary right third molar, lingual aspect.

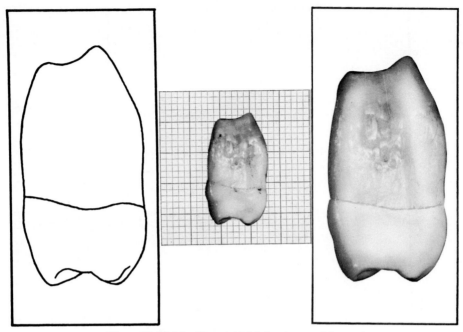

Figure 11–30. Maxillary right third molar, mesial aspect.

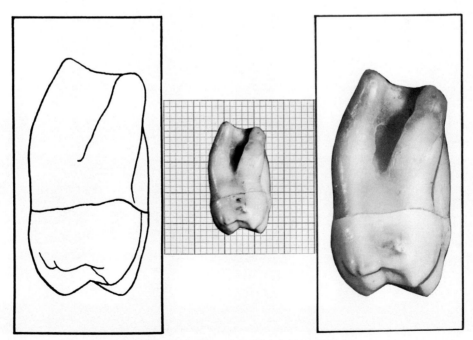

Figure 11–31. Maxillary right third molar, distal aspect.

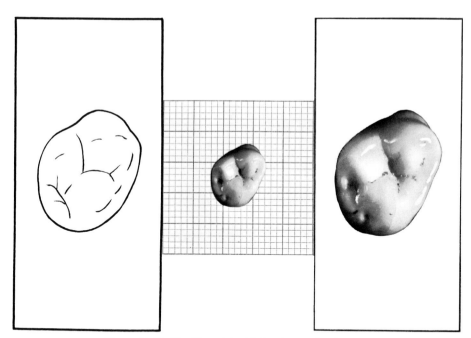

Figure 11–32. Maxillary right third molar, occlusal aspect.

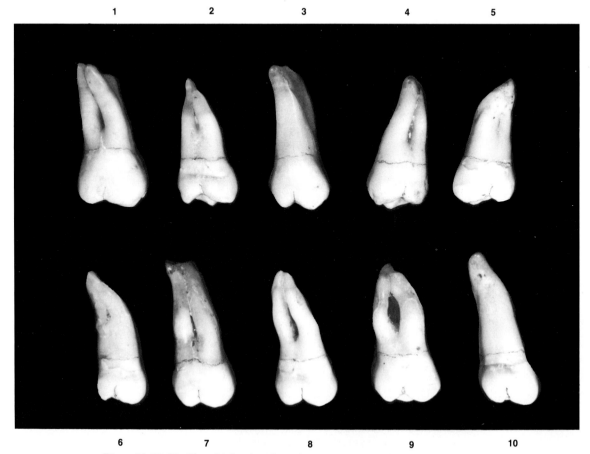

Figure 11–33. Maxillary third molars, buccal aspect. Ten typical specimens are shown.

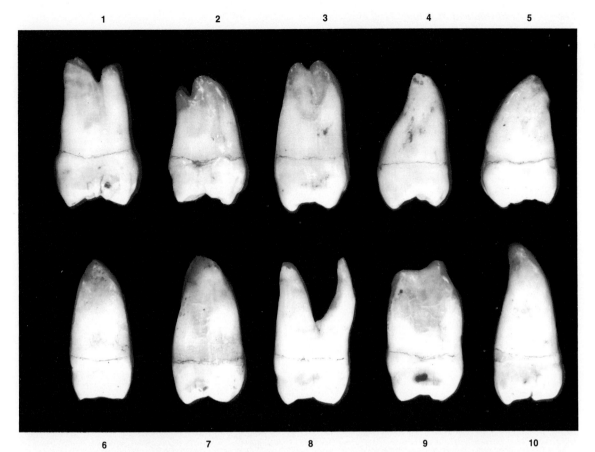

Figure 11–34. Maxillary third molars, mesial aspect. Ten typical specimens are shown.

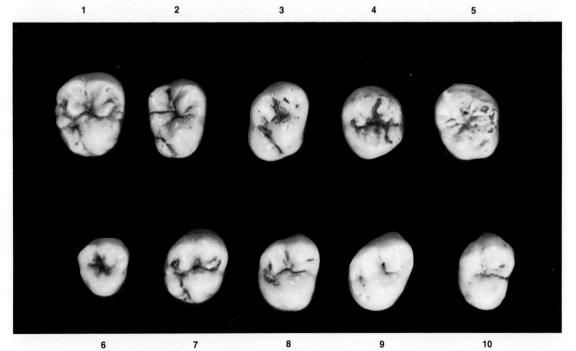

Figure 11–35. Maxillary third molars, occlusal aspect. Ten typical specimens are shown.

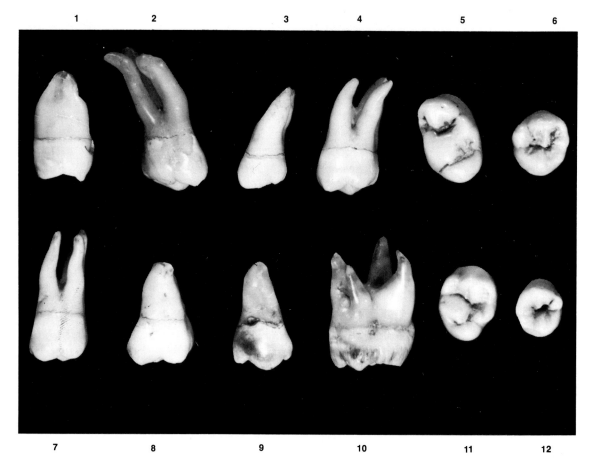

Figure 11-36. Maxillary third molars.
Twelve specimens with uncommon variations are shown.
  1, Very short fused root form.
  2, Extremely long roots with extreme distal angulation.
  3, Complete fusion of roots with extreme distal angulation.
  4, Three roots well separated; crown very wide at cervix.
  5, Extreme rhomboidal outline to crown, with developmental grooves oddly placed.
  6, Overdeveloped mesiobuccal cusp.
  7, Crown wide at cervix, with roots perpendicular.
  8, Very large crown; poorly developed root form.
  9, Complete absence of typical design.
  10, Specimen abnormally large, with four roots well separated.
  11, Five well-developed cusps, atypical in form.
  12, Small specimen, atypical cusp form.

Distal Aspect (Fig. 11–31)

From this aspect, most of the buccal surface of the crown is in view. More of the occlusal surface may be seen than can be seen on the second molar from this aspect because of the more acute angulation of the occlusal surface in relation to the long axis of the root. The measurement from the cervical line to the marginal ridge is short.

Occlusal Aspect (Figs. 11–32 and 11–35)

The occlusal aspect of a typical maxillary third molar presents a heart-shaped outline. The lingual cusp is large and well developed, and there is little or no distolingual cusp—which gives a semicircular outline to the tooth from one contact area to the other. On this type of tooth there are *three* functioning cusps; two buccal and one lingual.

The occlusal aspect of this tooth usually presents many supplemental grooves and many accidental grooves unless the tooth is very much worn.

The third molar may show four distinct cusps. This type may have a strong oblique ridge, a central fossa and a distal fossa, with a lingual developmental groove similar to that of the rhomboidal type of second molar. In most instances, the crown converges more lingually from the buccal areas than the second molar does, losing its rhomboidal outline. This is not, however, always true (compare specimens *1* and *3* in Figure 11–35).

References

Black, G. V. (1897). *Descriptive Anatomy of the Human Teeth*, 4th ed. Philadelphia: S. S. White Dental Manufacturing.

Carabelli, G. (1842). *Anatomie des Mundes*. Vienna: Braumuller and Seidel.

Carbonell, V. M. (1960). The tubercle of Carabelli in the Kish dentition. Mesopotamia, 3000 B.C. J. Dent. Res. 39:124.

Cope, F. D. (1888). On the tritubercular molar in human dentition. J. Morphol. 12:7.

Diamond, M. (1929). *Dental Anatomy*. New York: MacMillan.

Gregory, W. K. (1922). *The Origin and Evolution of the Human Dentition*. Baltimore, Md.: Williams & Wilkins.

Hopewell-Smith, A. (1913). *An Introduction to Dental Anatomy and Physiology*. Philadelphia: Lea & Febiger.

Kraus, B. S. (1951). Carabelli's anomaly of the maxillary molar teeth. Am. J. Hum. Genet. 3:348.

Osborn, H. F. (1907). Evolution of mammalian molar teeth. In Gregory, W. K. (ed.), *Biological Studies and Addresses*, Vol. 1. New York: MacMillan.

Tomes, C. S. (1894). *A Manual of Dental Anatomy*. London: Churchill.

12 *The Permanent Mandibular Molars*

The mandibular molars are larger than any other mandibular teeth. They are three in number on each side of the mandible: the first, second, and third mandibular molars. They resemble each other in functional form, although comparison of one with another shows variations in the number of cusps and some variation in size, occlusal design, and the relative length and positions of the roots.

The crown outlines exhibit similarities of outline from all aspects, and each mandibular molar has two roots, one mesial and one distal. Third molars and some second molars may show a fusion of these roots. All mandibular molars have crowns that are roughly quadrilateral, being somewhat longer mesiodistally than buccolingually. *Maxillary* molar crowns have their widest measurement buccolingually.

The mandibular molars perform the major portion of the work of the lower jaw in mastication and in the comminution of food. They are the largest and strongest mandibular teeth, both because of their bulk and because of their anchorage.

The crowns of the molars are shorter cervico-occlusally than those of the teeth anterior to them, but their dimensions are greater in every other respect. The root portions are not as long as those of some of the other mandibular teeth, but the combined measurements of the multiple roots, with their broad bifurcated root trunks, result in superior anchorage and greater efficiency.

Usually the sum of the mesiodistal measurements of mandibular molars is equal to or greater than the combined mesiodistal measurements of all the teeth anterior to the first molar and up to the median line.

The crowns of these molars are wider mesiodistally than buccolingually. The opposite arrangement is true of maxillary molars.

Mandibular First Molar

Normally, the mandibular first molar is the largest tooth in the mandibular arch. It has five well-developed cusps: two buccal, two lingual, and a distal cusp (Fig. 12–1). It has two well-developed roots, one mesial and one distal, which are very broad buccolingually. These roots are widely separated at the apices.

The dimension of the crown mesiodistally is greater by about 1 mm than the dimension buccolingually (Table 12–1). Although the crown is relatively short cervico-occlusally, it has mesiodistal and buccolingual measurements that provide a broad occlusal form.

Table 12–1. Mandibular First Molar

First evidence of calcification	At birth
Enamel completed	2½ to 3 years
Eruption	6 to 7 years
Root completed	9 to 10 years

Measurement Table

	Cervico-occlusal Length of Crown	Length of Root	Mesiodistal Diameter of Crown	Mesiodistal Diameter of Crown at Cervix	Labio- or Bucco-lingual Diameter of Crown	Labio- or Bucco-lingual Diameter of Crown at Cervix	Curvature of Cervical Line— Mesial	Curvature of Cervical Line— Distal
Dimensions suggested for carving technique	7.5*	14.0	11.0	9.0	10.5	9.0	1.0	0.0

*In millimeters.

275

The mesial root is broad and curved distally, with mesial and distal fluting that provides the anchorage of two roots (see Fig. 13–41). The distal root is rounder, broad at the cervical portion, and pointed in a distal direction. The formation of these roots and their positions in the mandible serve to brace efficiently the crown of the tooth against the lines of force that might be brought to bear against it.

Detailed Description of the Mandibular First Molar from All Aspects

Figures 12–1 through 12–17 present the mandibular first molar in various aspects.

Buccal Aspect (Figs. 12–3, 12–4, 12–12, 12–13, and 12–14)

From the buccal aspect, the crown of the mandibular first molar is roughly trapezoidal, with cervical and occlusal outlines representing the uneven sides of the trapezoid. The occlusal side is the longer.

If this tooth is posed vertically, all five of its cusps are in view. The two buccal cusps and the buccal portion of the distal cusp are in the foreground, with the tips of the lingual cusps in the background. The lingual cusps may be seen because they are higher than the others.

Two developmental grooves appear on the crown portion. These grooves are called the *mesiobuccal developmental groove* and the *distobuccal developmental groove*. The first-named groove acts as a line of demarcation between the mesiobuccal lobe and the distobuccal lobe. The latter groove separates the distobuccal lobe from the distal lobe (Figs. 12–2 and 12–3).

The mesiobuccal, distobuccal, and distal cusps are relatively flat. These cusp ridges show less curvature than those of any of the teeth described so far. The distal cusp, which is small, is more pointed than either of the buccal cusps. Flattened buccal cusps are typical of all mandibular molars. Most first molar specimens have the buccal cusps worn considerably, showing the buccal cusp ridges almost at the same level. Before they are worn, the buccal cusps and the distal cusp have curvatures that are characteristic of each one (Figs. 12–4 and 12–14, specimen *4*).

The mesiobuccal cusp is usually the widest mesiodistally of the three cusps. This cusp has some curvature but is relatively flat. The distobuccal cusp is almost as wide, with a cusp ridge of somewhat greater curvature. The two buccal cusps make up the major portion of the buccal surface of the crown. The distal cusp provides a very small part of the buccal surface, since the major portion of the cusp makes up the distal portion of the crown, providing the distal contact area on the center of the distal surface of the distal cusp. The distal cusp ridge is very round occlusally, being sharper than either of the two buccal cusps.

These three cusps have the mesiobuccal and distobuccal grooves as lines of demar-

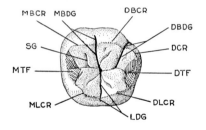

Figure 12–1. Mandibular right first molar, occlusal aspect. *DBCR*, Distobuccal cusp ridge; *DBDG*, distobuccal developmental groove; *DCR*, distal cusp ridge; *DTF*, distal triangular fossa (shaded area); *DLCR*, distolingual cusp ridge; *LDG*, lingual developmental groove; *MLCR*, mesiolingual cusp ridge; *MTF*, mesial triangular fossa (shaded area); *SG*, a supplemental groove; *MBCR*, mesiobuccal cusp ridge; *MBDG*, mesiobuccal developmental groove.

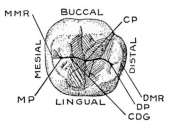

Figure 12–2. Mandibular right first molar, occlusal aspect. Shaded area—central fossa. *CP*, Central pit; *DMR*, distal marginal ridge; *DP*, distal pit; *CDG*, central developmental groove; *MP*, mesial pit; *MMR*, mesial marginal ridge.

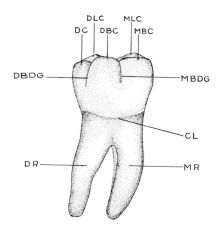

Figure 12–3. Mandibular right first molar, buccal aspect. *MBDG*, Mesiobuccal developmental groove; *CL*, cervical line; *MR*, mesial root; *DR*, distal root; *DBDG*, distobuccal developmental groove; *DC*, distal cusp; *DLC*, distolingual cusp; *DBC*, distobuccal cusp; *MLC*, mesiolingual cusp; *MBC*, mesiobuccal cusp.

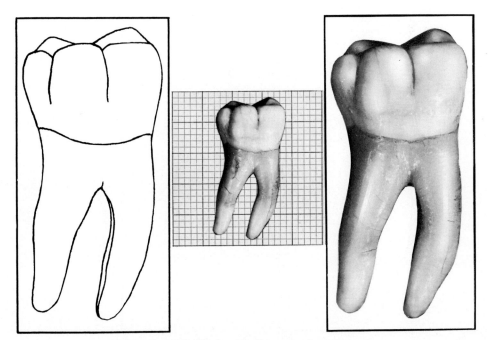

Figure 12–4. Mandibular right first molar, buccal aspect.

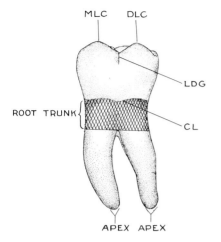

Figure 12–5. Mandibular right first molar, lingual aspect. *MLC,* Mesiolingual cusp; *DLC,* distolingual cusp; *LDG,* lingual developmental groove; *CL,* cervical line.

cation. The mesiobuccal groove is the shorter of the two, having its terminus centrally located cervico-occlusally. This groove is situated a little mesial to the root bifurcation buccally. The distobuccal groove has its terminus near the distobuccal line angle at the cervical third of the crown. It travels occlusally and somewhat mesially, parallel with the axis of the distal root.

The cervical line of the mandibular first molar is commonly regular in outline, dipping apically toward the root bifurcation.

The mesial outline of the crown is somewhat concave at the cervical third up to its junction with the convex outline of the broad contact area. The distal outline of the crown is straight above the cervical line to its junction with the convex outline of the distal contact area, which is also the outline of the distal portion of the distal cusp.

Text continued on page 283

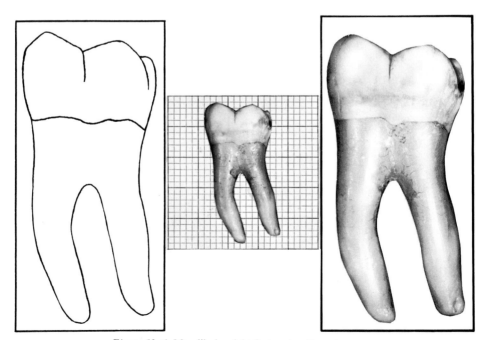

Figure 12–6. Mandibular right first molar, lingual aspect.

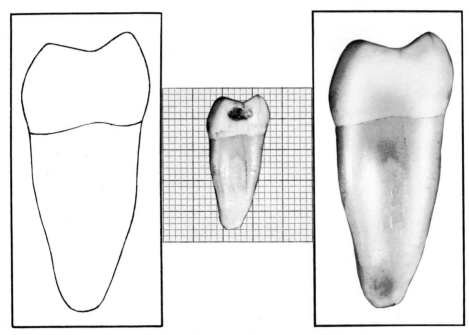

Figure 12–7. Mandibular right first molar, mesial aspect.

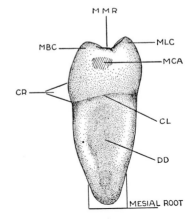

Figure 12–8. Mandibular right first molar, mesial aspect. *MMR,* Mesial marginal ridge; *MLC,* mesiolingual cusp; *MCA,* mesial contact area; *CL,* cervical line; *DD,* developmental depression; *CR,* cervical ridge; *MBC,* mesiobuccal cusp.

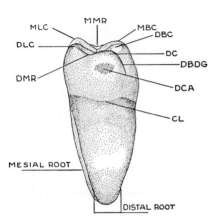

Figure 12–9. Mandibular right first molar, distal aspect. *MMR,* Mesial marginal ridge; *MBC,* mesiobuccal cusp; *DBC,* distobuccal cusp; *DC,* distal cusp; *DBDG,* distobuccal developmental groove; *DCA,* distal contact area; *CL,* cervical line; *DMR,* distal marginal ridge; *DLC,* distolingual cusp; *MLC,* mesiolingual cusp.

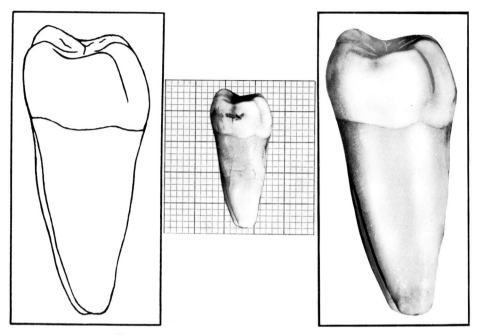

Figure 12–10. Mandibular right first molar, distal aspect.

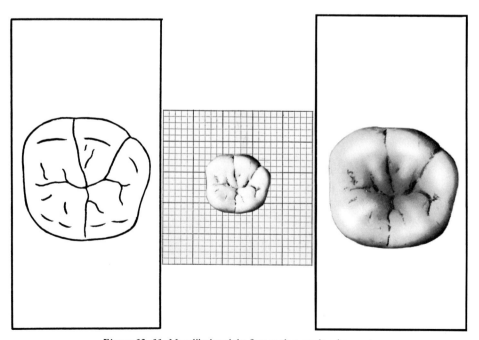

Figure 12–11. Mandibular right first molar, occlusal aspect.

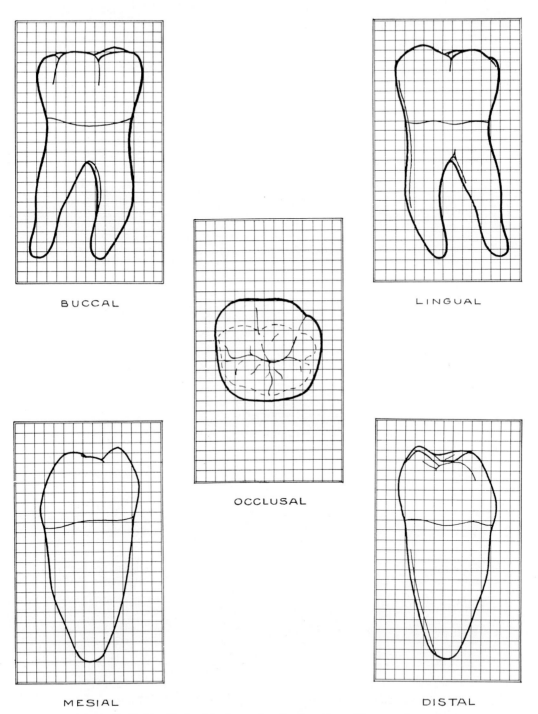

BUCCAL

LINGUAL

OCCLUSAL

MESIAL

DISTAL

Figure 12–12. Mandibular right first molar. Graph outlines of five aspects are shown.

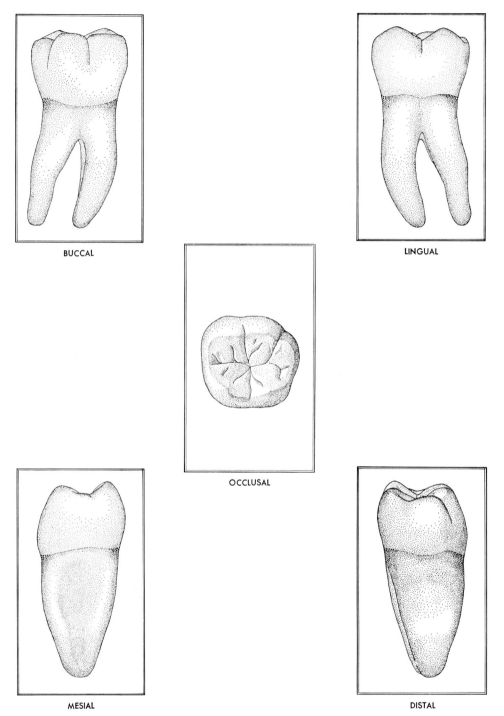

BUCCAL

LINGUAL

OCCLUSAL

MESIAL

DISTAL

Figure 12–13. Mandibular right first molar.

1   2   3   4   5

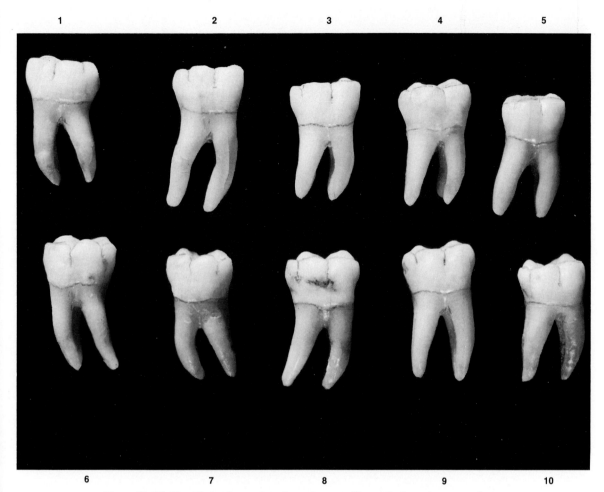

6   7   8   9   10

Figure 12–14. Mandibular first molars, buccal aspect. Ten typical specimens are shown.

The calibration of this tooth at the cervical line is 1.5 to 2 mm less mesiodistally than the mesiodistal measurement at the contact areas, which of course represents the greatest mesiodistal measurement of the crown.

The surface of the buccal portion of the crown is smoothly convex at the cusp portions with developmental grooves between the cusps. Approximately at the level of the ends of the developmental grooves, in the middle third, a developmental depression is noticeable. It runs in a mesiodistal direction just above the cervical ridge of the buccal surface (Fig. 12–14, specimens 6 and 8). This cervical ridge may show a smooth depression in it which progresses cervically, joining with the developmental concavity just below the cervical line, which is congruent with the root bifurcation buccally.

The roots of this tooth are, in most instances, well formed and constant in development.

When the tooth is posed so that the mesiobuccal groove is directly in the line of vision, part of the distal surface of the root trunk may be seen and, in addition, we may see part of the distal area of the mesial root because the lingual portion of the root is turned distally. These areas may be seen in addition to the buccal areas of the roots and root trunk.

The mesial root is curved mesially from a point shortly below the cervical line to the middle third portion. From this point it curves distally to the tapered apex, which is located

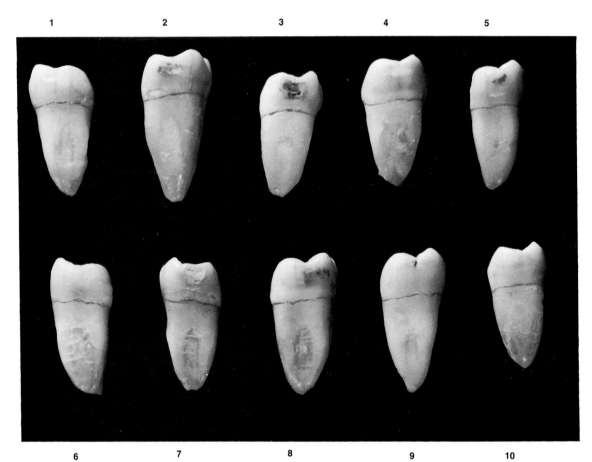

Figure 12–15. Mandibular first molars, mesial aspect. Ten typical specimens are shown.

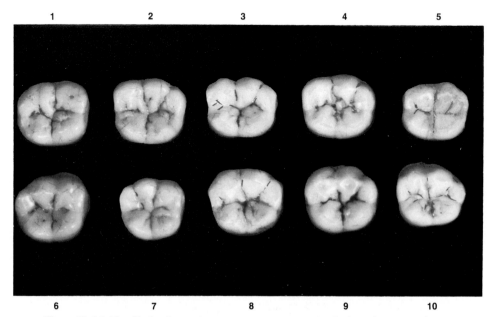

Figure 12–16. Mandibular first molars, occlusal aspect. Ten typical specimens are shown.

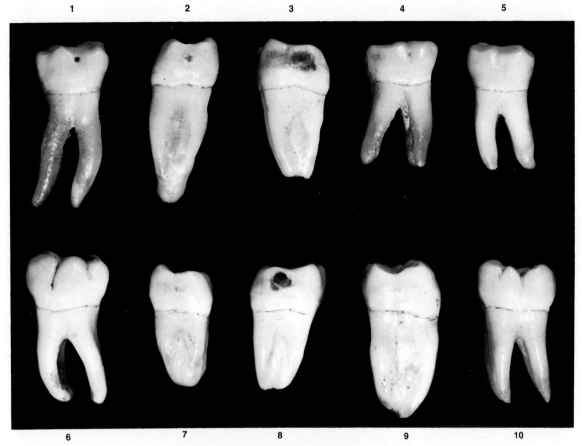

Figure 12–17. Mandibular first molars.
Ten specimens with uncommon variations are shown.
1, Root extremely long, crown small.
2, Mesial root longer than average with rounded apex.
3, Crown very wide buccolingually; roots short.
4, Roots short.
5, Crown has no buccal developmental grooves.
6, Crown and roots poorly formed.
7, Roots dwarfed.
8, Roots short; crown wide buccolingually.
9, Crown and root oversize buccolingually.
10, Extra tubercle or cusp attached to mesiolingual lobe.

directly below the mesiobuccal cusp. The crest of curvature of the root mesially is mesial to the crown cervix. The distal outline of the mesial root is concave from the bifurcation of the root trunk to the apex.

The distal root is less curved than the mesial root, and its axis is in a distal direction from cervix to apex. The root may show some curvature at its apical third in either a mesial or a distal direction (Fig. 12–14, specimens *1* and *8*). The apex is usually more pointed than that of the mesial root and is located below or distal to the distal contact area of the crown. There is considerable variation in the comparative lengths of mesial and distal roots (Fig. 12–14).

Both roots are wider mesiodistally at the buccal areas than they are lingually. Developmental depressions are present on the mesial and distal sides of both roots—a fact that lessens the mesiodistal measurement at those points. They are somewhat thicker at the lingual borders. This arrangement provides a secure anchorage for the mandibular first molar, preventing rotation. This I-beam principle increases the anchorage of each root (Chapter 13, Fig. 13–41).

The point of bifurcation of the two roots is located approximately 3 mm below the cervical line. There is a deep developmental depression buccally on the root trunk, which starts at the bifurcation and progresses cervically, becoming more shallow until it terminates at or immediately above the cervical line. This depression is smooth with no developmental groove or fold.

Lingual Aspect (Figs. 12–5, 12–6, 12–12, and 12–13)

From the lingual aspect, three cusps may be seen: two lingual cusps and the lingual portion of the distal cusp (Fig. 12–5). The two lingual cusps are pointed, and the cusp ridges are high enough to hide the two buccal cusps from view. The mesiolingual cusp is the widest mesiodistally, with its cusp tip somewhat higher than the distolingual cusp. The distolingual cusp is almost as wide mesiodistally as the mesiolingual cusp. The mesiolingual and distolingual cusp ridges are inclined at angles that are similar on both lingual cusps. These cusp ridges form obtuse angles at the cusp tips of approximately 100 degrees.

The *lingual developmental groove* serves as a line of demarcation between the lingual cusps, extending downward on the lingual surface of the crown for a short distance only. Some mandibular first molars show no groove on the lingual surface but show a depression lingual to the cusp ridges. The angle formed by the distolingual cusp ridge of the mesiolingual cusp and the mesiolingual cusp ridge of the distolingual cusp is more obtuse than the angulation of the cusp ridges at the tips of the lingual cusps.

The distal cusp is at a lower level than the mesiolingual cusp.

The mesial outline of the crown from this aspect is convex from the cervical line to the marginal ridge. The crest of contour mesially, which represents the contact area, is somewhat higher than the crest of contour distally.

The distal outline of the crown is straight immediately above the cervical line to a point immediately below the distal contact area; this area is represented by a convex curvature that also outlines the distal surface of the distal cusp. The junction of the distolingual cusp ridge of the distolingual cusp with the distal marginal ridge is abrupt; it gives the impression of a groove at this site from the lingual aspect. Sometimes there is a shallow developmental groove at this point (Fig. 12–10). Part of the mesial and distal surfaces of the crown and root trunk may be seen from this aspect because the mesial and distal sides converge lingually.

The cervical line lingually is irregular and tends to point sharply toward the root bifurcation and immediately above it.

The surface of the crown lingually is smooth and spheroidal on each of the lingual lobes. The surface is concave at the side of the lingual groove above the center of the crown lingually. Below this point, the surface of the crown becomes almost flat as it approaches the cervical line.

The roots of the mandibular first molar appear somewhat different from the lingual aspect. They measure about 1 mm longer lingually than buccally, but the length *seems* more extreme (Figs. 12–6 and 12–7). This impression is derived from the fact that the cusp ridges and cervical line are at a higher level (about 1 mm). This arrangement adds a millimeter to the distance from root bifurcation to cervical line. In addition, the mesiodistal measurement of the root trunk is less toward the lingual surface than toward the buccal surface. Consequently, this slenderness lingually, in addition to the added length, makes the roots appear longer than they are from the lingual aspect (Fig. 12–9).

As was mentioned, the root bifurcation lingually starts at a point approximately 4 mm below the cervical line. This developmental depression is quite deep at this point, although it is smooth throughout and progresses cervically and becomes more shallow until it fades out entirely immediately below the cervical line. The depression is rarely reflected in the cervical line or the enamel of the lingual surface of the crown as is found in many cases on the buccal surface of this tooth.

This bifurcation groove of the root trunk is located almost in line with the lingual developmental groove of the crown.

Mesial Aspect (Figs. 12–7, 12–12, 12–13, and 12–15)

When the mandibular first molar is viewed from the mesial aspect, the specimen being held with its mesial surface at right angles to the line of vision, two cusps and one root only are to be seen: the mesiobuccal and mesiolingual cusps and the mesial root (Fig. 12–7).

The buccolingual measurement of the crown is greater at the mesial portion than it is at the distal portion. The buccolingual measurement of the mesial root is also greater than the same measurement of the distal root. Therefore, since the mesial portions of the tooth are broader and the mesial cusps are higher, the distal portions of the tooth cannot be seen from this angle.

As mentioned before, all of the posterior mandibular teeth have crown outlines from the mesial aspect that show a characteristic relation between crown and root. The crown from the mesial or distal aspect is roughly rhomboidal, and the entire crown has a lingual tilt in relation to the root axis. It should be remembered that the crowns of maxillary posterior teeth have the center of the occlusal surfaces between the cusps in line with the root axes (Fig. 4–23, *e, f*).

It is interesting to note the difference between the *outline form of the mandibular first molar and the mandibular second premolar from the mesial aspect* (see Chapter 10). The first molar compares as follows:

1. The crown is a fraction of a millimeter to a millimeter shorter in the first molar.
2. The root is usually that much shorter also.
3. The buccolingual measurement of crown and root of the molar is 2 mm or more greater.
4. The lingual cusp is longer than the buccal cusp. (The opposite is true of the second premolar.)

Regardless of these differences, *the two teeth have the same functional form except for the added reinforcement given to the molar lingually.* Because of the added root width buccolingually, the buccal cusps of the first molar do not approach the center axis of the root as does the second premolar, and the lingual cusp tips are within the lingual outline of the roots instead of being on a line with them.

From the mesial aspect, the buccal outline of the crown of the mandibular first molar is convex immediately above the cervical line. Before occlusal wear has shortened the buccal cusps, this curvature is over the cervical third of the crown buccally, outlining the *buccal cervical ridge* (Fig. 12–8). This ridge is more prominent on some first molars than on others (Fig. 12–15). Just as on mandibular premolars, this ridge curvature does not exceed similar contours on other teeth as a rule when the mandibular first molar is posed in the position it assumes in the mandibular arch (Figs. 12–7 and Fig. 12–15, specimens *1* and *2*).

Above the buccal cervical ridge, the outline of the buccal contour may be slightly concave on some specimens (Fig. 12–15, specimens *1* and *2*); or the outline may just be less convex or even rather flat as it continues occlusally outlining the contour of the mesiobuccal cusp. The mesiobuccal cusp is located directly above the buccal third of the mesial root.

The lingual outline of the crown is straight in a lingual direction, starting at the cervical line and joining the lingual curvature at the middle third, the lingual curvature being pronounced between this point and the tip of the mesiolingual cusp. The crest of the lingual contour is located at the center of the middle third of the crown. The tip of the mesiolingual cusp is in a position directly above the lingual third of the mesial root.

The mesial marginal ridge is confluent with the mesial ridges of the mesiobuccal and mesiolingual cusps. The marginal ridge is placed about 1 mm below the level of the cusp tips.

The cervical line mesially is rather irregular and tends to curve occlusally about 1 mm toward the center of the mesial surface of the tooth (Fig. 12–15, specimens *1, 4, 9,* and *10*). The cervical line may assume a relatively straight line buccolingually (specimens *3, 6,* and *8*).

In all instances, the cervical line is at a higher level lingually than buccally, usually about 1 mm higher. The difference in level may be greater. This relation depends upon the assumption that the tooth is posed vertically. When the first molar is in its normal position in the lower jaw, leaning to the lingual, the cervical line is nearly level buccolingually.

The surface of the crown is convex and smooth over the mesial contours of the mesiolingual and mesiobuccal lobes. A flattened or slightly concave area exists at the cervical line immediately above the center of the mesial root. This area is right below the contact area and joins the concavity of the central portion of the root at the cervix. The contact area is almost centered buccolingually in the mesial surface of the crown, and it is placed below the crest of the marginal ridge about one third the distance from marginal ridge to cervical line. (See stained contact area on specimen, Fig. 12–9. Before contact wear has occurred, the contact area is not so broad. Refer also to Figure 12–4.)

The buccal outline of the mesial root drops straight down from the cervical line buccally to a point near the junction of cervical and middle thirds of the root. There is a gentle curve lingually from this point to the apex, which is located directly below the mesiobuccal cusp.

The lingual outline of the mesial root is slanted in a buccal direction, although the outline is nearly straight from the cervical line lingually to the point of junction of middle and apical thirds of the root. From this point, the curvature is sharply buccal to the bluntly tapered apex. On those specimens that show a short bifurcation at the mesial root end, the curvature at the apical third lingually is slight (Fig. 12–15, specimens *2* and *10*).

The mesial surface of the mesial root is convex at the buccal and lingual borders, with a broad concavity between these convexities the full length of the root from cervical line to apex. If a specimen tooth is held in front of a strong light so that we may see the distal side of the mesial root from the apical aspect, it is noted that the same contours exist on the root distally as are found mesially and the root is very thin where the concavities are superimposed. The root form appears to be two narrow roots fused together with thin hard tissue between.

The mesial surface of the distal root is smooth, with no deep developmental depressions.

Distal Aspect (Figs. 12–10, 12–12, and 12–13)

Since the gross outline of the distal aspect of crown and root of the mandibular first molar is similar to the mesial aspect, the description of outline form will not be repeated. When considering this aspect from the standpoint of a three-dimensional figure, however, we see more of the tooth from the distal aspect because the crown is shorter distally than mesially, and the buccal and lingual surfaces of the crown converge distally. The buccal surface shows more convergence than the lingual surface. The distal root is narrower buccolingually than the mesial root.

If a specimen of the first molar is held with the distal surface of the crown at right angles to the line of vision, a great part of the occlusal surface may be seen and some part of each of the five cusps also comparing favorably with the mandibular second premolar. This is caused in part by the placement of the crowns on the roots with a distal inclination to the long axes. The slight variation in crown length distally does not provide this view of the occlusal surface (Figs. 12–9 and 12–10).

From the distal aspect, the distal cusp is in the foreground on the crown portion. The distal cusp is placed a little buccal to center buccolingually, the distal contact area appearing on its distal contour.

The distal contact area is placed just below the distal cusp ridge of the distal cusp and at a slightly higher level above the cervical line than was found mesially when comparing the location of the mesial contact area.

The distal marginal ridge is short and is made up of the distal cusp ridge of the distal cusp and the distolingual cusp ridge of the distolingual cusp. These cusp ridges dip sharply in a cervical direction, meeting at an obtuse angle. Often a developmental groove or depression is found crossing the marginal ridge at this point. The point of this angle is above the lingual third of the distal root instead of being centered over the root as is true of the center of the mesial marginal ridge.

The distal contact area is centered over the distal root, which arrangement places it buccal to the center point of the distal marginal ridge.

The surface of the distal portion of the crown is convex on the distal cusp and the distolingual cusp. Contact wear may produce a flattened area at the point of contact on the distal surface of the distal cusp. Just above the cervical line, the enamel surface is flat where it joins the flattened surface of the root trunk distally.

The cervical line distally usually extends straight across buccolingually. It may be irregular, dipping rootwise just below the distal contact area (Fig. 12–10).

The end of the distobuccal developmental groove is located on the distal surface and forms a concavity at the cervical portion of the distobuccal line angle of the crown. The distal portion of the crown extends out over the root trunk distally at quite an angle (Fig. 12–4). The smooth flat surface below the contact area remains fairly constant to the apical third of the distal root. Sometimes a developmental depression is found here. The apical third portion of the root is more rounded as it tapers to a sharper apex than is found on the mesial root.

The lingual border of the mesial root may be seen from the distal aspect.

Occlusal Aspect (Figs. 12–1, 12–2, 12–11, 12–12, 12–13, and 12–16)

The mandibular first molar is somewhat hexagonal from the occlusal aspect (Fig. 12–2). The crown measurement is 1 mm or more greater mesiodistally than buccolingually. It must be remembered that the opposite arrangement is true of the maxillary first molar.

The buccolingual measurement of the crown is greater on the mesial than on the distal. Also, a measurement of the crown at the contact areas, which includes the two buccal cusps and the distal cusp, shows greater measurement than the mesiodistal measurement of the two lingual cusps. In other words, the crown converges lingually from the contact areas. This convergence varies in individual specimens (Fig. 12–16, specimens *1* and *4*).

It is interesting to note the degree of development of the individual cusps from the occlusal aspect. The mesiobuccal cusp is slightly larger than either of the two lingual cusps, which are almost equal to each other in size; the distobuccal cusp is smaller than any one of the other three mentioned, and the distal cusp is in most cases much the smallest of all.

There is more variance in the development of the distobuccal and distal lobes than in any of the others (Fig. 12–16, specimens *1, 7,* and *10*).

When the tooth is posed so that the line of vision is parallel with the long axis, a great part of the buccal surface may be seen, whereas only a small portion of the lingual surface may be seen lingual to the lingual cusp ridges. No part of the mesial or distal surfaces is in view below the outline of the mesial and distal marginal ridges. (Compare tooth outlines from the other aspects.)

All mandibular molars, including the first molar, are essentially quadrilateral in form. The mandibular first molar, in most instances, has a functioning distal cusp, although this is small in comparison with the other cusps. Occasionally four-cusp first molars are found, and more often one discovers first molars with distobuccal and distal cusps showing fusion with little or no trace of a distobuccal developmental groove between them (Fig. 12–16, specimen *1*; Fig. 12–17, specimens *4* and *5*). *From a developmental viewpoint, all mandibular molars have four major cusps, whereas maxillary molars have only three major cusps* (Fig. 11–11).

The occlusal surfaces of the mandibular first molar may be described as follows: There is a major fossa and there are two minor fossae. The major fossa is the *central fossa* (Fig. 12–2). It is roughly circular, and it is centrally placed on the occlusal surface between buccal and lingual cusp ridges. The two minor fossae are the *mesial triangular fossa,* immediately distal to the mesial marginal ridge, and the *distal triangular fossa,* placed immediately mesial to the distal marginal ridge (Fig. 12–1).

The developmental grooves on the occlusal surface are the *central developmental groove,* the *mesiobuccal developmental groove,* the *distobuccal developmental groove,* and the *lingual developmental groove.* Supplemental grooves, accidental short grooves and developmental pits are also found. Most of the supplemental grooves are tributary to the developmental grooves within the bounds of cusp ridges.

The *central fossa* of the occlusal surface is a concave area bounded by the distal slope of the mesiobuccal cusp, both mesial and distal slopes of the distobuccal cusp, the mesial slope of the distal cusp, the distal slope of the mesiolingual cusp, and the mesial slope of the distolingual cusp (Fig. 12–2).

All of the developmental grooves converge in the center of the central fossa at the *central pit.*

The *mesial triangular fossa* of the occlusal surface is a smaller concave area than the central fossa, and it is bounded by the mesial slope of the mesiobuccal cusp, the mesial marginal ridge and the mesial slope of the mesiolingual cusp. The mesial portion of the central developmental groove terminates in this fossa. Usually a buccal and a lingual supplemental groove join it at a *mesial pit* within the boundary of the mesial marginal ridge. Sometimes a supplemental groove crosses the mesial marginal ridge lingual to the contact area (Fig. 12–16, specimens *2, 8, 9,* and *10*).

The *distal triangular fossa* is in most instances less distinct than the mesial fossa. It is bounded by the distal slope of the distal cusp, the distal marginal ridge and the distal slope of the distolingual cusp. The central groove has its other terminal in this fossa. Buccal and lingual supplemental grooves are less common here. An extension of the central groove quite often crosses the distal marginal ridge, however, lingual to the distal contact area.

Starting at the central pit in the central fossa, the central developmental groove travels an irregular course mesially, terminating in the mesial triangular fossa. A short distance mesially from the central pit, it joins the mesiobuccal developmental groove. The latter groove courses in a mesiobuccal direction at the bottom of a sulcate groove separating the mesiobuccal and distobuccal cusps. At the junction of the cusp ridges of those cusps, the mesiobuccal groove of the occlusal surface is confluent with the mesiobuccal groove of the buccal surface of the crown. The lingual developmental groove of the occlusal surface is an irregular groove coursing in a lingual direction at the bottom of the lingual sulcate groove to the junction of lingual cusp ridges, where it is confluent with the lingual extension of the same groove. Again starting at the central pit, the central groove may be followed in a distobuccal direction to a point where it is joined by the distobuccal developmental groove of the occlusal surface. From this point, the central groove courses in a distolingual direction, terminating in the distal triangular fossa. The distobuccal groove passes from its junction with the central groove in a distobuccal course, joining its buccal extension on the buccal surface of the crown at the junction of the cusp ridges of the distobuccal and distal cusps.

The central developmental groove seems to be centrally located in relation to the buccolingual crown dimension. This arrangement makes the triangular ridges of lingual cusps longer than the triangular ridges of buccal cusps.

Note the relative position and relative size of the distal cusp from the occlusal aspect. The distal portion of it joins the distal contact area of the crown.

Mandibular Second Molar

The mandibular second molar supplements the first molar in function. Its anatomy differs in some details.

Normally, the second molar is smaller than the first molar by a fraction of a millimeter in all dimensions (Table 12–2). It does not, however, run true to form. It is not uncommon to find mandibular second molar crowns somewhat large than first molars, and although the roots are not as well formed, they may be longer.

The crown has four well-developed cusps: two buccal and two lingual, of nearly equal development. There is neither a distal nor a fifth cusp, but the distobuccal cusp is larger than that found on the first molar.

The tooth has two well-developed roots, one mesial and one distal. These roots are broad buccolingually, but they are not as broad as those of the first molar, nor are they as widely separated.

Detailed Description of the Mandibular Second Molar from all Aspects

In describing this tooth, direct comparisons will be made with the first mandibular molar. Figures 12–18 through 12–25 present the mandibular second molar in various aspects. Uncommon variations are shown in Figure 12–26.

Buccal Aspect (Figs. 12–18 and 12–23)

The crown is somewhat shorter cervico-occlusally and narrower mesiodistally than in the first molar. The crown and root show a tendency toward greater overall length, but are not always longer (Fig. 12–23, specimens *4, 7,* and *9*).

There is but one developmental groove buccally, the *buccal developmental groove.* This groove acts as a line of demarcation between the mesiobuccal and the distobuccal cusps, which are about equal in their mesiodistal measurements.

The cervical line buccally in many instances points sharply toward the root bifurcation (Fig. 12–23, specimens *1, 2, 3, 5,* and *9*).

Text continued on page 297

Table 12–2. Mandibular Second Molar

First evidence of calcification	2½ to 3 years
Enamel completed	7 to 8 years
Eruption	11 to 13 years
Root completed	14 to 15 years

Measurement Table

	Cervico-occlusal Length of Crown	Length of Root	Mesiodistal Diameter of Crown	Mesiodistal Diameter of Crown at Cervix	Labio- or Bucco-lingual Diameter of Crown	Labio- or Bucco-lingual Diameter of Crown at Cervix	Curvature of Cervical Line—Mesial	Curvature of Cervical Line—Distal
Dimensions suggested for carving technique	7.0*	13.0	10.5	8.0	10.0	9.0	1.0	0.0

*In millimeters.

292

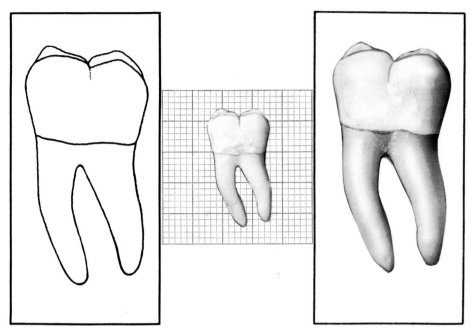

Figure 12–18. Mandibular left second molar, buccal aspect.

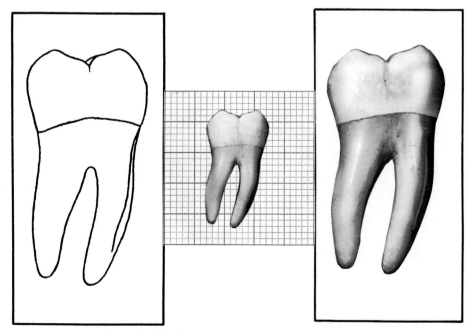

Figure 12–19. Mandibular left second molar, lingual aspect.

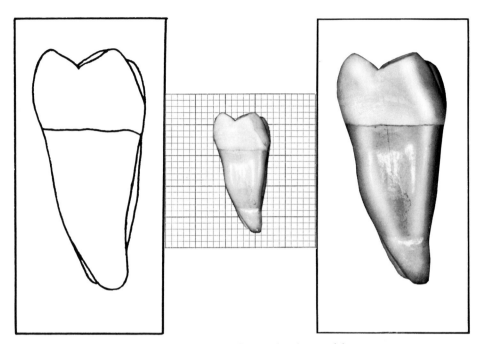

Figure 12–20. Mandibular left second molar, mesial aspect.

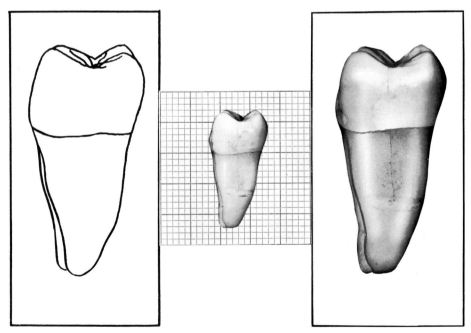

Figure 12–21. Mandibular left second molar, distal aspect.

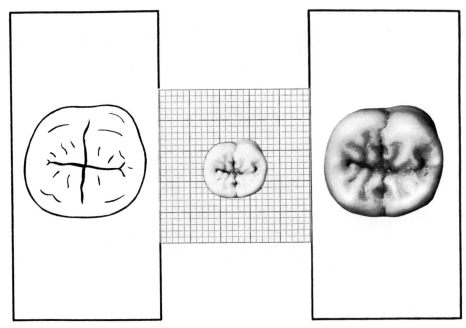

Figure 12–22. Mandibular left second molar, occlusal aspect.

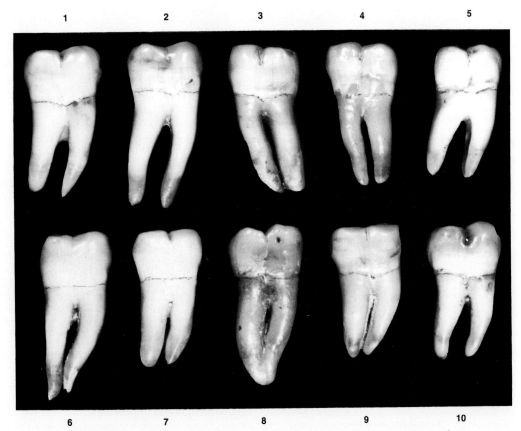

Figure 12–23. Mandibular second molars, buccal aspect. Ten typical specimens are shown.

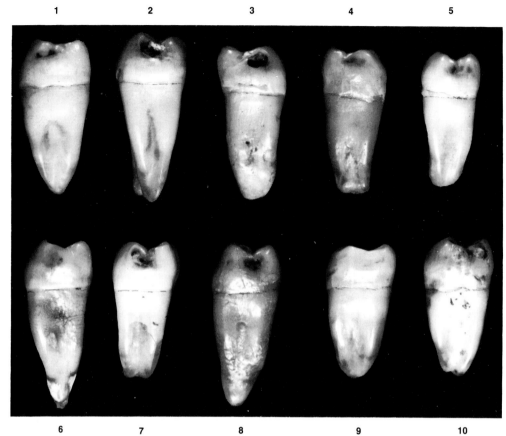

Figure 12–24. Mandibular second molars, mesial aspect. Ten typical specimens are shown.

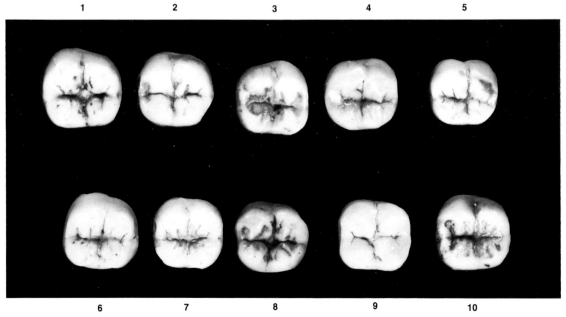

Figure 12–25. Mandibular second molars, occlusal aspect. Ten typical specimens are shown.

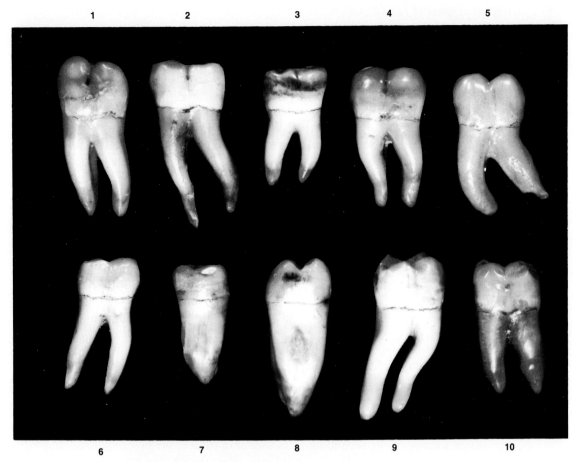

Figure 12–26. Mandibular second molars.
Ten specimens with uncommon variations are shown.
  1, Mesiodistal measurements at contact areas and cervix almost equal.
  2, Roots twisted and of extra length.
  3, Very small specimen; roots short.
  4, Roots short for such a large crown.
  5, Roots thick and malformed generally.
  6, Dwarfed crown, roots extra long.
  7, Mesial aspect, protective curvature buccally and lingually is absent.
  8, Roots of extra size; occlusal surface constricted buccolingually.
  9, Roots malformed.
  10, Crown wide mesiodistally at the cervix; roots short.

The roots may be shorter than those of the first molar, but they vary considerably in this as well as in their development generally. The roots are usually closer together, and their axes are nearly parallel. They may spread as much as those of the first molar (Fig. 12–23, specimen *5*), or they may be fused for all or part of their length (specimens *8* and *9*).

The roots are inclined distally in relation to the occlusal plane of the crown, their axes forming more of an acute angle with the occlusal plane than is found on the first molar. When one compares all of the mandibular molars, it may seem that the first molar shows one angulation of roots to occlusal plane, the second molar a more acute angle and the third molar an angle which is more acute still. (See Chapter 16, "Occlusion.")

Lingual Aspect (Fig. 12–19)

Differences in detail between the mandibular second molar and the mandibular first molar, to be noted from the lingual aspect, are these:

1. The crown and root of the mandibular second molar converge lingually but to a slight degree; little of the mesial or distal surfaces may therefore be seen from this aspect.
2. The mesiodistal calibration at the cervix lingually is always greater accordingly than that of the first molar.
3. The curvatures mesially and distally on the crown that describe the contact areas are more noticeable from the lingual aspect. They prove to be at a slightly lower level, especially in the distal area, than those of the first molar.

Mesial Aspect (Figs. 12–20 and 12–24)

Except for the differences in measurement from the mesial aspect, the second molar differs little from the first molar.

The cervical ridge buccally on the crown portion is in most instances less pronounced, and the occlusal surface may be more constricted buccolingually (Fig. 12–24, specimens *2*, *8*, and *10*).

The cervical line shows less curvature, being straight and regular in outline buccolingually.

The mesial root is somewhat pointed apically. If part of the distal root is in sight, it is seen buccally. In the first molar, when the distal root is in sight from the mesial aspect, it is in view lingually.

Distal Aspect (Fig. 12–21)

From the distal aspect, the second molar is similar in form to the first molar except for the absence of a distal cusp and a distobuccal groove. The contact area is centered on the distal surface buccolingually and is placed equidistant from cervical line and marginal ridge.

Occlusal Aspect (Figs. 12–22 and 12–25)

The occlusal aspect of the mandibular second molar differs considerably from the first molar. These variations serve as marks of identity. The small distal cusp of the first molar is not present, and the distobuccal lobe development is just as pronounced, and sometimes more so, than that of the mesiobuccal lobe. There is no distobuccal developmental groove occlusally or buccally. The buccal and lingual developmental grooves meet the central developmental groove at right angles at the central pit on the occlusal surface. These grooves form a cross, dividing the occlusal portion of the crown into four parts that are nearly equal.

In general, the cusp slopes on the occlusal surface are not as smooth as those found on first molars, since they are roughened by many supplemental grooves radiating from the developmental grooves.

The following characteristics of mandibular second molars from the occlusal aspect should be observed and noted:

1. Many of them are rectangular from the occlusal aspect (Fig. 12–25, specimens *7* and *9*).
2. Many show considerable prominence cervically on the mesiobuccal lobe only (Fig. 12–25, specimens *1*, *3*, and *6*).

3. Most second molars exhibit more curvature of the outline of the crown distally than mesially, showing a semicircular outline to the disto-occlusal surface in comparison with a square outline mesially.
4. The cusp ridge of the distobuccal cusp lies buccal to the cusp ridge of the mesiobuccal cusp (Fig. 12–25, specimens *2, 3, 8* and *10;* Fig. 12–22).

In anthropological studies, morphological categories used to describe the occlusal surfaces of the mandibular molars are based upon a topology developed by Gregory and Hellman (1926) and Hellman (1928): 5-Y refers to molars with five cusps arranged so that when viewed from the lingual edge of the tooth, the fissure pattern resembles a Y. The designation 4-Y is given to molars like 5-Y but with only four cusps. The category +5 designates molars with five cusps arranged in such a way that the fissure pattern resembles a cross. Similarly +4 refers to molars like +5 but having only four cusps. The criterion for determining whether a pattern is a Y or a + is contact of the metaconid with the hypoconid. If there is contact the pattern resembles a Y; if there is no contact, the pattern resembles a + (Fig. 12–27).

Mandibular Third Molar

The mandibular third molar varies considerably in different individuals and presents many anomalies both in form and in position. It supplements the second molar in function, although the tooth is seldom as well developed, the average mandibular third molar showing irregular development of the crown portion, with undersized roots, more or less malformed. Generally speaking, however, its design conforms to the general plan of all mandibular molars, conforming more closely to that of the second mandibular molar in the number of cusps and occlusal design than it does to the mandibular first molar. Occasionally, mandibular third molars are seen that are well formed and comparable in size and development to the mandibular first molar.

Many instances of mandibular third molars with five or more cusps are found, with the crown portions larger than those of the second molar (Table 12–3). In these cases, the alignment and occlusion with other teeth is not normal because insufficient room is available in the alveolar process of the mandible for the accommodation of such a large tooth and the occlusal form is too variable.

Although it is possible to find dwarfed specimens of mandibular third molars (Fig. 12–37, specimen *2*), most of them that are not normal in size are larger than normal in the crown portion particularly. Roots of these oversize third molars may be short and poorly formed.

The opposite situation is likely in maxillary third molars. Most of the anomalies are undersized. Mandibular third molars are the most likely to be impacted, wholly or partially, in the jaw. The lack of space accommodation is the chief cause.

If the third molar is congenitally absent from one side of the mandible or maxilla, it will most likely be absent from the other. However, there is probably not a significant association between third molar agenesis in the maxilla and mandible. Partial eruption of mandibular third molar teeth may result in periodontal defects on the distal aspects by the second molars, and in some instances resorption of distal root surfaces (Fig. 12–28). When third molars are to be restored, it should be remembered that the depth of the enamel on the occlusal surface is relatively greater than first or second molars.

Table 12–3. Mandibular Third Molar

First evidence of calcification	8 to 10 years
Enamel completed	12 to 16 years
Eruption	17 to 21 years
Root completed	18 to 25 years

Measurement Table

	Cervico-occlusal Length of Crown	Length of Root	Mesiodistal Diameter of Crown	Mesiodistal Diameter of Crown at Cervix	Labio- or Bucco-lingual Diameter of Crown	Labio- or Bucco-lingual Diameter of Crown at Cervix	Curvature of Cervical Line—Mesial	Curvature of Cervical Line—Distal
Dimensions suggested for carving technique	7.0*	11.0	10.0	7.5	9.5	9.0	1.0	0.0

*In millimeters.

300

Detailed Description of the Mandibular Third Molar from All Aspects

Figures 12–27 through 12–37 present the mandibular third molar in various aspects.

Buccal Aspect (Figs. 12–29 and 12–34)

From the buccal aspect, mandibular third molars vary considerably in outline. At the same time, they all have certain characteristics in common.

The outline of the crowns from this aspect is in a general way that of all mandibular molars. The crown is wider at contact areas mesiodistally than at the cervix, the buccal cusps are short and rounded, and the crest of contour mesially and distally is located a little more than half the distance from cervical line to tips of cusps. The type of third molar that is more likely to be in fair alignment and in good occlusion with other teeth is the four-cusp type; this is smaller and shows two buccal cusps only from this aspect (Fig. 12–34, specimens *1, 4, 5, 8, 9* and *10*).

The average third molar also shows two roots, one mesial and one distal. These roots are usually shorter, with a poorer development generally, than the roots of first or second molars, and their distal inclination in relation to the occlusal plane of the crown is greater. The roots may be separated with a definite point of bifurcation, or they may be fused for all or part of their length (Fig. 12–34).

Lingual Aspect (Fig. 12–30)

Observations from the lingual aspect add little to those already made from the buccal aspect. The mandibular third molar, when well developed, corresponds closely to the form of the second molar except for size and root development.

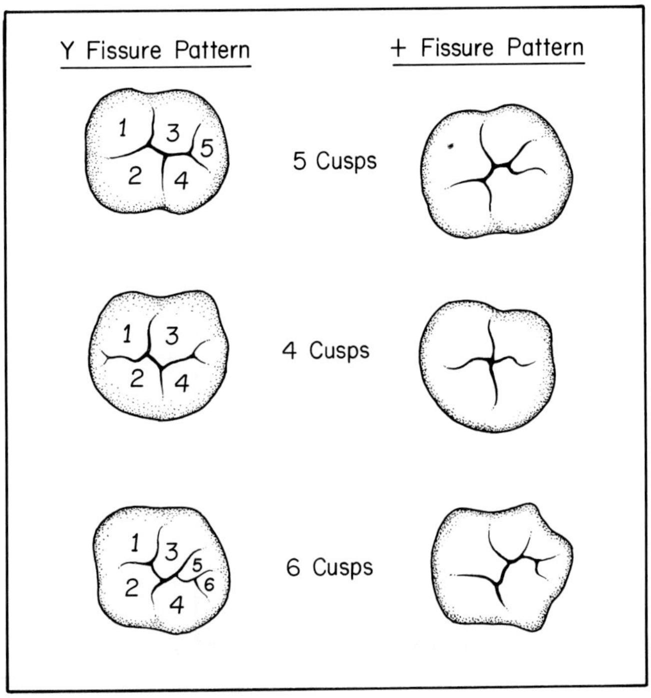

Figure 12–27. Mandibular molar patterns in the right lower molar. Y and + fissure patterns are shown. *1,* Protoconid; *2,* metaconid; *3,* hypoconid; *4,* entoconid; *5,* hypoconulid; *6,* sixth cusp.

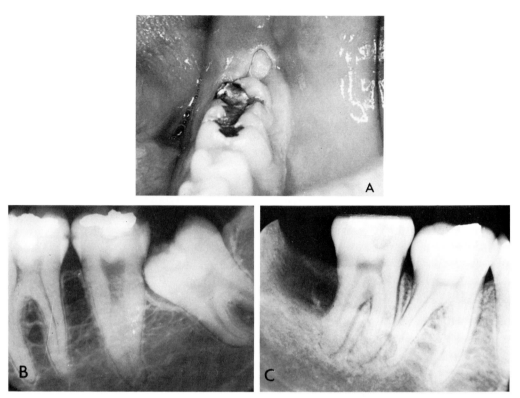

Figure 12–28. *A,* Partially erupted third molar. *B,* Impacted third molar. *C,* Defect immediately following extraction of a different third molar. Often the distal root surface of the second molar does not gain reattachment after a partially impacted third molar is extracted, especially if the surface has been exposed for some time prior to extraction.

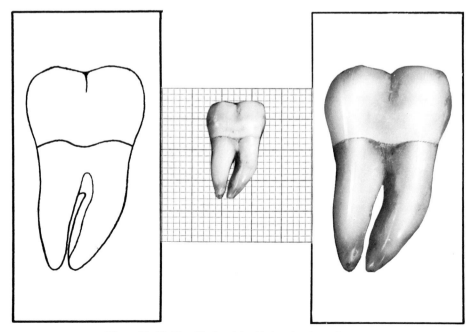

Figure 12–29. Mandibular right third molar, buccal aspect.

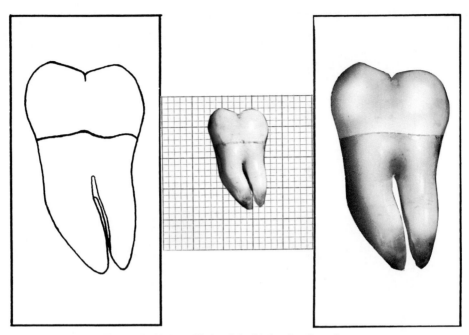

Figure 12–30. Mandibular right third molar, lingual aspect.

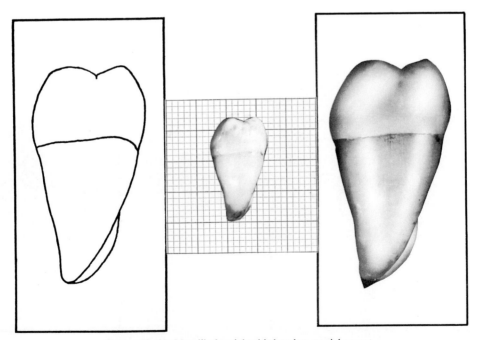

Figure 12–31. Mandibular right third molar, mesial aspect.

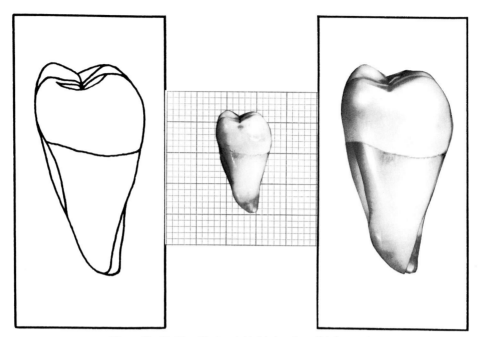

Figure 12–32. Mandibular right third molar, distal aspect.

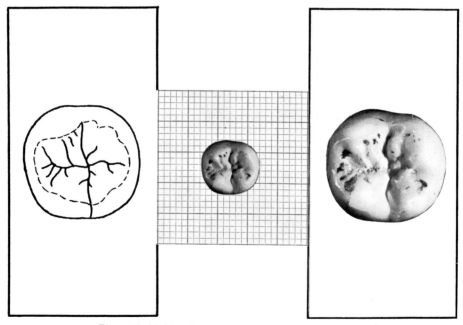

Figure 12–33. Mandibular right third molar, occlusal aspect.

1   2   3   4   5

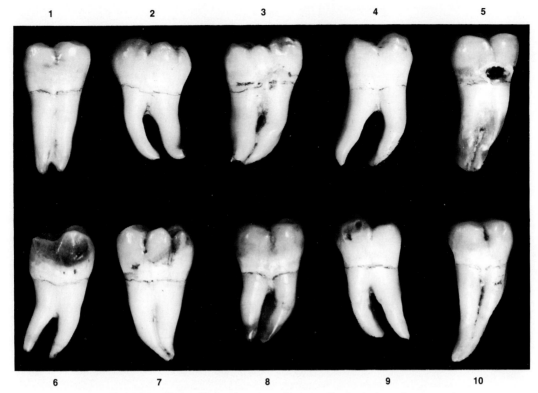

6   7   8   9   10

Figure 12–34. Mandibular third molars, buccal aspect. Ten typical specimens are shown.

Mesial Aspect (Figs. 12–31 and 12–35)

From the mesial aspect, this tooth resembles the mandibular second molar except in dimensions. The roots, of course, are shorter, with the mesial root tapering more from cervix to apex. The apex of the mesial root is usually more pointed.

Distal Aspect (Fig. 12–32)

The anatomic appearance of the distal portion of this tooth is much like that of the second molar except for size.

Those specimens that have oversize crown portions are much more spheroidal above the cervical line. The distal root appears small, both in length and in buccolingual measurement, when compared with the large crown portion.

Occlusal Aspect (Figs. 12–33 and 12–36)

The occlusal aspect is quite similar to that of the second mandibular molar when the development is such as to facilitate good alignment and occlusion (Fig. 12–36, specimens *2, 3, 4, 6, 7, 8,* and *9*). The tendency is toward a more rounded outline and a smaller buccolingual measurement distally.

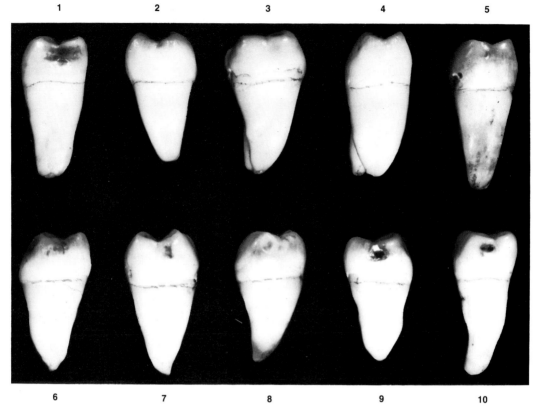

Figure 12–35. Mandibular third molars, mesial aspect. Ten typical specimens are shown.

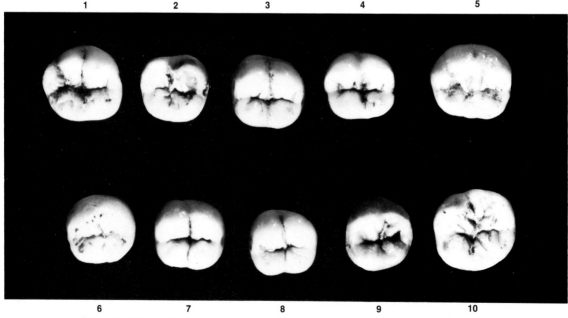

Figure 12–36. Mandibular third molars, occlusal aspect. Ten typical specimens are shown.

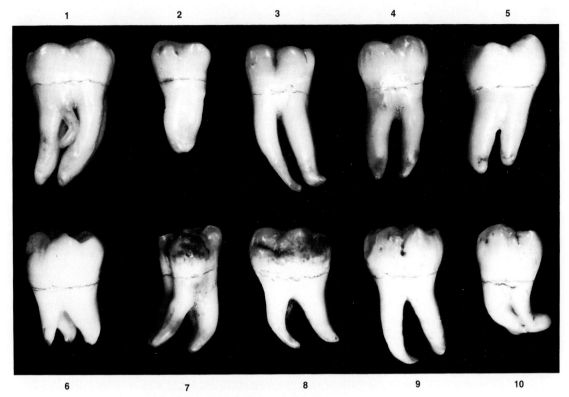

Figure 12–37. Mandibular third molars.
Ten specimens with uncommon variations are shown.
  1, Oversize generally, extra root lingually.
  2, Dwarfed specimen, odd extra cusp; fused roots.
  3, Crown resembling first molar; long slender roots.
  4, Formation closely resembling second molar.
  5, Large crown; malformed roots.
  6, Multicusp crown; dwarfed roots.
  7, No resemblance to typical functional form.
  8, Large crown; dwarfed roots.
  9, Odd crown form and root form.
  10, Crown long cervico-occlusally; roots fused and malformed.

References

Ash, M. M., et al. (1962). A study of periodontal hazards of third molars. J. Periodont. 33:209.

Banks, H. V. (1934). Incidence of third molar development. Angle Orthod. 4:223.

Comas, J. (1960). Manual of Physical Anthropology. Springfield, Ill.: Charles C. Thomas.

Garn, S. M., Arthur, B. L., and Vicinus, J. H. (1963). Third molar polymorphism and its significance to dental caries. J. Dent. Res. 42:1344.

Goblirsch, A. N. (1930). A study of third molar teeth. J. Am. Dent. Assoc. 17:1849.

Gregory, W. K., and Hellman, M. (1926). The crown patterns of fossils and recent human molar teeth and their meaning. Natural History 26:300.

Hellman, M. (1936). Our third molar teeth: Their eruption, presence and absence. Dental Cosmos 78:750.

Hellman, M. (1928). Racial characters in the human dentition. Proceedings of the American Philosophical Society 67:157.

Nanda, R. S. (1954). Agenesis of the third molar in man. Am. J. Orthodont. 40:698.

13 *The Pulp Cavities of the Permanent Teeth*

The dental pulp is the soft tissue component of the tooth. The pulp occupies the internal cavities of the tooth, i.e., the pulp chamber and pulp canal or root canal (Fig. 13–1). In general, the outline of the pulp tissue corresponds to the external outline form of the tooth; i.e., the outline form of the pulp chamber corresponds with the shape of the crown, whereas the outline form of the pulp canal corresponds with the shape of the roots of the teeth. The dental pulp within these cavities originates from the mesenchyme and has been assigned a number of different functions: formative, nutritive, sensory, and defensive. The primary function of the dental pulp is the formation of dentin. The complex sensory system within the dental pulp controls the blood flow and is responsible for at least mediation of the sensation of pain. The formation of reparative or irritation dentin is a defensive response to any form of irritation, whether it be mechanical, thermal, chemical, or bacterial in nature.

The primary function of the dentist is to prevent, intercept, and treat disease processes involving the dentition. The use of radiographs for the diagnosis and treatment of pulpal disease requires that the morphological features of the pulp chambers and root canals be known because images of a three-dimensional object are essentially compressed into a "one-dimensional" image. It is also essential that the clinician be aware of the location and size of the pulp cavities during operative procedures in order to prevent unnecessary encroachment upon the pulp.

The labial and buccal longitudinal sections of the teeth are clearly seen on standard radiographs (Fig. 13–2); however, the mesial and distal aspects of longitudinal sections are usually seen incidentally on radiographs of malposed teeth. Thus, the radiographic anatomy of the pulp cavity from the mesial-distal aspect is not well known.

The size of the pulp cavity depends on the age of the tooth and its history of trauma. Secondary dentin is formed continuously throughout the life of the tooth as a normal process, as long as the vitality of the tooth is maintained. The formation of secondary dentin is not uniform because the odontoblasts adjacent to the floor and roof of the pulp cavity produce greater quantities of secondary dentin than do the odontoblasts located adjacent to the walls of the pulp cavity. Therefore, the size of the pulp cavity is much larger in a young individual than in an adult (Fig. 13–3, *A* and *B*) and should be considered before extensive tooth reduction is accomplished.

Various traumatic injuries occur that, if severe enough, will initiate a different type of

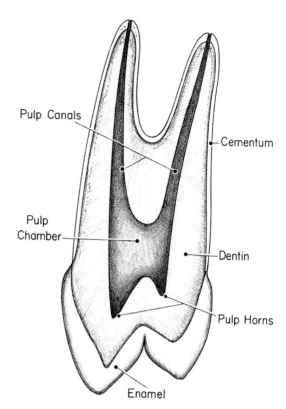

Figure 13-1. Buccolingual section of a maxillary premolar.

dentin formation. Irritation or reparative dentin may be formed in response to the carious process, abrasion, and attrition as well as to operative procedures. This response is protective in nature but may ultimately be detrimental in later years, because a finite amount of space is present within the pulp cavity. The size of the pulp cavity should be compared with that of the other teeth. If the calcification demonstrated is a localized phenomenon and is extensive, elective endodontic therapy is strongly suggested prior to any restorative procedure. Elective endodontics should be considered in the event that extreme calcification is present in a tooth scheduled for complex restorative procedures.

Endodontic procedures also require a thorough knowledge of the pulp cavity. Perforation during access preparation, failure to locate all the canals, or perforation of the apex or root surface may result in the ultimate loss of the tooth. Therefore, the clinician performing endodontics must know the size and location of the pulp chamber as well as the expected number of roots and canals. Radiographic detection of accessory roots or canals is not always possible. With a thorough knowledge of the pulp cavities in the permanent dentition, prevention, interception, and treatment of dentition-related disease processes will be accomplished with a greater degree of success.

The pulp cavity has been arbitrarily divided into the pulp chamber and the root canal (Fig. 13–1). The complexities of these cavities cannot be fully appreciated without studying longitudinal and transverse sections of each of the representative types of teeth (see Figs. 13–8 through 13–46).

The neurovascular bundle, which supplies the internal contents of the pulp cavity, enters through the apical foramen or foramina (Fig. 13–1). As the root begins to develop, the apical foramen is actually larger than the pulp chamber (Fig. 13–4), but it becomes more constricted at the completion of root formation (Fig. 13–4, *1, 2–5*).

It is possible for any root of a tooth to have a number of apical foramina. If these

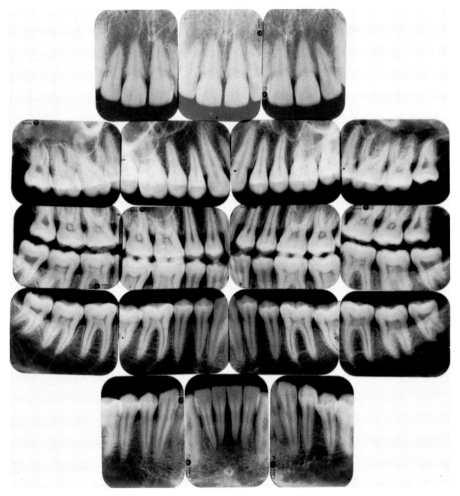

Figure 13–2. Dental radiographic examination.

openings are large enough, the space that leads to the main root canal is called a *supplementary* or *lateral canal* (Fig. 13–5). If the root canal breaks up into multiple tiny canals, it is referred to as a delta system because of its complexity (Fig. 13–6). The neurovascular bundle courses coronally through that portion of the pulp cavity known as the root canal.

The cementoenamel junction is approximately at the level at which the root canal becomes the pulp chamber (Fig. 13–1). This demarcation is mainly macroscopically based. Enamel covers the external surface of the dentin, which makes up part of the pulp chamber, whereas cementum covers all of the external dentinal surface of the root canal space. The demarcation is simpler in multirooted teeth because the pulp cavity within the root is the root canal and the remaining pulp cavity is the pulp chamber. Microscopically, the pulp within the chamber appears to be more cellular than the pulp found within the pulp of the root canal. The odontoblasts are cuboidal in the coronal pulp chamber but gradually flatten out as the apex is approached. The transition from the pulp chamber to the root canal is not sharply demarcated microscopically, and this demarcation is not sharply delineated macroscopically.

There are projections or prolongations in the roof of the pulp chamber that correspond to the various major cusps or lobes of the crown. The pulpal tissues that occupy these

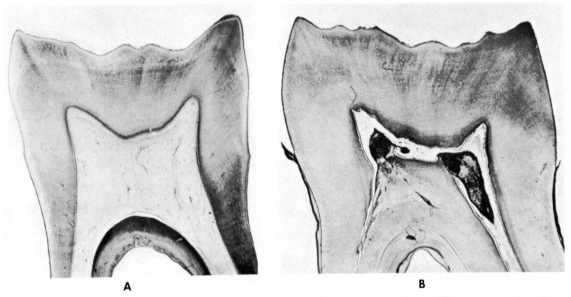

Figure 13–3. Comparison in size of the pulps of two intact lower first permanent molars at different ages. *A,* Age, 8 years. The pulp chamber is large. (Magnification ×8.) *B,* Age, 55 years. The pulp is greatly reduced in size. (Magnification ×8.) (From Kronfeld, R.: *Dental Histology and Comparative Dental Anatomy.* Philadelphia, Lea & Febiger, 1937.)

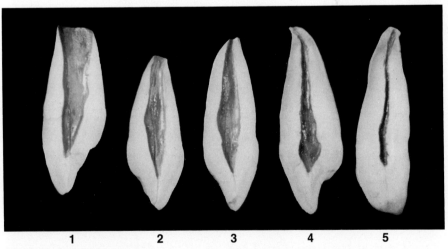

Figure 13–4. Maxillary canine.
Labiolingual sections show various stages of development.
1, Crown complete; root partially completed with large pulp cavity, wide open at apical end.
2, Tooth almost complete, except for lack of constriction of apical foramen.
3, Canine of young individual with large pulp cavity and completed root tip.
4, Typical canine of adult, demonstrating constriction of the foramen.
5, Canine of an elderly individual with a constricted pulp chamber and canal; this specimen has lost its original crown form because of wear during function.

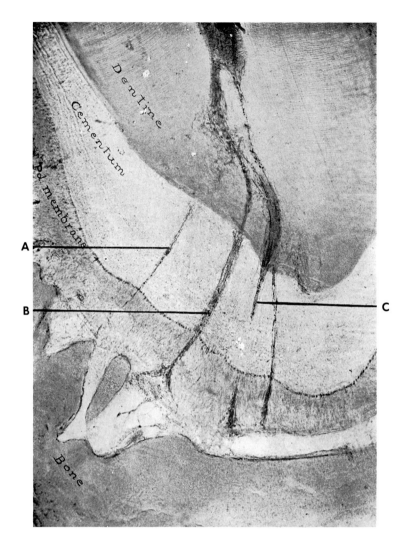

Figure 13–5. A section through the apex of a root showing multiple canals (*A–C*). Three canals are present within the dentin, but one canal divides at the cementum-dentin junction (*C*), making a total of four small canals that exit on the cemental surface of the tooth (Talbot).

prolongations are called pulp horns (Fig. 13–7). The prominence of the cusps or lobes corresponds with the development of the pulp horns. If the cusps or labial lobes are prominent (as in young individuals), we should expect to find equally prominent pulp horns underlying these structures (Fig. 13–8, *B, 5* and *6*). These projections become less prominent with time as a result of the formation of secondary dentin (Fig. 13–8, *B, 1*).

The Pulp Cavities of the Maxillary Teeth

Maxillary Central Incisors (Fig. 13–8, *A, B, C, D*)

Labiolingual Section (A)

The pulp cavity follows the general outline of the crown and root. The pulp chamber is very narrow in the incisal region. If a great amount of secondary or irritation dentin has been produced, this portion of the pulp chamber may be partially or completely obliterated (Fig.

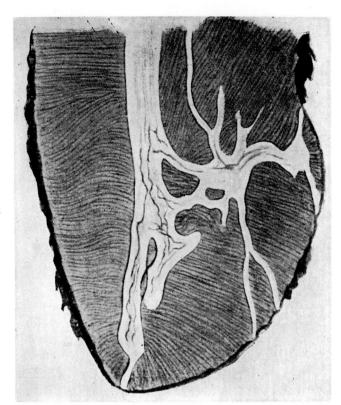

Figure 13-6. Apical end on root showing one main canal and an adjacent delta system. (From Riethmuller, R. H.: The filling of root canals with Prinz' paraffin compound. Dental Cosmos, 56:490, 1914.)

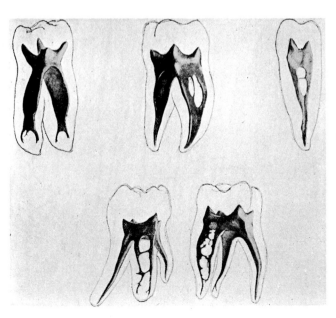

Figure 13-7. Molar and bicuspid pulp cavities. Note the prominence of the pulp horns and the complexities of the pulp chambers and root canal systems. (From Riethmuller, R. H.: The filling of root canals with Prinz' paraffin compound. Dental Cosmos, 56:490, 1914.)

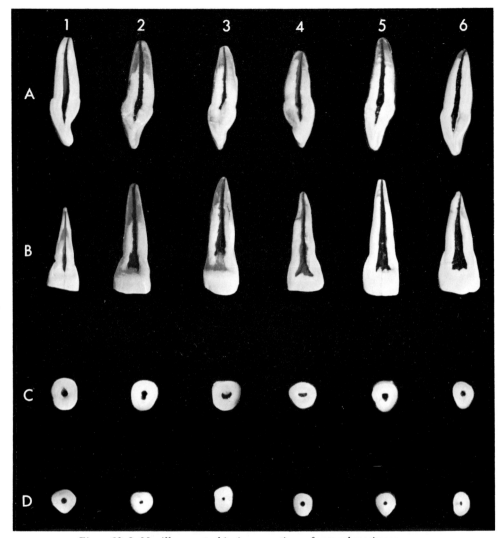

Figure 13–8. Maxillary central incisor—sections of natural specimens.
A, 1 to 6, Labiolingual sections. This aspect does not appear in radiographs.
B, 1 to 6, Mesiodistal sections.
C, 1 to 6, Cervical cross sections of root.
D, 1 to 6, Midroot cross sections.

13–8, *A, 3*). In the cervical region of the tooth, the pulp chamber increases to its largest labiolingual dimension.

Below the cervical area, the root canal tapers, gradually ending in a constriction at the apex of the tooth (apical constriction). The apical foramen is usually located near the very tip of the root but may be located slightly to the labial (Fig. 13–8, *A, 2, 3,* and *5*) or lingual aspect of the root (Fig. 13–8, *A, 6*). Because of this generalized phenomenon it has been suggested that the root canal filling should appear on radiographs to extend no closer than 1 mm from the radiographic apex of the tooth.

Mesiodistal Section (B)

The pulp chamber is wider in the mesiodistal dimension than in the labiolingual dimension. The pulp cavity conforms to the general shape of the outer surface of the tooth. If prominent mamelons (Fig. 1–9, *B*) are or have been present, it is not unusual to find definite prolongations or pulp horns in the incisal region of the tooth (Fig. 13–8, *B, 5* and *6*). The pulp cavity then tapers rather evenly along its entire length until reaching the apical constriction. The position of the apical foramen is usually slightly off center from the tip of the root, but some deviate drastically from the apex of the root (Fig. 13–8, *B, 6*).

Cervical Cross Section (C)

The pulp cavity is widest at the cervical level, and the pulp chamber is centered within the dentin of the root (Fig. 13–8, *C, 1–6*). In young individuals, the pulp chamber is roughly triangular in outline with the base of the triangle at the labial aspect of the root (Fig. 13–8, *C, 5*). As the amount of secondary or irritation dentin increases, the pulp chamber becomes more round or crescent-shaped (Fig. 13–8, *C, 3, 4,* and *6*). The outline form of the root at the cervical level is typically triangular with rounded corners (Fig. 13–8, *C, 4–6*), whereas some are more rectangular or angular with rounded corners (Fig. 13–8, *C, 1–3*). The root and pulp canal tend to be rounder at the midroot level (Fig. 13–8, *D, 1–6*) than at the cervical level. The anatomy at the midroot level is essentially the same as that found at the cervical level, just smaller in all dimensions. The importance of the location and shape of the pulp chamber and canal is shown in Figure 13–9, *A–C*.

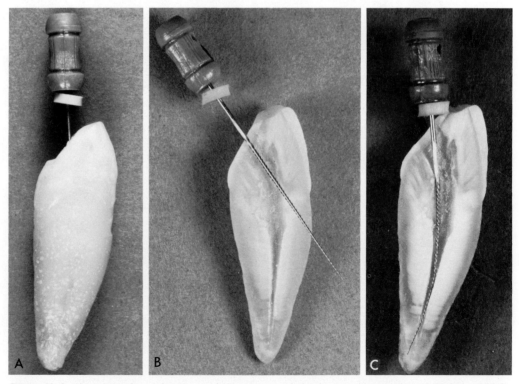

Figure 13–9. Access opening and root canal instrument angulation in a maxillary canine. *A,* Position of file in canal. *B,* Incorrect angulation for entrance into root canal. *C,* Flexible files are required to follow the difference in angulation between access to pulp chamber and entrance into the pulp canal.

Maxillary Lateral Incisor (Fig. 13–10, *A, B, C, D*)

Labiolingual Section (A)

The anatomy of the lateral incisor is very similar to that of the central incisor. The pulp cavity of the lateral incisor generally follows the outline form of the crown and the root. The pulp horns are usually prominent. The pulp chamber is narrow in the incisal region and may become very wide at the cervical level of the tooth (Fig. 13–10, *A, 3* and *5*). Those teeth lacking this cervical enlargement of the pulp chamber possess a root canal that tapers slightly to the apical constriction (Fig. 13–10, *A, 1, 4,* and *6*). Many of the apical foramina appear to be located at the tip of the root in the labiolingual aspect (Fig. 13–10, *A, 1, 3, 4,* and *6*), whereas some exit on the labial or lingual aspect of the root (Fig. 13–10, *A, 2,* and *5*).

Mesiodistal Cross Section (B)

The pulp cavity closely follows the external outline of the tooth. The pulpal projections or pulp horns appear to be blunted when viewed from the labial aspect of the tooth. The pulp chamber and root canal gradually taper toward the apex, which often demonstrates a significant curve in the apical region (Fig. 13–10, *B, 1, 2, 3,* and *6*).

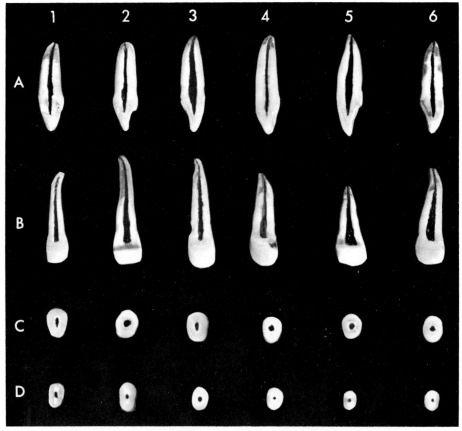

Figure 13–10. Maxillary lateral incisor—sections of natural specimens.
A, *1* to *6*, Labiolingual sections. This aspect does not appear in radiographs.
B, *1* to *6*, Mesiodistal sections.
C, *1* to *6*, Cervical cross sections of root.
D, *1* to *6*, Midroot cross sections.

Cervical Cross Section (C)

The cervical cross section shows the pulp chamber to be centered within the root. The root form of this tooth shows a large variation in shape (see the discussion of the lateral incisor, Chapter 6). The outline form of this tooth may be triangular, oval, or round (Fig. 13–10, *C*, *1, 3,* and *5*). The pulp chamber generally follows the outline form of the root, but secondary dentin may narrow the canal significantly (Fig. 13–10, *D, 4* and *6*). The anatomy of the pulp chamber of the various types of teeth must be known when performing endodontic access openings (Fig. 13–11). Figures 13–12 through 13–15 demonstrate the relationship of crown form to the pulp chamber and root canal.

Maxillary Canine (Fig. 13–16, *A, B, C, D, E*)

Labiolingual Section (A, D)

The maxillary canine has the largest labiolingual root dimension of any tooth in the mouth. Because the pulp cavity corresponds closely to the outline of the tooth, the size of the pulp chamber of this tooth may also be the largest in the mouth.

   The incisal aspect of the canine will correspond to the shape of the crown. If a prominent cusp is present, a long narrow projection from the pulp chamber (the pulp horn) will be present. The pulp chamber and incisal third or half of the root canal may be very wide, showing a very abrupt constriction of the root canal in the apical region, which then gently tapers toward the apex (Fig. 13–16, *A, 4–6* and *D, 16–18*). In other instances, a root canal may taper evenly from the pulp chamber to the apex of the root (Fig. 13–16, *A, 9; D, 10* and *12–14*).

   Some canines will possess severe curves in the apical aspect of the root (Fig. 13–16, *A, 3* and *7*). The apical foramen may appear to exit at the tip of the root (Fig. 13–16, *A, 2, 3,* and *5–9; D, 10, 11, 17,* and *18*) or labially to the apex of the root (Fig. 13–16, *D, 1, 4,* and *12–16*).

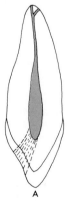
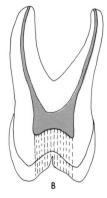

Figure 13–11. *A,* Drawing of a labiolingual section of a maxillary canine. Dotted lines represent the opening suggested for the approach to the pulp chamber.
B, Drawing of a buccolingual section of a maxillary molar. Dotted lines represent the opening suggested for the approach to the pulp chamber.

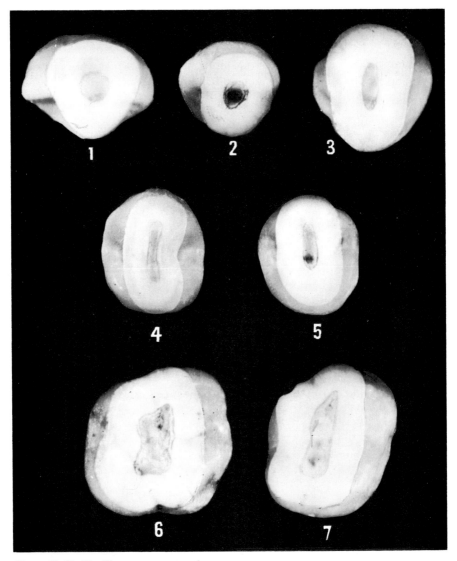

Figure 13–12. Maxillary permanent teeth.
    1, Central incisor.
    2, Lateral incisor.
    3, Canine.
    4, First premolar.
    5, Second premolar.
    6, First molar.
    7, Second molar.
    Interesting photographs of natural teeth made by a process of double exposure. Tooth specimens were sawed through at the cervical line; an exposure was made with the sections placed together, and one was made of occlusal and incisal views. Then the crown was removed and another exposure was made of the cross section at the cervix on the same film.
    The result is shown above, and the proportion of crown outline to cervical outline is accurately portrayed. The angulation of the field when such small specimens were exposed and the possibility of movement made standardization too difficult; consequently, some of the pictures do not have the crown and cervices centered in line with the long axis. Nevertheless, from an operative point of view, a comparison of the above photos makes an interesting study. (Courtesy of Dr. John T. Bird, Washington University School of Dentistry.)

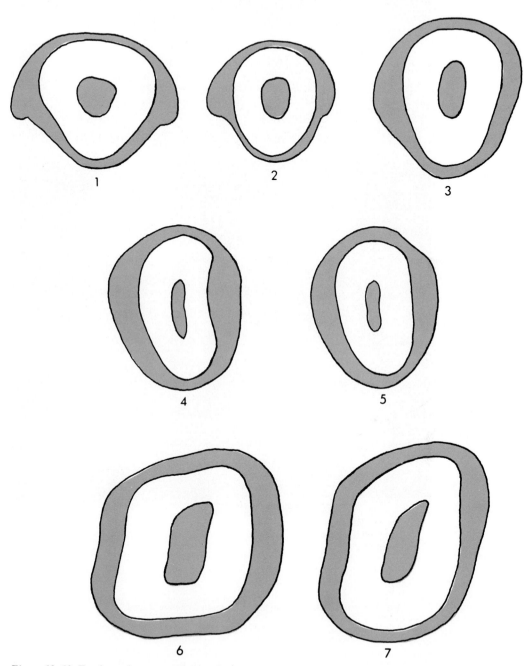

Figure 13–13. Tracings of crown outlines and root trunk outlines from Figure 13–12 placed in proper relation to each other. The photos of crowns and roots were correct in showing relative sizes, but the difficulties experienced in making double exposures prevented correct alignment at times.

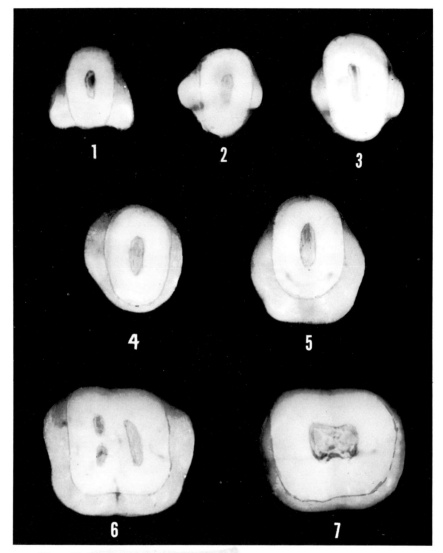

Figure 13–14. Mandibular permanent teeth.
1, Central incisor.
2, Lateral incisor.
3, Canine.
4, First premolar.
5, Second premolar.
6, First molar.
7, Second molar.
Double exposure photos of mandibular teeth to be compared with Figure 13–12.

Mesiodistal Section (B, E)

The pulp cavity is much narrower in the mesiodistal aspect. The dimension and degree of taper of the pulp canal of the maxillary canine are very similar to those of the central and lateral incisors; however, the cuspid has a much longer root. The pulp cavity gently tapers from the incisal aspect to the apical foramen. A mesial or distal curve of the apical root may be present (Fig. 13–16, *B, 1, 4, 6,* and *8; E, 14, 17,* and *18*). The apical foramen may appear

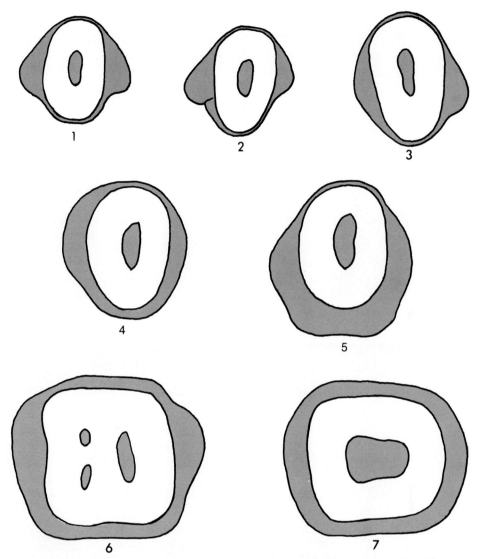

Figure 13–15. Tracings of crown outlines and root trunk outlines from Figure 13–14, placed in proper relation to each other. The photos of crowns and roots were correct in showing relative sizes, but the difficulties experienced in making double exposures prevented correct alignment at times.

to exit at the tip of the root (Fig. 13–16, *B, 1, 3–5, 7,* and *9; E, 10, 11, 13, 14, 17,* and *18*) or slightly to the mesial or distal aspect of the root (Fig. 13–16, *B, 2, 6,* and *8; E, 12, 15,* and *16*).

Cervical Cross Section (C)

The shape of the root and pulp cavity is oval (Fig. 13–16, *C, 6, 7,* and *9*), triangular (Fig. 13–16, *C, 8*), or elliptical (Fig. 13–16, *C, 1–5*). The pulp chamber and canal are usually centered within the crown and root (Fig. 13–16, *C, 1* and *3*).

The extent and location of openings for endodontic therapy are shown in Figures

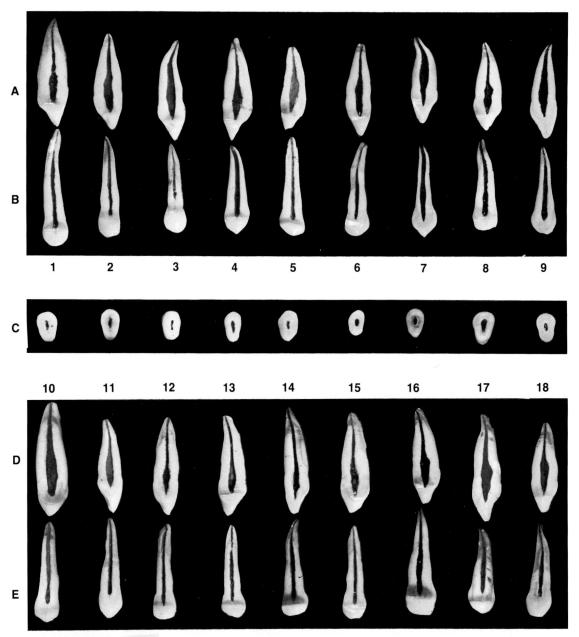

Figure 13–16. Maxillary canine.

A, Labiolingual section, exposing the mesial or distal aspect of the pulp cavity. This aspect does not appear in dental radiographs.

B, Mesiodistal section, exposing the labial or lingual aspect of the pulp cavity.

C, Cervical cross section at the cementoenamel junction exposing the pulp chamber. These are the openings to root canals that will be seen in the floor of the pulp chamber.

D, Labiolingual section, exposing the mesial or distal aspect of the pulp cavity.

E, Mesiodistal section, exposing the labial or lingual aspect of the pulp cavity.

13–17, *A*, and *B;* and 13–19. Figure 13–18 demonstrates the approximate locations of the canals.

Maxillary First Premolar (Fig. 13–20, *A, B, C, D, E*)

Buccolingual Section (A, D)

The maxillary first premolar may have two well-developed roots (Fig. 13–20, *A, 1, 2,* and *9; D, 10,* and *14*), two root projections which are not fully separated (Fig. 13–20, *A, 3, 5, 7,* and *8; D, 11–13* and *15–17*), or one broad root (Fig. 13–20, *A, 4* and *6; D, 18*). The majority of maxillary first premolars have two root canals (Fig. 13–20, *A* and *D*). A small percentage of maxillary first premolar teeth may have three roots that may be almost undetectable radiographically.

The pulp horn usually extends further incisally under the buccal cusp because this cusp is usually better developed than the lingual cusp. The pulp horns may be blunted (Fig. 13–20, *A, 1, 5,* and *6; D, 11*) in teeth possessing cusps that demonstrate a fair amount of attrition. The pulp chamber floor is below the cervical level of all the variations found in the maxillary first premolar. The pulp chamber of teeth having the least root separation usually shows the largest incisal apical dimension (Fig. 13–20, *A, 4; D, 18*). Those teeth possessing a partial root separation may also have this large dimension (Fig. 13–20, *A, 8*). Teeth having two separate canals usually demonstrate a rather small pulp chamber in the incisal-apical direction (Fig. 13–20, *A, 1, 2,* and *9; D, 10* and *14*). The shape of the pulp chamber (excluding the pulp horns) tends to be square (Fig. 13–20, *A, 1* and *8; D, 10, 12–14,* and *18*) or rectangular (Fig. 13–20, *A, 2–7; D, 11, 15–17*).

The root canal often appears to exit at the tip of the root (Fig. 13–20, *A, 1, 4, 6–8; B, 12, 13, 15–18*), slightly off center (Fig. 13–20, *A, 2, 3*), or a combination of the two locations (Fig. 13–20, *A, 3, 5,* and *9; B, 10, 11,* and *14*).

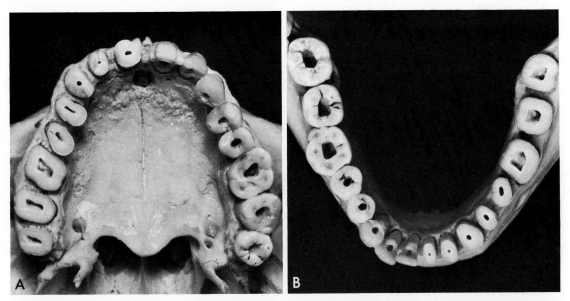

Figure 13–17. Access openings are shown for the left side of the maxillary arch (*A*) and for the right side of the mandibular arch (*B*). Cervical cross sections are shown for the right side of the maxillary arch and the left side of the mandibular arch.

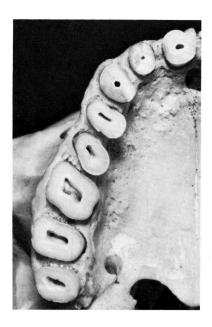

Figure 13–18. Enlargement of right maxillary arch of Figure 13–17, *A*, showing cervical cross sections. The alignment and relative shapes of the pulp chambers will help identify the number of canals that are present.

Mesiodistal Section (D, E)

The pulp horns appear blunted from the mesial or distal aspect. The pulp chamber cannot be differentiated from the root canal. The pulp cavity tapers slightly from the occlusal aspect to the apical foramen. If two canals are present, the radiopacity will increase in the apical half of the tooth because of an increased amount of dentin and bone and a decrease in volume of the pulp cavity.

The apical foramen appears to exit at the tip of the root most of the time (Fig. 13–20, *B*, *1–3*, and *6–9; E, 10, 12–18*), whereas some appear to exit on the buccal or lingual aspect of the root (Fig. 13–20, *4* and *5; E, 11*).

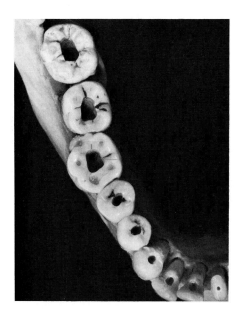

Figure 13–19. Enlargement of right mandibular arch of Figure 13–17, *B*, showing access openings. The alignment and relative shapes of the pulp chambers will help identify the number of canals that are present.

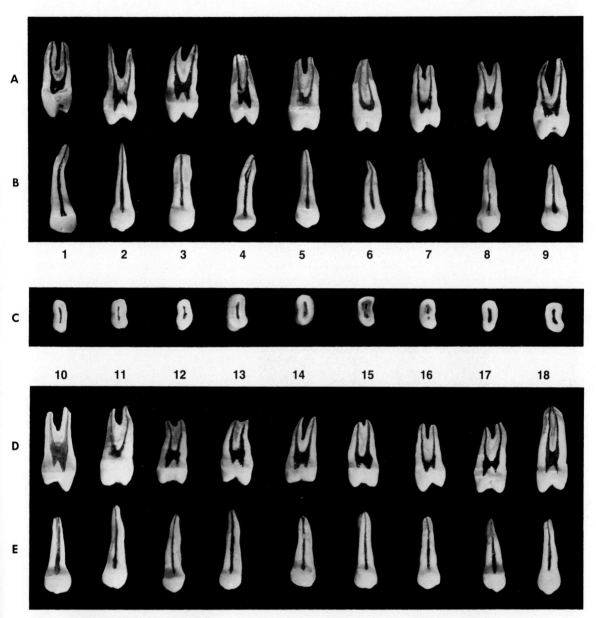

Figure 13–20. Maxillary first premolar.
  A, Buccolingual section, exposing the mesial or distal aspect of the pulp cavity. This aspect does not appear on dental radiographs.
  B, Mesiodistal section, exposing the buccal or lingual aspect of the pulp cavity.
  C, Cervical cross section at the cementoenamel junction exposing the pulp chamber. These are the openings to root canals that will be seen in the floor of the pulp chamber.
  D, Buccolingual section, exposing the mesial or distal aspect of the pulp cavity.
  E, Mesiodistal section, exposing the buccal or lingual aspect of the pulp cavity.

Cervical Cross Section (C)

The cross section of the cervical level shows the characteristic kidney-shaped outline form of the maxillary first premolar (Fig. 13–21, *B*). A mesial developmental groove is usually present, giving this tooth its classic indentation. The pulp cavity may demonstrate a constriction adjacent to the developmental groove (Fig. 13–20, *C, 2, 3, 6,* and *9*), or it may follow the general outline of the root surface (Fig. 13–20, *C, 1, 4, 5,* and *8*). Some roots will demonstrate two separate root canals (Fig. 13–20, *C, 7;* and Fig. 13–21), while a cross section of a three-rooted maxillary first premolar will show three separate canals (Fig. 13–20, *C, 3*).

Maxillary Second Premolar (Fig. 13–22, *A, B, C, D, E*)

Buccolingual Section (A, D)

Most maxillary second premolars have only one root and canal. Two roots are possible, although two canals within a single root may also be found. The pulp cavity may demonstrate well-developed pulp horns (Fig. 13–22, *A, 1, 2,* and *6–8; D, 10–12, 14, 16,* and *17*); others may have blunted or nonexistent pulp horns (Fig. 13–22, *A, 3–5, 9; D, 13, 15,* and *18*). The pulp chamber and root canal are very broad in the buccolingual aspect of single-canaled teeth. The pulp cavity does not show a well-defined demarcation between the root

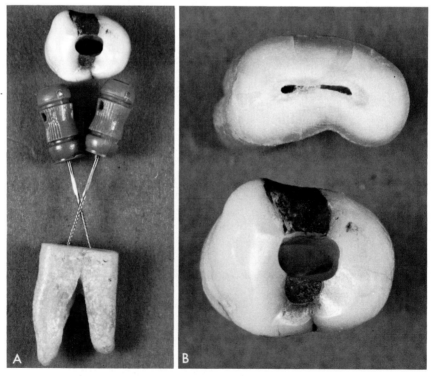

Figure 13–21. Maxillary first premolar. *A,* The access opening shown would allow instrumentation of the canal system. It should be noted that the files may cross in the cervical region in teeth possessing two separate canals. *B,* The access opening in the crown and a cross section at the cervical level demonstrate the relationship between their shapes.

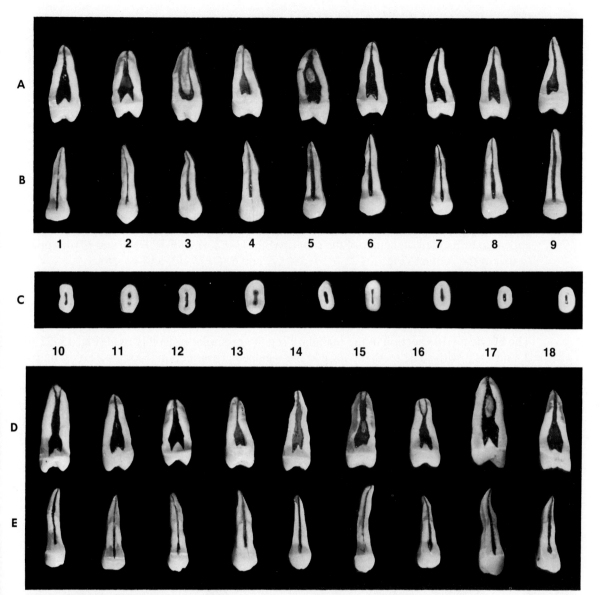

Figure 13–22. Maxillary second premolar.
    A, Buccolingual section, exposing the mesial or distal aspect of the pulp cavity. This aspect does not appear on the dental radiographs.
    B, Mesiodistal section, exposing the buccal or lingual aspect of the pulp cavity.
    C, Cervical cross section at the cementoenamel junction exposing the pulp chamber. These are the openings to root canals that will be seen in the floor of the pulp chamber.
    D, Buccolingual section, exposing the mesial or distal aspect of the pulp cavity.
    E, Mesiodistal section, exposing the buccal or lingual aspect of the pulp cavity.

cavity and the pulp cavity because of the large buccolingual extent of the pulp cavity in the upper half of the tooth. In the apical half or third of the tooth, the pulp cavity narrows abruptly (Fig. 13–22, *A, 1, 2, 4, 6, 8; D, 11–13,* and *18*) and then tapers gently toward the apex. Some teeth possess dentinal islands in the apical third of the root; this situation essentially forces the clinician to treat these as two-canaled teeth (Fig. 13–22, *A, 5; D, 15* and *17*). Other maxillary second premolars have a canal that bifurcates at the apical third of the root (Fig. 13–22, *D, 10, 15,* and *16*). It should also be noted that buccal and lingual pulpal projections or fins are present at the level of the cementoenamel junction (Fig. 13–22, *A, 2; D, 12* and *18*). Some teeth will show a constriction at this same level (Fig. 13–22, *D, 10*).

The apical foramen will often appear to exit at the tip of the root (Fig. 13–22, *A, 1, 2, 5, 6, 8; D, 11, 12,* and *14–18*). Some apical foramina appear to exit on the buccal aspect of the root (Fig. 13–22, *A, 4; D, 13*), on the lingual aspect of the root (Fig. 13–22, *A, 7* and *9*), or on both sides of the root tip (Fig. 13–22, *A, 3; D, 10, 15,* and *16*).

Mesiodistal Section (B, E)

The view of the pulp cavity in the mesiodistal section of the second maxillary premolar does not vary from that found in the maxillary first premolar. The pulp horns are blunted, and the pulp cavity tapers slightly from the occlusal aspect to the apex. The apical foramen may appear to be located off center of the root tip (Fig. 13–22, *A, 2, 6, 9; D, 10* and *13*) or appear to exit at the root tip (Fig. 13–22, *A, 1, 3–5, 7,* and *8; D, 11, 12,* and *14–18*).

Cervical Cross Section (C)

The cervical cross section of the maxillary second premolar is usually oval (Fig. 13–22, *C, 2,* and *4–9*), with some teeth having a kidney-shaped cross section (Fig. 13–22, *C, 1* and *3*). The pulp cavity will be centered in the root and may have a constriction in the middle of the canal space (Fig. 13–22, *C, 1, 4, 6,* and *9*), an entire separation (Fig. 13–22, *C, 2*) or an elliptical pulp cavity (Fig. 13–22, *C, 3, 5, 7,* and *8*). The similarities of the maxillary first and second premolar chambers are easily seen in cervical cross sections (Fig. 13–23, *B;* and Fig. 13–21).

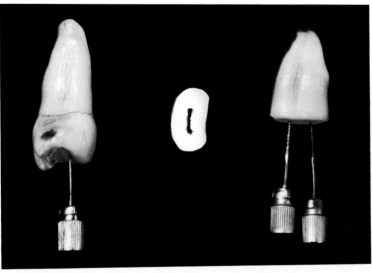

Figure 13–23. Maxillary second premolar.

1, Position of instrument as it enters single broad canal through a comparatively wide occlusal opening buccolingually. Sometimes the broad canal buccolingually will branch as it progresses apically. (See No. 16, Figure 13–22).

2, Cross section of root at cementoenamel junction is slightly kidney-shaped with elongated pulp chamber, but it is less extreme in this respect than the maxillary first premolar.

3, Two root canal instruments placed partially parallel in the broad canal with the crown removed for clarity of observation.

1   2   3

Maxillary First Molar (Fig. 13–24, *A, B, C, D, E*)

Buccolingual Section (A, D)

The buccolingual section of the maxillary first molar shows the pulp cavities of the mesio-buccal and palatal root. These roots were chosen to demonstrate the pulp cavity anatomy because of the complexity of the mesiobuccal root. The distobuccal root is straighter and

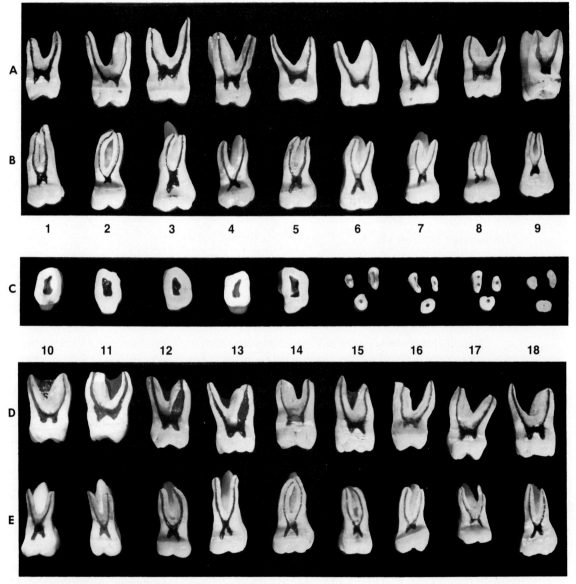

Figure 13–24. Maxillary first molar.
    A, Buccolingual section, exposing the mesial or distal aspect of the pulp cavity. This aspect does not appear on dental radiographs.
    B, Mesiodistal section, exposing the buccal or lingual aspect of the pulp cavity.
    C, Five cross sections at cervical line and four cross sections at midroot.
    D, Buccolingual section, exposing the mesial or distal aspect of the pulp cavity.
    E, Mesiodistal section, exposing the buccal aspect of the pulp cavity.

smaller and presents fewer variations in shape. The entire removal of the pulp is an impossibility in many maxillary first molar teeth because of the complexities of the root canal system (Fig. 13–7).

The maxillary first molar usually has three roots and three canals. The palatal root usually has the largest dimensions, followed by the distobuccal and mesiobuccal roots, respectively. The mesiobuccal root is often very wide buccolingually and often possesses an accessory canal, which usually is the smallest of all the canals in this tooth.

The pulp horns are usually prominent in this tooth (Fig. 13–24, *A, 1* and *4–8; D, 10–13,* and *15–18*). The pulp chamber is somewhat rectangular in shape (excluding the pulp horns) when viewed from the mesial aspect of the tooth. The palatal root canal usually has the largest canal (Fig. 13–24, *A, 1–3, 5,* and *6; D, 10, 15, 17,* and *18*). The mesiobuccal canal is often very small (Fig. 13–24, *A, 2,* and *6; D, 10, 14,* and *17*), but some mesiobuccal canals may be very wide within a very wide root (Fig. 13–24, *A, 9; D, 12* and *13*).

The root canals of the wide mesiobuccal roots are widest at the midroot level and taper to a very fine diameter at the apical foramen. The palatal root canal and the mesiobuccal root canal of most teeth taper gently to the apical region where they terminate at or near the apex. The apical foramen of the palatal canal may appear to exit at the apex (Fig. 13–24, *A, 1* and *4–9; D, 11–18*), slightly lingually (Fig. 13–24, *A, 2; D, 10*), or buccally to the root tip (Fig. 13–24, *A, 3; D, 17*).

The apical foramen of the mesiobuccal canal may appear to exit on the tip of the root (Fig. 13–24, *A, 2–5* and *7–9; D, 10, 12, 13, 17,* and *18*), on the buccal (Fig. 13–24, *A, 1* and *6; D, 11, 14,* and *15*) or on the lingual (Fig. 13–24, *D, 16*) aspect of the root.

Mesiodistal Section **(B, E)**

The mesiodistal section of the maxillary first molar includes the distobuccal root, which was not visible on the buccolingual section. The mesiobuccal root has a great tendency to possess a more curved root and canal than the distobuccal root (Fig. 13–24, *B, 1–3,* and *5–8; E, 12, 14,* and *15*). Some of the buccal canals are relatively straight (Fig. 13–24, *E, 10, 11,* and *13*).

The pulp horns are very distinct from this view, with the mesiobuccal pulp horn usually appearing a little larger than the distobuccal pulp horn (Fig. 13–24, *B, 1,* and *3–9; E, 10–13,* and *15–18*). In some teeth, the pulp horns are of equal size (Fig. 13–24, *B, 2; E, 14*). The pulp chamber is somewhat square (if the pulp horns are excluded) when viewed from the buccal aspect. The demarcation of the root canal is much more distinct in the mesiodistal section. The root canals appear much smaller when viewed from the buccal or lingual aspect. The canals taper slightly as they approach the apical foramen. The apical foramen often appears to be located at the tip of the root (Fig. 13–24, *B, 1–7* and *9; E, 11, 14, 16,* and *18*), but the apical foramen may appear to be located on the mesial (Fig. 13–24, *E, 15,* and *17,* mesial roots only) or distal aspect of the root (Fig. 13–24, *A, 8; D, 10, 12,* and *13,* distal root only).

Cervical Cross Section **(C)**

The cervical outline form of the maxillary first molar is rhomboidal in shape with rounded corners (Fig. 13–24, *C, 1–5;* and Fig. 13–26). The mesiobuccal angle has an acute angle, the distobuccal angle is obtuse, and the lingual angles are essentially right angles. The orifices of the root canals have the following relation to the floor of the pulp chamber: The palatal canal is centered lingually; the distobuccal canal is near the obtuse angle of the pulp chamber; the mesiobuccal root canal is buccal and mesial to the distobuccal canal, in what seems to be the extreme corner, positioned within the acute angle of the pulp chamber. If an accessory mesiobuccal canal is present, it will be located lingual to the mesiobuccal canal or distolingually. The canals of this tooth form a triangular pattern; a line drawn between the mesiobuccal canal and the palatal canal makes the base of the triangle, and the distobuccal canal (which is slightly closer to the palatal canal) makes the third point of the triangle. If a mesiobuccal accessory canal is present, it will be between the mesiobuccal and palatal canal just off the imaginary line between the two canals (Fig. 13–24, *C, 7–9*).

Midroot Cross Section (C)

The midroot sections were added to the molar descriptions because some molars possess more than one canal within the root (Fig. 13–24, *C, 6–9*). The palatal root is usually the largest root having a round outline form. The distobuccal canal is oval to round in shape but much smaller than the palatal root. The mesiobuccal root is an elongated oval- to kidney-shaped root with the indentation located toward the furcation. The root canals of the palatal and distobuccal root are oval to round, whereas the mesiobuccal canals are elongated (Fig. 13–24, *C, 6 and 9*), elliptical (Fig. 13–24, *C, 7*), or round (Fig. 13–24, *C, 8 and 9*). The pulp canals may be extremely difficult to locate and instrument if secondary or irritation dentin is abundant (Fig. 13–24, *C, 9*). A thorough knowledge of the anatomy of the pulp chambers and canals is necessary if endodontic procedures are to be accomplished (Figs. 13–25 through 13–27).

Maxillary Second Molar (Fig. 13–28, *A, B, C, D, E*)

Buccolingual Section (A, D)

The buccal roots of the maxillary second molar are straighter and closer together than those of the maxillary first molar. The tendency for root fusion is greater in the second maxillary molar than in the first maxillary molar, but the palatal root is usually separate. Most maxillary second molars possess three roots and three canals. The mesiobuccal root of the maxillary second molar is not as complex as that formed in the maxillary first molar. The tendency for a very wide mesiobuccal canal is not present in the maxillary second molar.

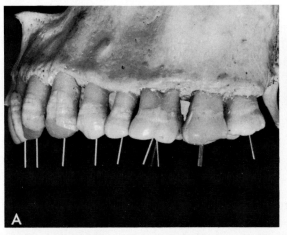 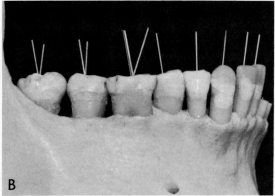

Figure 13–25. Maxillary (*A*) and mandibular (*B*) arches. A silver cone has been inserted into every canal through the access opening, demonstrating the angle of approach for each of the root canals within each type of tooth.

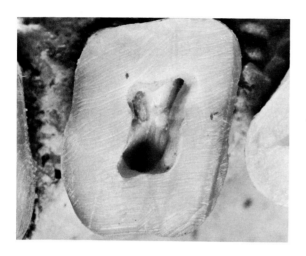

Figure 13–26. This cervical cross section demonstrates the relationship between the pulp chamber and the outline form of the tooth.

Although the presence of two canals in the mesiobuccal root of the maxillary second molar is not common, it does occur (Fig. 13–28, *A, 5* and *7*).

The pulp horns may be well developed (Fig. 13–28, *A, 1–5, 8,* and *9; D, 10–18*) or virtually absent (Fig. 13–28, *A, 4, 6,* and *7*). The pulp chamber appears somewhat rectangular (excluding the pulp horns) in shape. The pulp canals gradually taper toward the apex until reaching the apical constriction, which occurs just before the apical foramen.

The mesiobuccal root canal of the maxillary second molar does not have the tendency to be extremely large, as is demonstrated in the mesiobuccal canal of the maxillary first molar. The apical foramen of the palatal root often appears to exit at the tip of the root (Fig. 13–28, *A, 1–3* and *5–8; D, 11, 13, 14, 16–18*), but it may exist on the lingual (*A, 4* and *9; D, 1* and *5*) or buccal aspect of the root (Fig. 13–28, *D, 10* and *12*).

Mesiodistal Section (B, E)

The mesiodistal section of the maxillary second molar is similar to that of the maxillary first molar. The buccal roots of the second molar are not separated as far apart as they are in the maxillary first molar, and their buccal roots have a greater tendency to be fused.

The pulp horns are usually well developed (Fig. 13–28, *B, 1–5, 8,* and *9; E, 10–15* and *17*). Some teeth demonstrate an obvious blunting or absence of the pulp horns (Fig. 13–28, *B, 6* and *7; E, 18*). The mesiobuccal pulp horn is often larger than the distobuccal pulp horn (Fig. 13–28, *B, 1, 4, 5, 8,* and *9; E, 10, 12, 13, 15, 17,* and *18*).

The pulp chamber is much smaller in the mesiodistal section than in the buccolingual section. The pulp chamber is square (excluding the pulp horns) when viewed from the buccal aspect. The pulp canals gently taper from the pulp chamber to the apical constriction. The mesiobuccal pulp canal has a greater tendency to be curved than the distobuccal canal. The majority of the apical foramen appears to exit at the tip of the root (Fig. 13–28, *B, 1–9; E, 10–16* and *18*).

Cervical Cross Section (C)

The cervical cross section of the maxillary second molar demonstrates angulations of the outline form that are more extreme than those found in the maxillary first molar. The mesiobuccal angle is more acute and the distobuccal angle is more obtuse than that found in the maxillary first molar and the outline form of the pulp chamber reflects these differences.

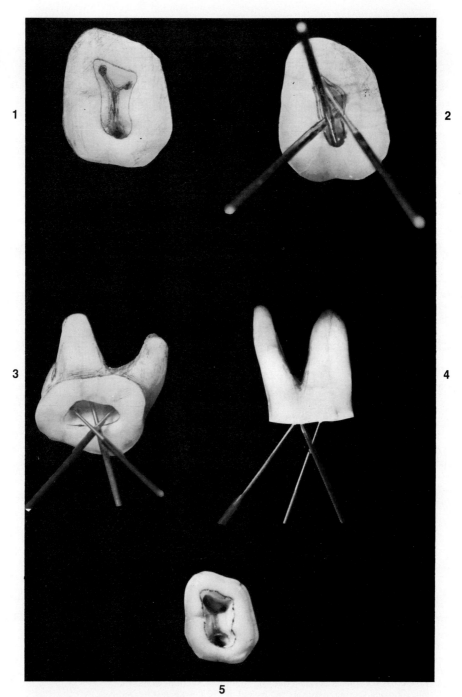

1   2

3   4

5

Figure 13–27. Maxillary first molar.

    1, The exposed pulp chamber looks somewhat enlarged when the crown is removed at the cementoenamel junction. Note the relative location of the entrances to pulp canals. The distobuccal and the palatal canal openings are in line buccolingually, but the mesiobuccal canal opening is in a rather extreme mesiobuccal direction toward the mesiobuccal line angle of the tooth crown.

    2, The same subject with probes in the canals, demonstrating the varied directions traveled.

    3, The same subject as *2,* with the tooth over on its side, presenting a different perspective.

    4, The same specimen as *3,* providing still another view for comparison.

    5, An unretouched photograph of another specimen of maxillary first molar showing rather graphically the open pulp chamber with its entrances to pulp canals.

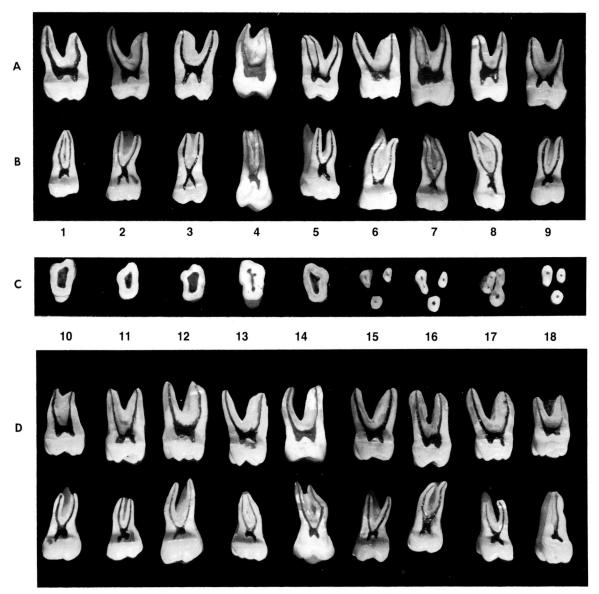

Figure 13–28. Maxillary second molar.
   A, Buccolingual section, exposing the mesial or distal aspect of the pulp cavity. This aspect does not appear in dental radiographs.
   B, Mesiodistal section, exposing the buccal or lingual aspect of the pulp cavity.
   C, Five cross sections at cervical line and four cross sections at midroot.
   D, Buccolingual section, exposing the mesial or distal aspect of the pulp cavity.
   E, Mesiodistal section, exposing the buccal or lingual aspect of the pulp cavity.

The mesiobuccal canal orifice is located farther to the buccal and mesial aspect of the pulp chamber (Fig. 13–28, *C, 4* and *5*). The distobuccal canal more nearly approaches the midpoint between the mesiobuccal and palatal canal (Fig. 13–28, *C, 4*). The palatal canal is located at the most lingual aspect of the root. Because of the tendency for the roots to be fused or at least closer together, the orifices of the root canals in the maxillary second molar are much closer together than in the maxillary first molar (Fig. 13–28, *C, 4*). In the cervical cross section, the triangularity of the floor of the pulp chamber is clearly demonstrated.

Midroot Cross Section (C)

The palatal root of the maxillary second molar may be the largest of the three roots (Fig. 13–28, *C, 6–9*). The mesiobuccal root may have a larger buccolingual dimension, but it has a narrower mesiodistal dimension. The distobuccal canal is the smallest root of the three. The distobuccal root and the palatal root have a round or oval outline form. The mesiobuccal root is usually rectangular in shape with rounded corners. If one canal is present, the canal follows the outline form of the root and is usually narrower at the middle of the root, making the canal appear as two canals (Fig. 13–28, *C, 7*). If two separate canals are present, they are usually round (Fig. 13–28, *C, 8*). Anatomical similarities are present between the first and second maxillary molars, but differences do exist and should be acknowledged while performing endodontic procedures (Fig. 13–29).

Maxillary Third Molar (Fig. 13–30, *A, B, C, D, E*)

The maxillary third molar has the most variable anatomy of any of the maxillary teeth. A description of the pulpal anatomy will not be provided because of the tremendous variability of the maxillary third molar. A sample of longitudinal and cross sections, displayed in the same manner as all the other maxillary teeth, shows a comparison of this molar with the other maxillary molars (Fig. 13–30). When the maxillary third molar is compared in development and eruption with findings in the other maxillary molars, it is evident that the third molar is smaller than the other molars. The crown is usually triangular or round rather than quadrilateral. The roots are shorter, more curved, and have a greater tendency for root

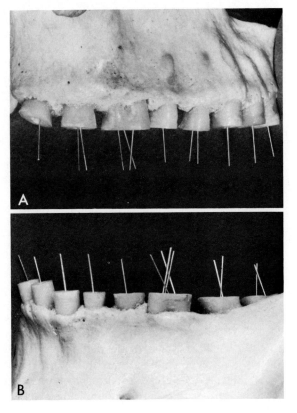

Figure 13–29. Maxillary (*A*) and mandibular (*B*) arches. A silver cone was inserted into every canal after the crown was removed, demonstrating the angle of approach for the root canals within each type of tooth.

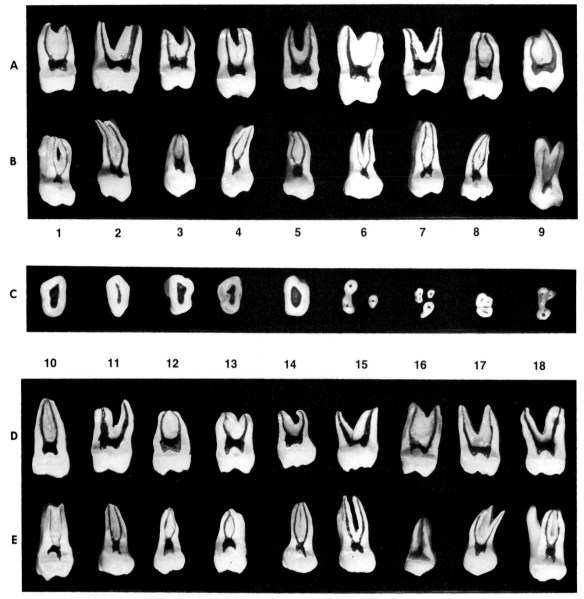

Figure 13–30. Maxillary third molar.
    A, Buccolingual section, exposing the mesial or distal aspect of the pulp cavity. This aspect does not appear in dental radiographs.
    B, Mesiodistal section, exposing the buccal or lingual aspect of the pulp cavity.
    C, Five cross sections at cervical line and four cross sections at midroot.
    D, Buccolingual section, exposing the mesial or distal aspect of the pulp cavity.
    E, Mesiodistal section, exposing the buccal or lingual aspect of the pulp cavity.

fusion, which makes these teeth appear to be single-rooted (Fig. 13–30, *A, 8; B, 3, 5,* and *8; D, 10,* and *12; E, 11–14,* and *16*). Because the maxillary third molar is 8 or 9 years younger than the first molar, the pulp chamber will have less secondary dentin than the "older" first and second molars. This allows easier access to the canals. However, because of the higher incidence in malformations of the roots, the endodontic procedure may be very difficult. Third molars have generally been condemned without fully appreciating their possible usefulness in later years. If these teeth can be cleansed well and are functioning, they should be maintained since they could provide suitable support for restorative procedures in later years.

The Pulp Cavities of the Mandibular Teeth

Mandibular Central Incisor (Fig. 13–31, *A, B, C, D, E*)

Labiolingual Section (A, D)

The mandibular central incisor is the smallest tooth in the mouth, but its labiolingual dimension is very large. This tooth usually has one canal, but two canals may be found quite frequently. The pulp horn is well developed in this tooth (Fig. 13–31, *A, 1–6* and *8; D, 10–18*). As attrition occurs, irritation dentin is produced that will essentially move the pulp tissue farther from the original location of the external surface of the tooth (Fig. 13–31, *A, 9*). The pulp chamber may be very large (Fig. 13–31, *A, 2, 4, 5,* and *8; D, 10, 11, 13,* and *16–18*); intermediate in size (Fig. 13–31, *A, 1, 3, 6, 7,* and *9; D, 12*); or very small in size (Fig. 13–31, *D, 14, 15*). The pulp canal may taper gently to the apex (Fig. 13–31, *A, 2, 3,* and *7; D, 10, 11, 14, 16,* and *18*) or narrow abruptly in the apical 3 or 4 mm of the root (Fig. 13–31, *A, 1, 4, 5, 6,* and *8; D, 12, 13, 15,* and *17*). The apical foramen may appear to exit at the apex (Fig. 13–31, *A, 1, 4–7,* and *9; D, 11, 12, 15, 16,* and *18*) or on the buccal aspect of the root (Fig. 13–31, *A, 2, 3,* and *8; D, 10, 13,* and *14*).

Mesiodistal Section (B, E)

A buccal or facial view of a mesiodistal section of the mandibular central incisor demonstrates the narrowness of the pulp cavity. A small endodontic file can usually be used to negotiate these canals in spite of this narrowness because of the wide labiolingual dimension of the pulp chamber. However, secondary or tertiary (irritation) dentin may interfere with endodontic treatment (Fig. 13–31, *B, 7; D, 16* and *18; E, 13* and *18*). The pulp horn is usually prominent, but single. The canal also appears narrow, having a gentle taper from the pulp chamber to the apical constriction. The canal may exit at the apex (Fig. 13–31, *A, 2, 5,* and *8; E, 12, 14, 16,* and *17*), or mesially or distally to the apex of the root (Fig. 13–31, *A, 1, 3, 4, 6, 7,* and *9; D, 10, 11, 13, 15,* and *18*).

Cervical Cross Section (C)

The cervical cross section demonstrates the proportions of the root. The mesiodistal dimension is small, whereas the labiolingual dimension is very large. The external shape is variable; some are round, oval, or elliptical. The rounder the root, the rounder the canal. Two separate canals may be present, or a dentinal island may make it appear as though two canals are present (Fig. 13–32, *B*).

Mandibular Lateral Incisor (Fig. 13–33, *A, B, C, D, E*)

Labiolingual Section (A, D)

The mandibular lateral incisor tends to be a little larger than the mandibular central incisor in all dimensions, and the pulp chamber is also larger. The form and function of the mandibular lateral incisor are identical to those of the central incisor.

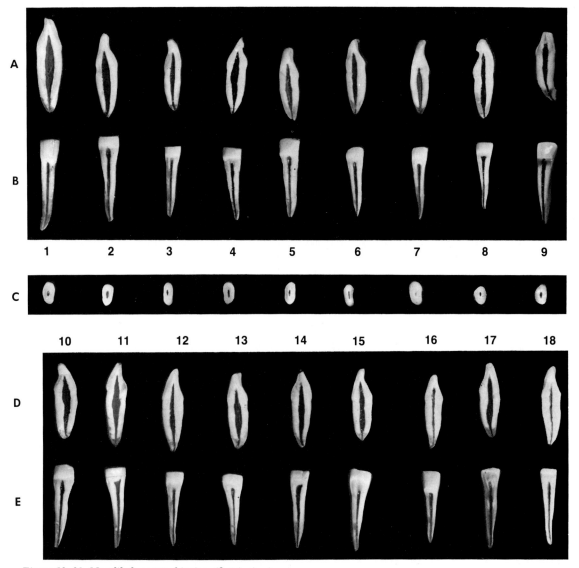

Figure 13–31. Mandibular central incisor (first incisor).

 A, Labiolingual section, exposing the mesial or distal aspect of the pulp cavity. This aspect does not appear on dental radiographs.

 B, Mesiodistal section, exposing the labial or lingual aspect of the pulp cavity.

 C, Cervical cross section at the cementoenamel junction exposing the pulp chamber. These are the openings to root canals that will be seen in the floor of the pulp chamber.

 D, Labiolingual section, exposing the mesial or distal aspect of the pulp cavity.

 E, Mesiodistal section, exposing the labial or lingual aspect of the pulp cavity.

  The pulp horn is usually prominent. The pulp chamber may possess a dimension that is very large (Fig. 13–33, *A, 2, 4, 5, 8,* and *9; D, 10–12,* and *16–18*), intermediate in size (Fig. 13–33, *A, 1, 3, 6, 7; D, 12*), or small in size (Fig. 13–33, *D, 14* and *15*). The pulp canal may taper gently from the apex (Fig. 13–33, *A, 1, 2, 4, 6, 7,* and *9; D, 12, 14–17*)or narrow abruptly in the last 3 to 4 mm of the canal (Fig. 13–33, *A, 3, 5,* and *8; D, 10–14*). The apical foramen appears to exit at the tip of the root (Fig. 13–33, *A, 1–6, 8,* and *9; D, 12–15, 17,* and *18*) or on the buccal or lingual aspect of the root tip (Fig. 13–33, *A, 7; D, 10, 11,* and *16*).

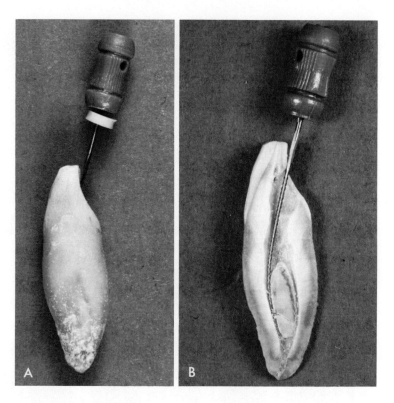

Figure 13–32. Mandibular central incisor. *A,* This view demonstrates the angle of a file, seen with adequate access. *B,* This longitudinal section demonstrates the need for flexible files and the presence of two canals.

Mesiodistal Section (B, E)

The pulp chamber and canal, as viewed from this aspect, will demonstrate a slender cavity. The mandibular lateral incisor resembles the mandibular incisor, but it may appear a little wider and have a pulpal dimension that is larger. The pulp horns are prominent, and the pulp chamber and canal gently taper to the apex. The apical foramen may appear to the exit at the tip (Fig. 13–33, *A, 1–4, 6, 7,* and *9; D, 10–15, 17,* and *18*) or on the mesial or distal aspect of the root tip (Fig. 13–33, *A, 5,* and *8; D, 16*).

Cervical Cross Section (C)

The cervical cross section of the mandibular lateral incisor will show the pulp canal centered in the root. A comparison of several of the sections demonstrates a root somewhat larger than the mandibular central incisor. There is considerable variation in the form of the root. The root outline form is oval to elliptical. Some cross sections of the larger teeth will resemble the cervical cross sections of small mandibular canines (Fig. 13–33, *C, 2–4*). The root canal will follow the outline form of the root, and some roots will demonstrate root grooves (Fig. 13–33, *C, 6*).

Mandibular Canine
(Fig. 13–34, *A, B, C, D, E*)

Labiolingual Section (A and D)

The pulp cavity of the mandibular canine is similar in size and shape to that of the maxillary canine. The mandibular canine tends to be a little shorter, although the opposite can be found. It is not uncommon to find two roots or at least two canals in the mandibular canine.

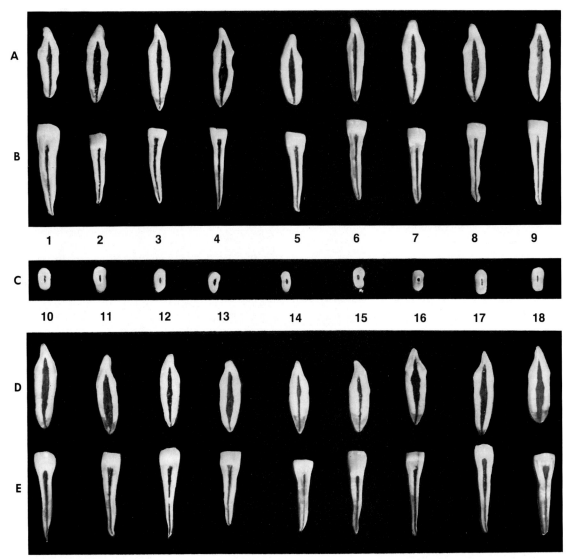

Figure 13–33. Mandibular lateral incisor (second incisor).

A, Labiolingual section, exposing the mesial or distal aspect of the pulp cavity. This aspect does not appear on the dental radiograph.

B, Mesiodistal section, exposing the labial or lingual aspect of the pulp cavity.

C, Cervical cross section at the cementoenamel junction, exposing the pulp chamber. These are the openings to root canals that will be seen in the floor of the pulp chamber.

D, Labiolingual section, exposing the mesial or distal aspect of the pulp cavity.

E, Mesiodistal section, exposing the labial or lingual aspect of the pulp cavity.

A dental "island" may be found in any tooth that demonstrates an extremely wide labiolingual dimension and a narrow mesiodistal dimension. Because the presence of two canals cannot be easily detected radiographically, their presence must be ruled out clinically as well.

The pulp cavity in a tooth of this kind varies according to where the section is examined (see Fig. 8–24, *1, 2, 5,* and *6*). The pulp horn is prominent in the mandibular canine unless an extensive amount of attrition has taken place (Fig. 13–34, *A, 1* and *3*). The pulp chamber usually is very wide (Fig. 13–34, *A, 1, 3–5, 7,* and *8; D, 10, 12, 14, 15, 17,* and

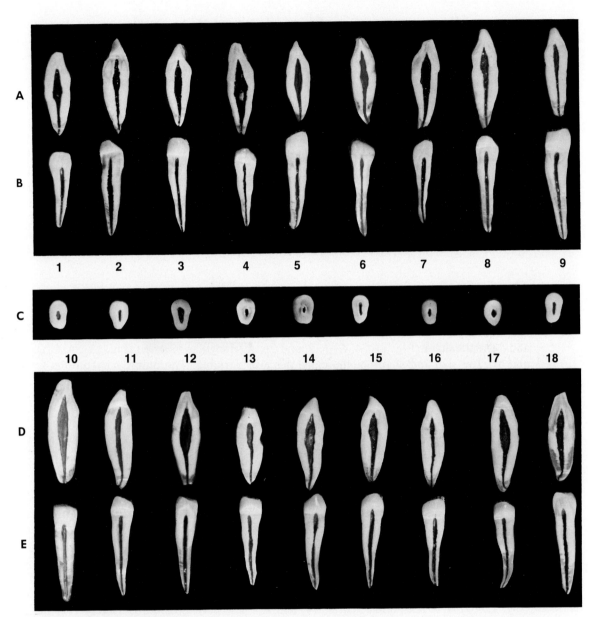

Figure 13–34. Mandibular canine.

A, Labiolingual section, exposing the mesial or distal aspect of the pulp cavity. This aspect does not appear on dental radiographs.

B, Mesiodistal section, exposing the labial or lingual aspect of the pulp cavity.

C, Cervical cross section at the cementoenamel junction, exposing the pulp chamber. These are the openings to root canals that will be seen in the floor of the pulp chamber.

D, Labiolingual section, exposing the mesial or distal aspect of the pulp cavity.

E, Mesiodistal section, exposing the labial or lingual aspect of the pulp cavity.

18,) but may be average to small in size (Fig. 13–34, *A, 2, 6,* and *9; D, 11, 13,* and *16*). Some mandibular canines demonstrate an abrupt narrowing of the pulp cavity when passing from the region of the pulp chamber to the region of the pulp canal (Fig. 13–34, *A, 1, 2, 6,* and *8; D, 13*). Other mandibular canines demonstrate an abrupt narrowing of the pulp canal in the apical region (Fig. 13–34, *A, 3,* and *4; D, 11, 12,* and *18*), after which the canal gently tapers to the apex. If an abrupt narrowing of the canal is absent, the tooth will demonstrate a canal that gently tapers to the apical foramen. The apical foramen often appears to exit at the tip of the apex (Fig. 13–34, *A, 3–5, 7*, and *9; D, 10*, and *12–16*), or slightly buccally (Fig. 13–34, *A, 1, 2, 6*, and *8; D, 11*, and *17*), or lingually to the root tip (Fig. 13–34, *D, 18*).

Mesiodistal Section (B, E)

The mesiodistal cross section of the mandibular canine appears very similar to that of the maxillary canine. The mesiodistal section demonstrates how narrow this tooth is in the mesiodistal aspect. This view also shows the degree of curvature of the apical portion of the root. The curvature of the root canal is usually in the mesial direction (Fig. 13–34, *E, 17*). The pulp horn is usually prominent but appears blunted in this view. The pulp chamber and canal show a continuous gentle taper to the apex where the apical foramen appears to exit at the tip of the root (Fig. 13–34, *A, 1–4*, and *6–8; D, 10–18*) or slightly mesially or distally to the root tip (Fig. 13–34, *A, 5*).

Cervical Cross Section (C)

A cervical cross section of the mandibular canine shows considerable variation in size and shape (Fig. 13–34, *C, 1–9*). The outline form of the root may be oval (Fig. 13–34, *C, 4, 7*, and *8*), rectangular (Fig. 13–34, *C, 1, 5*, and *9*), or triangular in shape (Fig. 13–34, *C, 2, 3*, and *6*). The size and shape of the canal are also variable. The pulp cavity outline form closely resembles the root form.

Mandibular First Premolar
(Fig. 13–35, A, B, C, D, E)

Buccolingual Section (A, D)

The mandibular first premolar looks like a small mandibular canine with an extra small cusp. The pulp cavity also looks similar to the mandibular canine. The majority of these teeth have one canal, but two canals are possible (Fig. 13–35, *A, 9; D, 18*).

   The pulp horn of the buccal cusp is prominent in some teeth (Fig. 13–35, *A, 1, 2, 4*, and *6–9; D, 10–18*). The pulp horn of the lingual cusp may be prominent but small (Fig. 13–35, *D, 15–17*), vestigial (Fig. 13–35, *A, 1, 4, 7*, and *9; D, 10, 11*, and *13*), or completely absent (Fig. 13–35, *A, 2, 3, 5*, and *6; D, 12, 14*, and *18*). The pulp chamber is usually very large. The pulp cavity may taper gently toward the apex (Fig. 13–35, *A, 2, 3, 5*, and *6; D, 12* and *13*), taper abruptly as the root canal starts (Fig. 13–35, *A, 1, 4*, and *7; D, 11* and *18*), or taper gently and abruptly constrict in the apical region (Fig. 13–35, *A, 8; D, 10*, and *14–16*).

   The apical foramen usually appears to exit at the apex (Fig. 13–35, *A, 1–9; D, 10–13* and *18*), or slightly to the buccal (Fig. 13–35, *D, 14* and *15*) or lingual aspect of the root tip (Fig. 13–35, *D, 17*).

Mesiodistal Section (B, E)

The pulp horn is prominent and may be very fine at its occlusal extent (Fig. 13–35, *A, 6* and *9; D, 12* and 18). The pulp chamber and root canal taper gently to the apex. The apical foramen may appear to exit at the tip of the root (Fig. 13–35, *A, 3, 5, 8*, and *9; D, 11, 14, 17*,

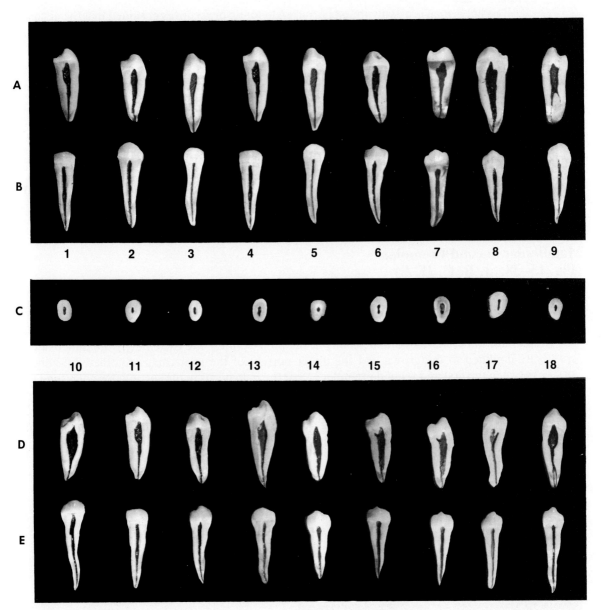

Figure 13–35. Mandibular first premolar.

    A, Buccolingual section, exposing the mesial or distal aspect of the pulp cavity. This aspect does not appear in a dental radiograph.

    B, Mesiodistal section, exposing the buccal or lingual aspect of the pulp cavity.

    C, Cervical cross section at the cementoenamel junction, exposing the pulp chamber. These are the openings to root canals that will be seen in the floor of the pulp chamber.

    D, Buccolingual section, exposing the mesial or distal aspect of the pulp cavity.

    E, Mesiodistal section, exposing the buccal or lingual aspect of the pulp cavity.

and *18*) or on the buccal or lingual aspect of the root (Fig. 13–35, *A, 1, 2, 4, 6,* and *7; D, 10, 12, 13, 15,* and *16*).

The pulp canal is usually found during endodontic procedures provided that the access opening is made in the long access of the tooth and not perpendicular to the cusps (Figs. 13–36 and 13–37).

Cervical Cross Section (C)

The crown and root size of the mandibular premolars vary considerably, and the pulp cavities vary proportionately. The outline form of the root may be oval (Fig. *13–35, C, 2, 3, 6,* and *9*), rectangular (Fig. 13–35, *C, 1* and *4*), or triangular (Fig. 13–35, *C, 5, 7,* and *8*). The pulp cavity may be round, elliptical, or triangular, depending on the external shape of the root. If two separate canals are present and the cross section is below the bifurcation level, two round canals would be seen rather than an elliptical- or ribbon-shaped canal.

Mandibular Second Premolar
(Fig. 13–38, *A, B, C, D, E*)

Buccolingual Section (A, D)

The mandibular second premolar has a larger crown and root than the first premolar. In addition to the increased dimensions of the pulp cavities, the extremely wide dimensions are confined to the crown and the upper portion of the root canal. Another difference between the first and second premolar is that the pulp horns in the second premolar tend to be more prominent and the lingual pulp horn is present more often. The pulp horns are prominent in most of the teeth (Fig. 13–38, *A, 1–3, 7,* and *9; D, 10, 13, 16–18*), but the lingual pulp horn may be vestigial (Fig. 13–38, *A, 4–6; D, 11, 12, 14,*and *15*) or nonexistent (Fig. 13–38, *A, 8*). The pulp chambers are usually large and may abruptly constrict (Fig. 13–38, *A, 1, 2, 4, 5, 7,* and *8; D, 11, 13, 14, 16,* and *18*) or gently taper into the pulp canal (Fig. 13–38, *A, 1, 3, 6,* and *9; D, 10, 12,* and *17*). The apical foramen may appear to exit at

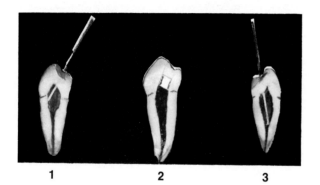

1   2   3

Figure 13–36. Mandibular first premolar.
    1, A small opening made in the central groove of the occlusal surface will not allow access to the root canal because of the angulation of the occlusal surface with long axis of the root.
    2, A cut-out that indicates the minimum of occlusal access permissible.
    3, Even with the generous opening into the occlusal surface, care will be required in approaching the apical third of the root.
    Compare with Figure 13–37.

Figure 13–37. Mandibular first premolar.
1, Occlusal view of occlusal opening necessary to facilitate entrance of root canal instruments.
2, The root outline and pulp chamber opening to be found at the level of cementoenamel junction.
3, Profile view buccolingually, showing relationship of the alignment of the instrument to the opening in the crown.
The cusp of the mandibular first premolar leans lingually so that it is almost centered over the root. The occlusal opening must approach the cusp tip in order to allow easy access to instruments. In this respect this tooth is similar to the mandibular canine.

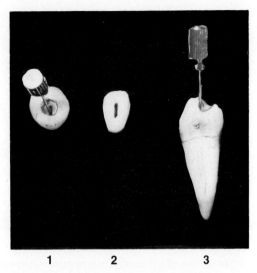

1   2   3

the apex (Fig. 13–38, *A, 1–6, 8,* and *9; D, 10–17*) or on the buccal or lingual aspect of the tip of the root (Fig. 13–38, *A, 7; D, 18*).

Mesiodistal Section (B, E)

The mandibular second premolar is very similar to the first mandibular premolar, except that the overall dimensions of the second premolar are slightly larger. In general, the mesiodistal cross section of the mandibular premolars and the canine are similar. The mandibular second premolar usually has one root and canal that may be curved, but usually in the distal direction.

The pulp horns are prominent, and the pulp chamber and root canal gently taper toward the apex. The apical foramen appears to exit at the tip of the root in the majority of cases.

Cervical Cross Section (C)

The amount of root structure is substantial in the mandibular second premolar as clearly demonstrated in the cervical cross section. The outline form of the root is rectangular (Fig. 13–38, *C, 1, 3, 6, 8,* and *9*), oval (Fig. 13–38, *C, 4* and *7*), or triangular in shape (Fig. 13–38, *C, 2* and *5*). The pulp cavity will generally follow the outline of the tooth unless two canals are present (Fig. 13–38, *C, 6*).

Access to the pulp chamber of the second mandibular premolar is similar to that of the first mandibular premolar, but the angle at which the file enters the pulp cavity of the second premolar is less pronounced, making it more perpendicular to the occlusal surface of the tooth (Figs. 13–39 and 13–40).

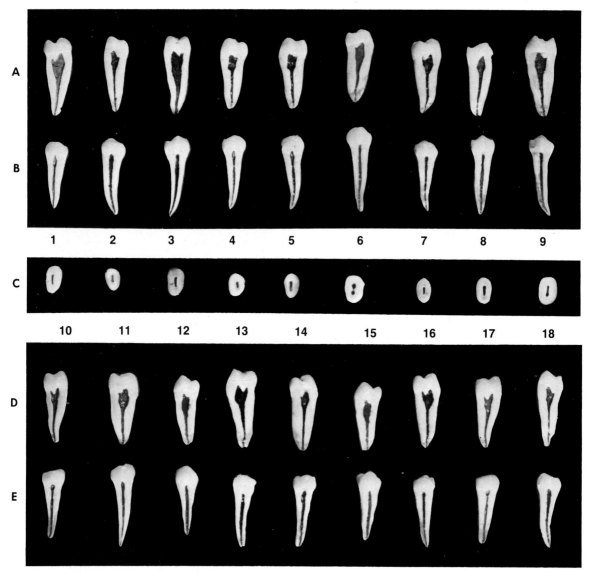

Figure 13–38. Mandibular second premolar.
   A, Buccolingual section, exposing the mesial or distal aspect of the pulp cavity. This aspect does not appear in a dental radiograph.
   B, Mesiodistal section, exposing the buccal or lingual aspect of the pulp cavity.
   C, Cervical cross section exposing the pulp chamber. These are the openings to root canals that will be seen in the floor of the pulp chamber.
   D, Buccolingual section, exposing the mesial or distal aspect of the pulp cavity.
   E, Mesiodistal section, exposing the buccal or lingual aspect of the pulp cavity.

Mandibular First Molar
(Fig. 13–41, *A, B, C, D, E*)

Buccolingual Section (A, D)

The buccolingual cross section of the mandibular first molar demonstrates a generous pulp chamber that may extend well down into the root formation (Fig. 13–41, *A, 1* and *2; D, 16* and *18*). The mesial root usually has a more complicated root canal system because of the

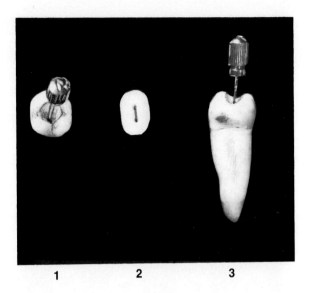

Figure 13–39. Mandibular second premolar.
1, Occlusal view of canal instrument entering the root canal occlusally. Note the size of the opening necessary to properly approach the pulp chamber.

2, Cross section of this tooth at the cervical line that exposes the pulp chamber.

3, Profile view buccolingually, showing the angle at which the instrument enters the root canal.

Compare this picture with its counterpart showing the mandibular first premolar (Fig. 13–37).

presence of two canals. The distal root usually has one large canal, but two canals are often present. Occasionally there may be a fourth canal that has its own separate root, but this is infrequent.

The pulp horns are quite prominent in most of the mandibular first molars (Fig. 13–41, *A, 1, 2, 5, 6, 8,* and *9; D, 10–12, 14, 15, 17,* and *18*), whereas the pulp horns of some of the mandibular first molars are quite small (Fig. 13–41, *A, 3, 4,* and *7; D, 13* and *16*). The pulp chambers of the mesial roots are rectangular in shape (excluding the pulp horns) (Fig. 13–41, *A, 1, 2, 4, 6, 7,* and *9; D, 10–12, 14, 16,* and *18*), but this demarcation is not seen in the single-canaled distal root (Fig. 13–41, *A, 3, 5,* and *8; D, 13, 15,* and *17*).

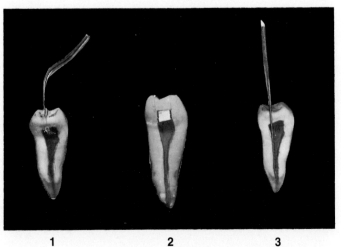

Figure 13–40. Mandibular second premolar (actual cross sections).
1, A small opening in the center of the occlusal surface will leave undercuts in the pulp chamber roof.

2, A window in the side of the specimen indicates the width of opening necessary to obliterate undercuts.

3, A probe placed over the photo to show the straight approach possible when dealing with the mandibular second premolar. Nevertheless, it must be noted that the lingual wall only is in line with the center of the occlusal surface.

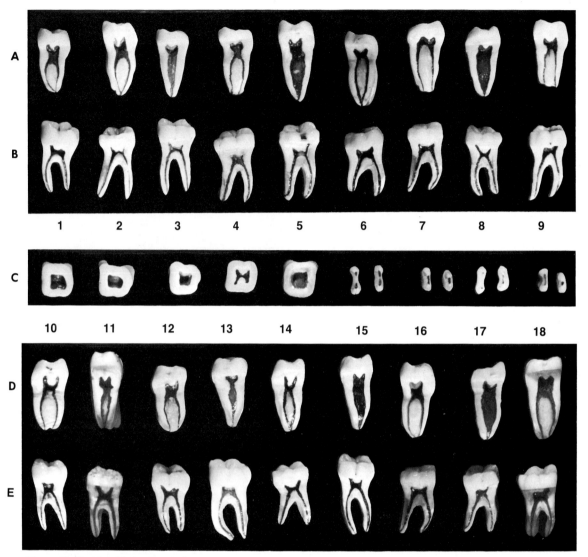

Figure 13–41. Mandibular first molar.

   A, Buccolingual section, exposing the mesial or distal aspect of the pulp cavity. This aspect does not appear in a dental radiograph.

   B, Mesiodistal section, exposing the buccal or lingual aspect of the pulp cavity.

   C, Five cross sections at cervical line and four cross sections at midroot.

   D, Buccolingual section, exposing the mesial or distal aspect of the pulp cavity.

   E, Mesiodistal section, exposing the buccal or lingual aspect of the pulp cavity.

   The mesial canals may be severely curved (Fig. 13–41, *A*, *1* and *7; D, 16* and *18*), moderately curved (Fig. 13–41, *A*, *4* and *6; D, 10, 12,* and *14*), or relatively straight (Fig. 13–41, *A*, *7* and *9*). The two canals may join each other in the apical region to exit in a common foramen (Fig. 13–41, *A*, *1, 2,* and *6; D, 14*), or they may have a separate apical foramen (Fig. 13–41, *A*, *4, 7,* and *9; D, 10, 12, 16,* and *18*).

   The apical foramen usually appears to exit on the tip of the broad mesial root (Fig. 13–41, *A*, *1, 2, 4, 6, 7,* and *9; D, 10, 14,* and *16*), but some roots have one of the two canals exit on the side of the root tip (Fig. 13–41, *D, 12,* and *18*). The diameter of the mesial canals is usually very small and demonstrates a slight taper.

The distal root usually has one large pulp chamber, which is very wide in the buccolingual dimension (Fig. 13–41, *A, 3, 5,* and *8; D, 15* and *17*), whereas other distal roots may possess a pulp chamber that is more constricted (Fig. 13–41, *D, 11* and *13*). The distal root usually has one large pulp canal, which may show a considerable buccolingual dimension until the canal constricts abruptly a few millimeters from the apex of the root (Fig. 13–41, *A, 3, 5,* and *8; D, 17*). The constriction of the canal, in the last few millimeters of the root, is not always present (Fig. 13–41, *D, 15*). When two canals are present, they will be partially or completely separated by a dentinal island (Fig. 13–41, *D, 11*). The apical foramen of the single-canaled distal root usually appears to be located at the apex of the root (Fig. 13–41, *A, 3* and *8; D, 13* and *17*), but it may be slightly buccal or lingual to the apex of the root (Fig. 13–41, *A, 5* and *15*).

Mesiodistal Section (B, E)

The mesiodistal section of the mandibular first molar will present few variations in the form of the pulp chamber or canals. The mesial and distal pulp cavities have canals and chambers that are centered within the roots and crowns. The pulp horns may be prominent (Fig. 13–41, *A, 8; E, 8, 11, 14,* and *15*), moderately evident (Fig. 13–41, *A, 2, 3, 6,* and *7; E, 12*), barely detectable (Fig. 13–41, *A, 4; E, 13* and *16*), or possibly demonstrating a combination of these variations (Fig. 13–41, *A, 1, 5,* and *9; E, 10, 17,* and *18*). The pulp chambers are usually rectangular in shape (excluding the pulp horns) and may be large (Fig. 13–41, *A, 1, 4–7,* and *9; E, 10–18*) or very small (Fig. 13–41, *A, 2, 3,* and *8*). Mandibular first molars showing a very small pulp chamber should be approached with caution while gaining access for endodontic purposes, as a furcation perforation can occur quite easily.

The mesial root and canal usually show considerable curvature (Fig. 13–41, *B, 1, 3–5,* and *7–9; E, 12, 13, 15, 16,* and *18*). Those that are not curved may be easier to negotiate with an endodontic file (Fig. 13–41, *B, 6; E, 10, 11, 14,* and *17*) unless the canal is calcified (extensive secondary or irritation dentin deposition) (Fig. 13–41, *B, 2*).

The apical foramen usually appears to exit at the tip of the root (Fig. 13–41, *A, 1, 5, 7,* and *8; E, 10–15, 17,* and *18*), whereas others appear to exit on the mesial (Fig. 13–41, *B, 2, 4, 6,* and *9; E, 16*) or distal (*B, 3*) aspect of the root.

The distal root is usually straighter and tends to be a little shorter than the curved mesial root (Fig. 13–41, *B, 1, 3, 6,* and *8; E, 12, 14,* and *15*); however, it may be the same length (Fig. 13–41, *B, 2, 4,* and *7; E, 10, 11, 13,* and *16–18*) or even slightly longer (Fig. 13–41, *B, 5* and *9*). The distal canal is usually a little larger than the mesial canal (Fig. 13–41, *B, 2* and *4–7; E, 11, 14, 15,* and *18*), but the canals may look very similar in size when viewed from the buccal aspect (Fig. 13–41, *B, 1, 3, 8,* and *9; E, 10, 12, 13, 16,* and *17*).

The distal canal usually tapers gently to the apical constriction. The apical foramen often appears to be located on the distal aspect of the root (Fig. 13–41, *B, 2, 3, 5, 7,* and *8; E, 13, 16,* and *17*). In some teeth, this distal deviation will be quite marked (Fig. 13–41, *B, 5* and *7; E, 17*). Although mesial deviation of the canal is rare, it does occur (Fig. 13–41, *B, 6*); however, it is usually only a minor deviation. The apical foramen will often appear to be located at the tip of the root (Fig. 13–41, *B, 1; E, 10–12, 14, 15,* and *18*).

Access to the canals of the mandibular first molar should allow the endodontic instruments to pass freely into and out of the canals. Because of the root canal's curvature or angle, the files will cross one another in the cervical region of the tooth (Fig. 13–42 and 13–43).

Cervical Cross Section (C, 1, 2, 3, 4, 5)

The cervical cross section of the mandibular first molar is generally quadrilateral in form. Distally, it tapers a little from the wider buccolingual measurement of the mesial aspect of the tooth. The pulp chamber outline generally follows that of the root (Fig. 13–41, *C, 1, 2,* and *5*) but may show buccal (Fig. 13–41, *C, 3*) and/or lingual (Fig. 13–41, *C, 4*) projections of dentin if the pulp chamber is excessively narrowed by secondary or irritation dentin. The pulp chamber floor has two small funnel-shaped openings into the mesial root (one buccal and one lingual), whereas the distal aspect of the pulp chamber shows a single opening that is less constricted.

Midroot Cross Section (C, 6, 7, 8, 9)

The midroot view of the mandibular molar will usually demonstrate the root canal form, which is consistent with the major form of this tooth. The mesial root will usually be somewhat kidney-shaped, with two separate canals (Fig. 13–41, *C, 7*), but a figure-8 shape of the root is also very common (Fig. 13–41, *C, 6* and *8*). The two canals may be totally separate (Fig. 13–41, *C, 6* and *8*) or confluent with the other canal (Fig. 13–41, *C, 7* and *9*). The distal root is usually rounder than the mesial root (Fig. 13–41, *C, 7* and *9*), but a very wide root is also common (Fig. 13–41, *C, 6* and *8*). Those roots that tend to be round usually demonstrate only one canal, whereas the broader distal roots tend to have two canals (Fig. 13–41, *C, 6*) or a very thin canal that is single; or they may possess a dentinal ''island'' (Fig.

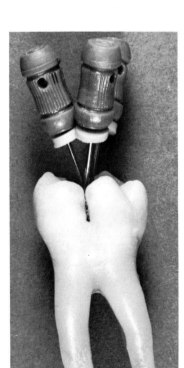

Figure 13–42. Mandibular first molar. A file is present in every canal, demonstrating the angles of the files in relationship to the roots.

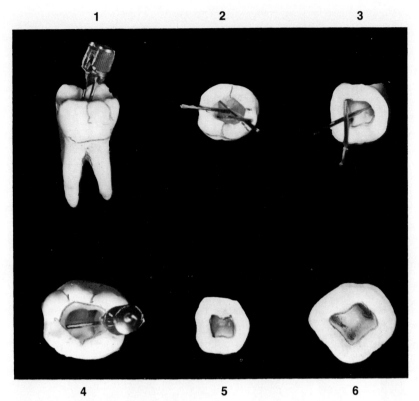

Figure 13–43. Mandibular first molar.
1, Root canal instruments placed in two mesial canals. Note the angulation and the parallelism.
2, An occlusal view showing an access opening which is larger than necessary for convenience in approaching the root canals in the pulp chamber. Three probes in place indicate the variation in the directions the canals traverse.
3, The same illustration with the crown portion of the tooth removed and the image enlarged somewhat.
4, Occlusal view of the occlusal opening. Note the extreme angle of the instrument entering the distal root canal. A narrower occlusal opening would not permit ease of access.
5, 6, Two views, one enlarged, show the design of the pulp chamber with canal entrances at a cervical cross section of the mandibular first molar. Usually, there are two canals or their equivalent in the mesial root, whereas the distal root normally contains one broad canal.

13–41, *C, 8*). Even the single-canaled distal canal tends to show a developmental depression or concavity on the mesial aspect of the root (Fig. 13–41, *C, 7* and *9*), and this should be considered when postpreparations are being considered.

Mandibular Second Molar (Fig. 13–44, *A, B, C, D, E*)

Anatomically, the mandibular second molar has many similarities with the mandibular first molar. The proportions of the crown and root are very similar to the mandibular first molar. The roots of the second molar may be straighter with less divergence from the furcation than in the first molar. The roots may be shorter, but there is no assurance that any of these differences will be manifested in any one case.

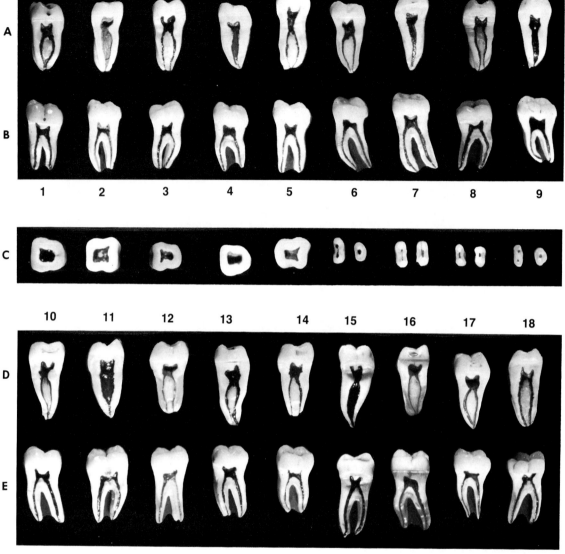

Figure 13–44. *Mandibular second molar.*
   A, Buccolingual section, exposing the mesial or distal aspect of the pulp cavity. This aspect does not appear on the dental radiograph.
   B, Mesiodistal section, exposing the buccal or lingual aspect of the pulp cavity.
   C, Five cross sections at cervical line and four cross sections at midroot.
   D, Buccolingual section, exposing the mesial or distal aspect of the pulp cavity.
   E, Mesiodistal section, exposing the buccal aspect of the pulp cavity.

Buccolingual Section (A, D)

The buccolingual section of the mandibular second molar demonstrates a pulp chamber and pulp canals that tend to be more variable and complex than those found in the mandibular first molar.

   The pulp horns of the mandibular second molar are usually rather prominent (Fig. 13–44, *A, 1, 3, 5, 6, 8,* and *9; D, 10, 13–15, 17,* and *18*), but some pulp horns may be small to nonexistent (Fig. 13–44, *A, 2, 4,* and *7; D, 11, 12,* and *16*). The pulp chamber of the mesial root (Fig. 13–44, *A, 1, 3, 5, 6,* and *8; D, 12–14, 16–18*) is well demarcated because of the presence of two small canals. The pulp chamber (excluding the pulp horns) may be somewhat square (Fig. 13–44, *A, 1, 3,* and *8; D, 10, 12, 14,* and *16–18*) or rectangular (Fig. 13–44, *A, 5* and *6; D, 13*) in shape.

Two root canals are usually present in the mesial root, but only one may be present. The mesial canals may show a large (Fig. 13–44, *A, 1; D, 17* and *18*), medium (Fig. 13–44, *A, 3, 5, 6,* and *8; D, 13*), or small (Fig. 13–44, *D, 12, 14,* and *16*) dimension. The curvature of these canals may be severe (Fig. 13–44, *A, 1; D, 13*), moderate (Fig. 13–44, *5* and *8; D, 12* and *16*), virtually absent (Fig. 13–44, *D, 14* and *18*), or a combination of the aforementioned variations (Fig. 13–44, *A, 1* and *6; D, 17*). Most of the canals will appear to exit from the mesial root separately (Fig. 13–44, *A, 3, 5, 6,* and *8; D, 12–14, 16,* and *18*), but some will join just prior to reaching the apex so that there is a common canal that exits from the apex (Fig. 13–44, *A, 1; D, 17*). The apical foramen usually appears to be located at the tip of the root (Fig. 13–44, *A, 1, 3, 5,* and *6; D, 12, 14, 17,* and *18*), but some appear to exit slightly to the buccal or lingual aspect of the apex of the root (Fig. 13–44, *A, 8; D, 14* and *16*).

The pulp chamber of the distal root of the mandibular second molar (Fig. 13–44, *A, 2, 4, 7,* and *9; D, 10, 11,* and *15*) is not as easily identified because of the extremely large pulp canal that is usually present (Fig. 13–44, *A, 2, 4, 7,* and *9; D, 11,* and *15*). One canal is usually present in the distal root, but two totally or partially separate canals are possible (Fig. 13–44, *D, 10*). The pulp horns may be present, but they are not nearly as prominent as in the mesial root (Fig. 13–44, *A, 2, 4, 7,* and *9; D, 11* and *15*) unless two canals are present (Fig. 13–44, *D, 10*). The pulp canal is usually very large in the mesiobuccal sections. The pulp canal may taper gently from the pulp chamber until the apical constriction (Fig. 13–44, *A, 2* and *7; D, 10* and *15*) or an abrupt constriction of the canal may occur in the last 2 or 3 mm of the canal (Fig. 13–44, *A, 4* and *9; D, 11*). The apical foramen usually appears to be located at the tip of the root (Fig. 13–44, *A, 1, 4, 7,* and *9; D, 10, 11,* and *15*), but this is not always the case.

Mesiodistal Section (**B, E**)

The mesiodistal sections of the mandibular second molar are very similar to those of the mandibular first molar. However, the roots of the mandibular first molar tend to be straighter and closer together (less furcation deviation).

The pulp horns are usually prominent (Fig. 13–44, *B, 1–5, 7–9; E, 10, 11, 13, 15,* and *18*), but some are small or absent (Fig. 13–44, *B, 4* and *6; E, 12, 14, 16,* and *17*). The pulp chamber is rectangular in shape (excluding the pulp horns). The size of the chamber varies from very large (Fig. 13–44, *B, 1, 3–5, 7,* and *9; E, 13* and *16*) to very small (Fig. 13–44, *B, 2, 8,* and *9; E, 11, 14, 17,* and *18*). The curvature of the mesial canal may be severe (Fig. 13–44, *B, 3, 6, 8,* and *9; E, 11, 14,* and *16*), moderate (Fig. 13–44, *B, 2, 4,* and *7; E, 10, 13, 15, 17,* and *18*), or essentially straight (Fig. 13–44, *B, 1* and *5; E, 12*). The canals gently taper from the pulp chamber to the apical constriction. The apical foramen usually appears to be located at the tip of the root (Fig. 13–44, *B, 1, 2, 4–7, 8; E, 11, 12, 15, 17,* and *18*), but the foramen may appear to be located mesially (Fig. 13–44, *B, 3; E, 10, 13,* and *16*) or distally (Fig. 13–44, *B, 9* and *14*) on the root tip. The distal canal may be slightly curved (Fig. 13–44, *B, 1–5* and *7; E, 11* and *14–16*) or straight (Fig. 13–44, *B, 4, 6, 8,* and *9; E, 10, 12, 13, 17,* and *18*). The distal root may be slightly shorter than (Fig. 13–44, *B, 1, 2, 4,* and *7*), equal to (Fig. 13–44, *B, 3, 5,* and *6; E, 10, 13, 14, 16,* and *17*), or longer than (Fig. 13–44, *B, 8* and *9; E, 11, 12, 15,* and *18*) the mesial root. The distal canal is usually larger than the mesial canals (Fig. 13–44, *B, 3, 4, 6–9; E, 11, 13, 15,* and *16*) but may be equal to the mesial canals (Fig. 13–44, *B, 1, 2,* and *5; E, 12, 14,* and *18*). The distal canal tapers gently to the apex. The apical foramen usually appears to be located at the tip of the root (Fig. 13–44, *B, 1–7; E, 10–13, 16,* and *18*), but the foramen may appear to exit mesially (Fig. 13–44, *B, 9*) or distally (Fig. 13–44, *B, 8; E, 14, 15,* and *17*) to the apex of the root.

Cervical Cross Section (C, 1, 2, 3, 4, 5)

The cervical cross section of the mandibular second molar is similar to that of the mandibular first molar (Fig. 13–44, *C, 1–5*). The outline form of the mandibular second molar is more triangular (rather than square like the mandibular first molar) because of the smaller dimensions that are usually seen in the distal aspect of this tooth. The pulp chamber also tends to be triangular in form. The floor of the pulp chamber may have two openings, one mesially and one distally, which are centered within the dentin. If only one canal is present in the distal root, it will be centered within the dentin.

Midroot Cross Section (C, 6–9)

Midroot cross sections of the mandibular molars will demonstrate the very broad (buccolingually) and narrow (mesiodistally) mesial root (Fig. 13–44, *C, 6–9*). The outline form will be kidney-shaped (Fig. 13–44, *C, 6* and *7*) or slightly in the form of a figure 8 (Fig. 13–44, *C, 8* and *9*). The canals may be totally separate (Fig. 13–44, *C, 9*) or confluent (Fig. 13–44, *C, 6–8*), making it difficult to determine the presence of two mesial canals (Fig. 13–44, *C, 8*). The distal root may be rounder than the mesial root because the outline form of this root is usually oval (Fig. 13–44, *C, 6* and *9*), but broad distal roots are also seen (Fig. 13–44, *C, 7* and *8*). One canal is usually present in the distal canal, but two canals are possible.

Access to the pulp chamber and canals of the mandibular second molar is similar to that of the mandibular first molar. Because of these similarities, the departure of the files from the tooth will be the same as found in the mandibular first molar (Fig. 13–45).

Mandibular Third Molar (Fig. 13–46, A, B, C, D, E)

The mandibular third molar pulp cavities vary greatly. The pulp cavity will resemble the second mandibular molar most, but the crown will look too large for the roots, which may be shorter and curved and tend to be fused together.

Buccolingual Section (A, D)

The pulp cavities of the mandibular third molar show a great deal of variation. Two roots and three canals are often present (Fig. 13–46, *6* and *7*), but two canals in one or two roots (Fig. 13–46, *C, 8* and *9*) are also possible. The presence of one canal and one root can also be found, but usually these teeth are not of much value for restorative purposes because they have short roots that taper quickly. The pulp horns of the mandibular third molar are usually prominent (Fig. 13–46, *A, 1, 2,* and *4–9; D, 10–12, 14, 15, 17,* and *18*), although others demonstrate small to nonexistent pulp horns (Fig. 13–46, *A, 3; D, 13* and *16*).

The mesial roots of mandibular third molars (Figs. 13–46, *A, 2, 5,* and *9; D, 10, 11, 13,* and *14*) usually demonstrate a square-shaped pulp chamber (excluding the pulp horns). The mesial root usually has two canals (Fig. 13–46, *A, 2, 5,* and *9; D, 10, 11, 13,* and *14*), but a single mesial root can be found (Fig. 13–46, *D, 14*). The canals may be very curved (Fig. 13–46, *A, 5* and *9; D, 10* and *14*) or straight (Fig. 13–46, *A, 2; D, 11* and *13*) as they taper gently toward the apical constriction. The apical foramen usually appears to be located on the tip of the root (Fig. 13–46, *A, 1* and *5; D, 10, 11,* and *13*), but it may be located buccally

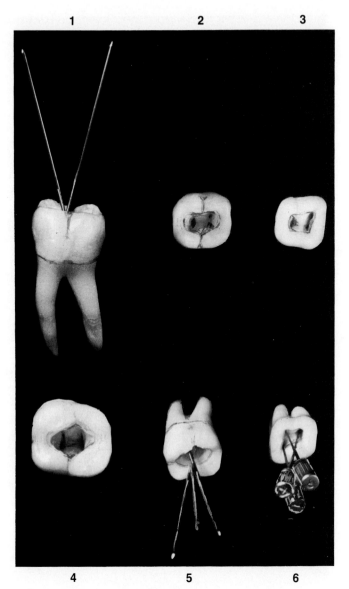

Figure 13–45. Mandibular second molar.

1, Buccal view of the mandibular second molar with probes in canals showing the direction of insertion. The picture continues to prove the lack of parallelism existing in multirooted posterior teeth by the directions traversed by pulp canals. Also, root canals seldom follow a course at right angles to the occlusal surfaces of crowns.

2, Occlusal opening of the left second molar showing easy access to the pulp chamber.

3, A cervical cross section of this molar, which shows graphically in an actual photograph of a natural specimen the shape and location of the canal openings and an anatomically correct outline of the pulp chamber.

4, A closeup of the occlusal opening in the second molar and the approach to the pulp canals.

5, An odd angle of the whole tooth showing the direction taken by probes in the three canals.

6, Instruments placed in the canals with the crown portion of the tooth removed to permit a closer survey of the situation.

(Fig. 13–46, *A, 9; D, 14*) or lingually to the tip of the root. If two canals are present, they will usually possess separate apical foramen (Fig 13–46, *A, 2* and *5; D, 10, 11,* and *13*), whereas others will join in the apical region exiting through a common foramen (Fig. 13–46, *A, 9*).

The distal root of mandibular third molars possesses a very large pulp chamber and canal that are difficult to delineate into separate areas (Fig. 13–46, *A, 1, 3, 4,* and *6–8; D, 12* and *15–18*). The pulp chambers are rectangular in shape (excluding the pulp horns). The pulp canals, which are very large (Fig. 13–46, *A, 1, 4, 6,* and *7; D, 12, 15,* and *18*), may taper gently to the root tip (Fig. 13–46, *A, 4, 6,* and *7; D, 16* and *18*) or demonstrate an abrupt constriction of the canal in the last few millimeters (Fig. 13–46, *A, 1; D, 12, 15,* and *17*). The pulp chambers, which are very small (Fig. 13–46, *A, 3* and *8*), tend to show a constriction at the junction of the pulp chamber and canal, after which they taper gently to the apical constriction. The apical foramen usually appears to be located at the tip of the root (Fig.

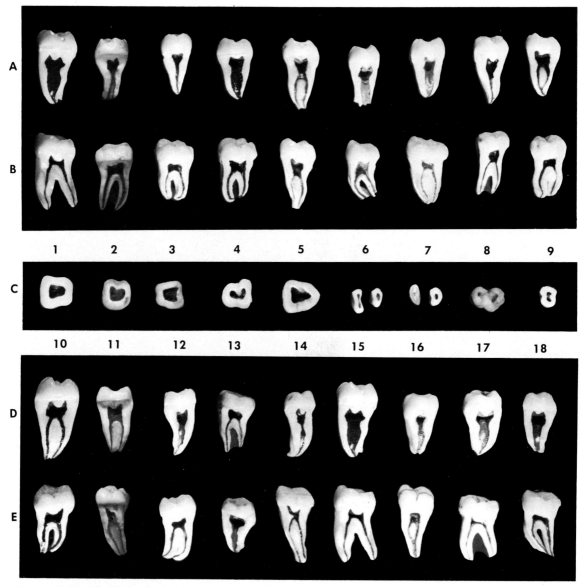

Figure 13–46. Mandibular third molar.

A, Buccolingual section, exposing the mesial or distal aspect of the pulp cavity. This aspect does not appear on the dental radiograph.

B, Mesiodistal section, exposing the buccal or lingual aspect of the pulp cavity.

C, Five cross sections at cervical line and four cross sections at midroot.

D, Buccolingual section, exposing the mesial or distal aspect of the pulp cavity.

E, Mesiodistal section, exposing the buccal or lingual aspect of the pulp cavity.

13–46, *A, 3, 6, 7,* and *8; D, 16* and *17*), but it may be located buccally or lingually to the root tip (Fig. 13–46, *A, 1* and *4; D, 15* and *18*).

Mesiodistal Section (B, E)

The pulp horns of the mandibular third molar may be prominent (Fig. 13–46, *B, 1* and *5; E, 10–12, 14,* and *15*), small (Fig. 13–46, *A, 4, 6,* and *7; D, 17*), or virtually absent (Fig. 13–46, *B, 2, 3, 8,* and *9; E, 13, 16,* and *18*). The pulp chambers are usually rectangular when viewed from the buccal aspect (Fig. 13–46, *B, 1–4, 7,* and *9; E, 10, 12, 13, 15, 17,* and *18*), but they may be somewhat square (excluding the pulp horns). The degree of curvature of the mesial root may be slight (Fig. 13–46, *E, 13* single-rooted), moderate (Fig. 13–46, *B, 1, 2, 5, 8,* and *9; E, 11, 15,* and *17*), or severe (Fig. 13–46, *B, 3, 4, 6,* and *7; E, 10, 12, 14, 16,* and *18*). The canal within the mesial root may be large (Fig. 13–46, *B, 2* and *4; E, 10*) or very small (Fig. 13–46, *B, 1* and *3–9; E, 11, 12* and *14–18*), making endodontic procedures more difficult to accomplish. The canals usually taper gently to the apical constriction. The apical foramen may appear to be located at the apex of the root (Fig. 13–46, *B, 1–3, 5, 6, 8,* and *9; E, 11, 12, 14, 17, 18*) or mesially (Fig. 13–46, *B, 7*) to the apex of the root (Fig. 13–46, *B, 4; E, 10* and *15*). The length of the mesial roots may be equal to (Fig. 13–46, *B, 2, 3,* and *8; E, 10* and *11*), shorter than (Fig. 13–46, *B, 5* and *9; E, 18*), or longer than (Fig. 13–46, *B, 1, 4, 6,* and *7; E, 12, 14, 15,* and *17*) the distal root. The distal canal may be larger than the mesial canal (Fig. 13–46, *B, 2–5* and *9; E, 14* and *18*), but many will be equal in size (Fig. 13–46, *B, 1* and *6–8; E, 10–12, 15,* and *17*). The distal canal gently tapers to the apical constriction. The apical foramen may appear to be located at the apex of the root (Fig. 13–46, *B, 1–5, 7,* and *9; E, 10, 11, 12, 15, 17,* and *18*) or mesially (Fig. 13–46, *B, 8*) or distally (Fig. 13–46, *B, 6; E, 14*) to the apex of the root. Some teeth will show only one root with one or two canals. If only one canal is present (Fig. 13–46, *E, 13*), the canal will be very large. If the third molar is multirooted, the canals will be much smaller (Fig. 13–46, *E, 16*).

Cervical Cross Section (C, 1, 2, 3, 4, 5)

The cervical cross section demonstrates a variable outline form that may be rectangular (Fig. 13–46, *C, 1–4*) or triangular in shape (Fig. 13–46, *C, 5*).

Midroot Cross Section (C, 6, 7, 8, 9)

The mesial root when present is oval to figure-8 in shape (Fig. 13–46, *C, 6* and *7*). The distal root is oval (Fig. 13–46, *C, 6*) or kidney-shaped (Fig. 13–46, *C, 7*). If the roots are fused (Fig. 13–46, *C, 8*) or if only one root is present (Fig. 13–46, *C, 9*), the canals are usually larger. The canals in the roots that are kidney-shaped or are in the form of a figure 8 are more elliptical.

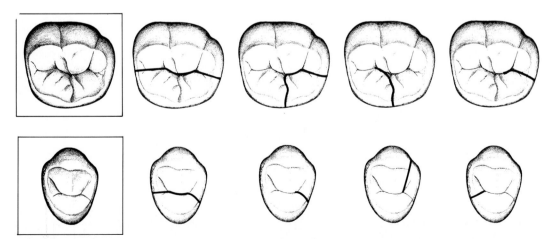

Figure 13–47. Fracture lines most commonly seen in first maxillary premolar and first mandibular molar.

Cuspal Fractures (Fig. 13–47)

Of particular interest to the clinician is the fracture of cusps. Fractures of cusps of the maxillary first premolar and mandibular first molars often occur along developmental grooves or stress lines as shown (Fig. 13–47). Such fractures may occur relative to bruxism and/or restorations. It is not uncommon for the distolingual cusp to fracture in relation to a large restoration leading to disease of the pulp.

References

Acosta Vigouroux, A. S., et al. (1978). Anatomy of the pulp chamber floor of the permanent maxillary first molar. J. Endod. 4:214.

Barker, B. C., et al. (1973). Anatomy of root canals: I. Permanent incisors, canines and premolars. Aust. Dent. J. 18:320.

Barker, B. C., et al. (1974). Anatomy of root canals. II. Permanent maxillary molars. Aust. Dent. J. 19:46.

Barker, B. C., et al. (1974). Anatomy of root canals. III. Permanent mandibular molars. Aust. Dent. J. 19:408.

Burah, J. G., et al. (1974). A study of the presence of accessory foramina and the topography of molar furcations. Oral Surg. 38:451.

Gardner, D. G., et al. (1978). Taurodontism, shovel-shaped incisors and the Klinefelter syndrome. Dent. J. 44:372.

Grossman, L. I. (1946). *Root Canal Therapy*. Philadelphia: Lea & Febiger.

Harris, W. E. (1980). Unusual root canal anatomy in the maxillary molar. J. Endod. 6:573.

Hess, W., and Zurcher, E. (1925). *The Anatomy of Root Canals*. London: John Bale Sons and Danielsson.

Ibrahim, S. M., et al. (1977). Pulp cavities of permanent teeth. Egypt Dent. J. 23:83.

Kerekes, K., et al. (1977). Morphometric observations on the root canals of human molars. J. Endod. 3:114.

Kirkham, D. B. (1975). The location and incidence of accessory pulp canals in periodontal pockets. J. Am. Dent. Assoc. 91:353.

Mageean, J. F. (1972). The significance of root canal morphology in endodontics. J. Br. Endod. Soc. 6:67.

Middleton-Shaw, J. C. (1931). *The Teeth, the Bony Palate and the Mandible in Bantu Races of South Africa*. London: John Bale Sons and Danielsson.

Okumura, T. (1927). Anatomy of the root canals. J. Am. Dent. Assoc. 14:632.

Senyurek, M. S. (1939). Pulp cavities of molars in primates. Am. J. Phys. Anthropol. 25:119.

Stone, L. H., et al. (1981). Maxillary molars demonstrating more than one palatal root canal. Oral Surg. 51:649.

Sutalo, J., et al. (1980). Morphologic characteristics of root canals in upper and lower premolars. Acta. Stomatol. Croat. 14:23.

Tidmarsh, B. G. (1980). Micromorphology of pulp chambers in human molar teeth. Int. Endod. J. 13:69.

Vertucci, F. J., and Williams, R. G. (1974). Furcation canals in the human mandibular first molar. Oral Surg. 38:308.

Vertucci, F. J., et al. (1974). Root canal morphology of the human maxillary second premolar. Oral Surg. 88:456.

Vertucci, F. J., et al (1979). Root canal morphology of the human maxillary first premolar. Oral Surg. 99:194.

Warren, E. M. (1981). The relationship between crown size and the incidence of bifid root canals in mandibular incisor teeth. Oral Surg. 52:425.

14 *Dento-Osseous Structures*

The osseous structures that support the teeth are the maxilla and the mandible. The maxilla, or upper jaw, consists of two bones: a *right maxilla* and a *left maxilla* sutured together at the median line. Both maxillae in turn are joined to other bones of the head. The *mandible,* or lower jaw, has no osseous union with the skull and is movable.

A description of the maxilla and the mandible must include the normally developed framework encompassing the teeth in complete dental arches. *This establishes the teeth as foundation tissues to be included with the bones for jaw support and as a part of the framework for the mobile portion of the face. The root forms with their size and angulation will govern the shape of the alveoli in the jaw bones, and this in turn shapes the contour of the dento-osseous portions facially.*

The Maxillae

The maxillae make up a large part of the bony framework of the facial portion of the skull. They form the major portion of the roof of the mouth, or hard palate, and assist in the formation of the floor of the orbit and the sides and base of the nasal cavity. They bear the 16 maxillary teeth.

Each maxilla is an irregular bone somewhat cuboidal in shape which consists of a body and the four processes: the *zygomatic, frontal, palatine,* and *alveolar processes.* The maxilla is hollow and contains the *maxillary sinus* air space, also called the *antrum of Highmore.* From the dental viewpoint, in addition to its general shape and the processes mentioned, the following landmarks on this bone are among those most important:

1. Incisive fossa
2. Canine fossa
3. Canine eminence
4. Infraorbital foramen
5. Posterior alveolar foramina
6. Maxillary tuberosity
7. Pterygopalatine fossa
8. Incisive canal

The *body* of the maxilla has four surfaces:

1. Anterior or facial surface
2. Infratemporal surface
3. Orbital surface
4. Nasal surface

Anterior Surface

The *anterior* or *facial surface* (Figs. 14–1 and 14–2) is separated above from the orbital aspect by the *infraorbital ridge*. Medially it is limited by the margin of the nasal notch, and posteriorly it is separated from the posterior surface by the anterior border of the zygomatic process, which has a confluent ridge directly over the roots of the first molar. The ridge corresponding to the root of the canine tooth is usually the most pronounced and is called the *canine eminence*.

Anterior to the canine eminence, overlying the roots of the incisor teeth, is a shallow concavity known as the *incisive fossa*. Posterior to the canine eminence on a higher level is a deeper concavity called the *canine fossa*. The floor of this canine fossa is formed in part by the projecting zygomatic process. Above this fossa and below the infraorbital ridge is the *infraorbital foramen,* the external opening of the infraorbital canal. The major portion of the canine fossa is directly above the roots of the premolars.

Posterior Surface

The *posterior* or *infratemporal surface* (Figs. 14–2 and 14–3) is bounded above by the posterior edge of the orbital surface. Inferiorly and anteriorly it is separated from the anterior surface by the zygomatic process and the zygomatic ridge, which runs from the inferior border of the zygomatic process to the alveolus of the maxillary first molar. This

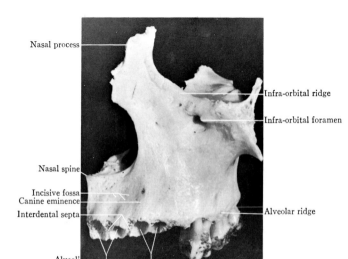

Nasal process

Infra-orbital ridge

Infra-orbital foramen

Nasal spine

Incisive fossa
Canine eminence
Interdental septa

Alveolar ridge

Alveoli

Figure 14–1. Frontal view of left maxilla.

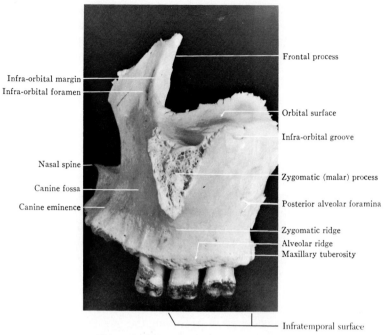

Infra-orbital margin
Infra-orbital foramen

Nasal spine

Canine fossa

Canine eminence

Frontal process

Orbital surface

Infra-orbital groove

Zygomatic (malar) process

Posterior alveolar foramina

Zygomatic ridge
Alveolar ridge
Maxillary tuberosity

Infratemporal surface

Figure 14–2. Lateral view of left maxilla.

surface is more or less convex and is pierced in a downward direction by two or more *posterior alveolar foramina*. These two canals are on a level with the lower border of the zygomatic process and are somewhat distal to the roots of the third molar.

The inferior portion of this surface is more prominent where it overhangs the root of the third molar and is called the *maxillary tuberosity*. Medially this tuberosity is limited by a

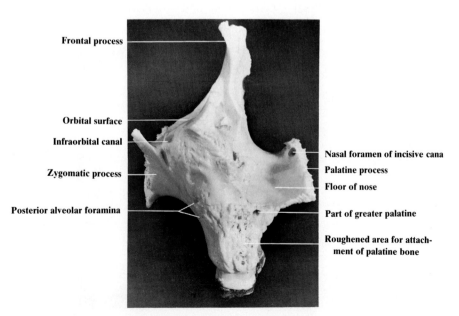

Frontal process

Orbital surface

Infraorbital canal

Zygomatic process

Posterior alveolar foramina

Nasal foramen of incisive cana

Palatine process

Floor of nose

Part of greater palatine

**Roughened area for attach-
ment of palatine bone**

Figure 14–3. Posterior view of left maxilla.

sharp, irregular margin that articulates with the pyramidal process of the palatine bone and, in some cases, the lateral pterygoid plate of the sphenoid bone. The maxillary tuberosity is the origin for some fibers of the medial pterygoid muscle.

A portion of the infratemporal surface superior to maxillary tuberosity is the anterior boundary to the pterygomaxillary fissure.

Orbital Surface

This surface is smooth and together with the orbital surface of the zygomatic bone forms the floor of the orbit. The junction of this surface and the anterior surface forms the infraorbital margin or ridge, which runs superiorly to form part of the nasal process. Its posterior border or edge coincides with the inferior boundary of the inferior orbital fissure.

The thin medial edge of the orbital surface is notched anteriorly, forming the *lacrimal groove*. Behind this groove it articulates with the lacrimal bone for a short distance, then for a greater length with a thin portion of the ethmoid bone, and terminates posteriorly in a surface which articulates with the orbital process of the palatal bone. Its lateral area is continuous with the base of the zygomatic process (Fig. 14–2).

Traversing the posterior portion of the orbital surface is the *infraorbital groove*. This groove begins at the center of the posterior surface and runs anteriorly. The anterior portion of this groove is covered, becoming the *infraorbital canal,* the anterior opening of which is located directly below the infraorbital ridge on the anterior surface.

If the covered portion of this canal were to be laid open, the orifices of the middle and anterior superior alveolar canal would be seen transmitting the corresponding vessels and nerves to the premolars, canines, and the incisor teeth.

Nasal Surface

This surface (Figs. 14–4 and 14–5) is directed medially toward the nasal cavity. It is bordered below by the superior surface of the palatine process; anteriorly it is limited by the sharp edge of the nasal notch. Above and anteriorly, it is continuous with the medial

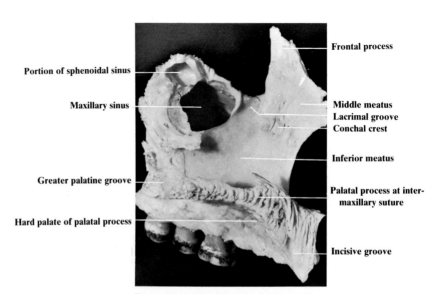

Portion of sphenoidal sinus

Maxillary sinus

Greater palatine groove

Hard palate of palatal process

Frontal process

Middle meatus
Lacrimal groove
Conchal crest

Inferior meatus

Palatal process at inter-maxillary suture

Incisive groove

Figure 14–4. Medial view of left maxilla.

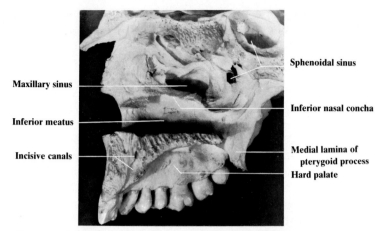

Figure 14–5. Medial view of right maxilla. This specimen has not been disarticulated completely and has the maxillary teeth in situ.

surface of the frontal process; behind this it is deeply channeled by the lacrimal groove, which is converted into a canal by articulation with the lacrimal and inferior turbinate bones.

Behind this groove the upper edge of the nasal surface corresponds to the medial margin of the orbital surface, and the maxilla articulates in this region with the lacrimal bone, a thin portion of the ethmoid bone and the orbital process of the palatine bone.

The posterior border of the maxilla, which articulates with the palatine bone, is traversed obliquely from above downward and slightly medially by a groove which, by articulation with the palate bone, is converted into the *greater palatine canal.*

Toward the posterior and upper part of this nasal surface a large, irregular opening into the maxillary sinus (antrum of Highmore) may be seen. In an articulated skull, this opening is partially covered by the uncinate process of the ethmoid bone and the inferior nasal concha.

Anterior to the lacrimal groove, the nasal surface is ridged for the attachment of the *inferior nasal concha.* Below this the bone forms a lateral wall of the *inferior nasal meatus.* Above the ridge for a small distance on the medial side of the nasal process, the smooth lateral wall of the *middle meatus* appears.

Zygomatic Process

The *zygomatic process* may be seen in the lateral views of the maxillary bone as a roughly triangular eminence whose apex is placed inferiorly directly over the first molar roots. The lateral border is rough and spongelike in appearance where it has been disarticulated from the zygomatic or cheek bone (Fig. 14–2).

Frontal Process

The *frontal process* (Figs. 14–1 through 14–4) arises from the upper and anterior body of the maxilla.

Part of this process is formed by the upward continuation of the infraorbital margin medially. Its edge articulates with the nasal bone. Superiorly the process articulates with the frontal bone. The medial surface of the frontal process forms part of the lateral wall of the nasal cavity. Anteriorly the frontal process articulates with the nasal bone.

Palatine Process

The palatine process (Figs. 14–1 through 14–7) is a horizontal ledge extending medially from the nasal surface of the maxilla. Its superior surface forms a major portion of the nasal floor. The inferior surfaces of the combined left and right palatine processes form the hard palate as far posteriorly as the second molar where they articulate with the horizontal parts of the palatine bone (Figs. 14–6 and 14–7) at the transverse palatine suture.

The inferior surface of the palatine process is rough and pitted for the palatine mucous glands in the roof of the mouth and pierced by numerous small foramina for the passage of blood vessels and nerve fibers. At the posterior border of the process is a groove or canal which passes the greater palatine nerve and vessels to the palatal soft tissues. The posterior edge of the palatine process becomes relatively thin where it joins the palatine bone at the point of the greater palatine foramen. The palatine process becomes progressively thicker anteriorly from the posterior border. Anteriorly, the palatal process is confluent with the alveolar process surrounding the roots of the anterior teeth.

Immediately posterior to the central incisor alveolus, when looking at the medial aspect of the maxilla, we see a smooth groove that is half of the *incisive canal,* when the two maxillae are joined together. The *incisive fossa* into which the canals open may be seen immediately lingual to the central incisors at the median line, or *intermaxillary suture,* when the maxilla are joined. Two canals open laterally into the incisive foramen, the foramina of Stenson, carrying the nasopalatine nerves and vessels. Occasionally, two midline foramina are present, the foramina of Scarpi.

Extending laterally from the incisive foramen to the space between the lateral incisor and canine alveoli are the remnants of the suture between the maxilla and premaxilla. In most mammals the premaxilla remains an independent bone.

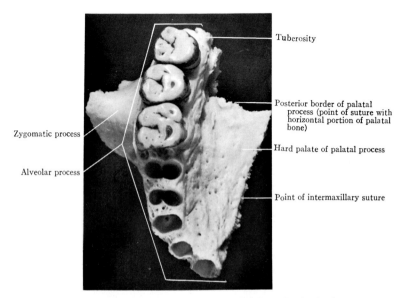

Figure 14–6. Palatal view of maxilla. Note the dental foramina in the deepest portion of the canine alveolus.

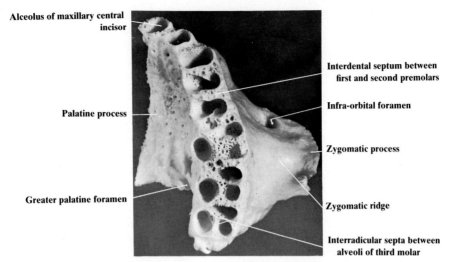

Alceolus of maxillary central incisor

Palatine process

Greater palatine foramen

Interdental septum between first and second premolars

Infra-orbital foramen

Zygomatic process

Zygomatic ridge

Interradicular septa between alveoli of third molar

Figure 14–7. View of inferior surface of the maxilla showing alveolar process and alveoli.

Alveolar Process

The *alveolar process* makes up the inferior portion of the maxilla; it is that portion of the bone which surrounds the roots of the maxillary teeth and which gives them their osseous support. The process extends from the base of the tuberosity posterior to the last molar to the median line anteriorly, where it articulates with the same process of the opposite maxilla (Figs. 14–6 and 14–7). It merges with the palatine process medially and with the zygomatic process laterally (Fig. 14–7).

When we look directly at the inferior aspect of the maxilla toward the alveoli with teeth removed, it is apparent that the alveolar process is curved to conform with the dental arch. It completes, with its fellow of the opposite side, the alveolar arch supporting the roots of the teeth of the maxilla.

The process has a facial (labial and buccal) surface and a lingual surface with ridges corresponding to the surfaces of the roots of the teeth supported by it. It is made up of labiobuccal and lingual plates of very dense but thin cortical bone separated by interdental septa of cancellous bone.

The facial plate is thin, and the positions of the alveoli are well marked on it by visible ridges as far posteriorly as the distobuccal root of the first molar (Fig. 14–1). The margins of these alveoli are frail, and their edges sharp and thin. The buccal plate over the second and third molars, including the alveolar margins, is thicker. Generally, the lingual plate of the alveolar process is heavier than the facial plate. In addition, the alveolar process is longer where it surrounds the anterior teeth, sometimes extending posteriorly to include the premolars. In short, it extends farther down in covering the lingual portion of the roots.

The bone is very thick lingually, over the deeper portions of the alveoli of the anterior teeth and premolars. This formation is brought about by the merging of the alveolar process with the palatal process. The lingual plate is paper-thin over the lingual alveolus of the first molar, however, and rather thin over the lingual alveoli of the second and third molars. This thin lingual plate over the molar roots is part of the formation of the *greater palatine canal* (Fig. 14–7).

The alveolar process is maintained by the presence of the teeth. Should any tooth be lost, that portion of the alveolar process which supported the missing tooth will be subject to atrophic reduction. Should all of the teeth be lost, the alveolar process will eventually cease to exist.

The Alveoli (Tooth Sockets)

These cavities are formed by the facial and lingual plates of the alveolar process and by connecting septa of bone placed between the two plates. The form and depth of each alveolus are determined by the form and length of the root it supports (Table 1–1).

The *alveolus* nearest the median line is that of the *central incisor* (Figs 14–7 and 14–8). The periphery is regular and round, and the interior of the alveolus is evenly tapered and triangular in cross section, with the apex toward the lingual.

The second *alveolus* in line is that of the *lateral incisor*. It is generally conical and egg-shaped, or ovoid, with the widest portion to the labial. It is narrower mesiodistally than labiolingually and is smaller on cross section, although it is often deeper than the central alveolus. Sometimes it is curved at the upper extremity (Figs. 14–7 and 14–9).

The *canine alveolus* is the third from the median line. It is much larger and deeper than those just described. The periphery is oval and regular in outline with the labial width greater than the lingual. The socket extends distally. It is flattened mesially and somewhat concave distally. The bone is so frail at the canine eminence on the facial surface of the alveolus that the root of the canine is often exposed on the labial surface near the middle third (Fig. 14–1).

The *first premolar alveolus* (Figs. 14–7 and 14–9) is kidney-shaped in cross section with the cavity partially divided by a spine of bone which fits into the mesial developmental groove of the root of this tooth. This spine divides the cavity into a buccal and a lingual portion. If the tooth root is bifurcated for part of its length, as is often the case, the terminal portion of the cavity is separated into buccal and lingual alveoli. The socket is flattened distally and much wider buccolingually than mesiodistally (see Table 1–1).

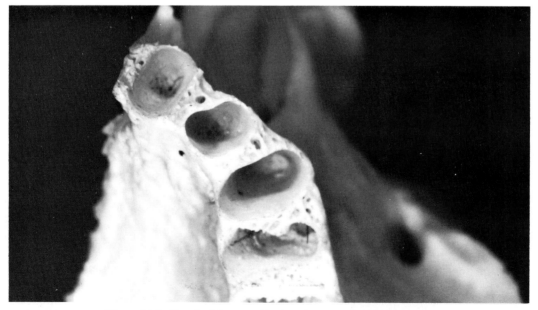

Figure 14–8. Alveoli of the central incisor, lateral incisor, and canine.

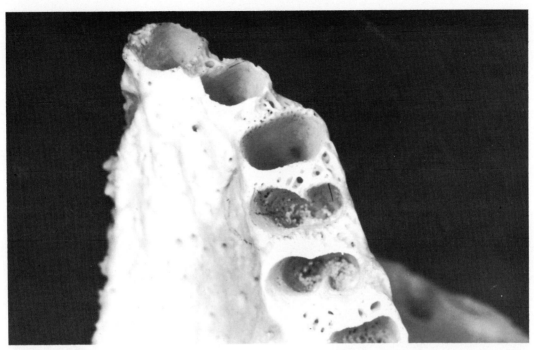

Figure 14–9. Alveoli of the premolar area.

The *second premolar alveolus* is also kidney-shaped, but the curvatures are in reverse to those of the first premolar alveolus. The proportions and depth are almost the same. The septal spine is located on the distal side instead of the medial, since the second premolar root is inclined to have a well-defined developmental groove distally. This tooth usually has one broad root with a blunt end, but it is occasionally bifurcated at the apical third.

The *first molar alveolus* (Figs. 14–7 and 14–10) is made up of three distinct alveoli widely separated. The *lingual alveolus* is the largest; it is round, regular, and deep. The cavity extends in the direction of the hard palate, having a lingual plate over it which is very thin. The lingual periphery of this alveolus is extremely sharp and frail. This condition may contribute to tissue recession often seen at this site.

The *mesiobuccal* and *distobuccal alveoli* of the first molar have no outstanding characteristics except that the buccal plates are thin. The bone is somewhat thicker at the peripheries than that found on the lingual alveolus. Nevertheless, it is thinner farther up on the buccal plate. It is not uncommon for one to find the roots uncovered by bone in spots when examining dry specimens.

The forms of the buccal alveoli resemble the forms of the roots they support. The mesiobuccal alveolus is broad buccolingually, with the mesial and distal walls flattened. The distobuccal alveolus is rounder and more conical.

The *septa* that separate the three alveoli (interradicular septa) are broad at the area which corresponds to the root bifurcation, and they become progressively thicker as the peripheries of the alveoli are approached. The bone septa are very cancellous, denoting a rich blood supply, as is true of all the septa, including those separating the various teeth as well.

A general description of the alveoli of the *second molar* would coincide with that of the first molar; these alveoli are closer together, since the roots of this tooth do not spread as much. As a consequence, the septa separating the alveoli are not so heavy.

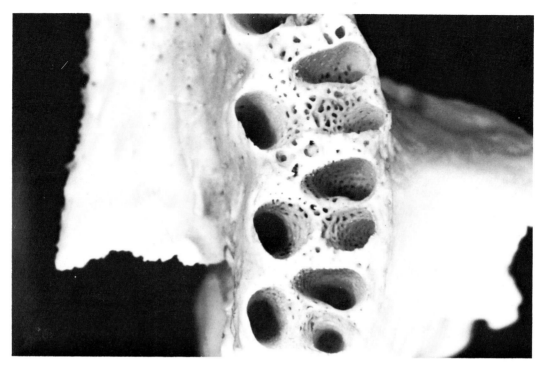

Figure 14-10. Alveoli of the molar area. Note the thinness of buccal plates over the first molar roots when compared with those of the second and third maxillary molars. The third alveoli are rarely separated as distinctly as in this specimen.

Figures 14-8, 14-9, and 14-10 demonstrate a number of significant observations concerning the maxillary alveoli:

1. The facial cortical plate of bone is thin over the anterior teeth and is considerably thicker over the posterior teeth, expecially the molars. Cancellous bone seems to exist buccal to some of the posterior roots.

2. Inter-radicular septa are thick but with numerous nutrient canals.

3. Cancellous bone, furnishing numerous opportunities for blood supply, is evident in the apical portions of the alveoli. The anterior alveoli are lined laterally with a layer of smooth cortical bone. This lining is less prominent in the posterior alveoli.

The *third molar alveolus* is similar to that of the second molar, except that it is somewhat smaller in all dimensions. Figure 14-7 shows a third molar socket to accommodate a tooth with three well-defined roots, a rare occurrence. Usually, the two buccal (and often all three) roots will be fused. The interradicular septum changes accordingly. If the roots of the tooth are fused, a septal spine will appear in the alveolus at the points of fusion on the roots marked by deep developmental grooves.

Maxillary Sinus

The maxillary sinus lies within the body of the bone and is of corresponding pyramidal form; the base is directed toward the nasal cavity. Its summit extends laterally into the root of the zygomatic process. It is closed in laterally and above by the thin walls that form the anterolateral, posterolateral, and orbital surfaces of the body. The sinus overlies the alveolar process in which the molar teeth are implanted, more particularly the first and second molars, the alveoli of which are separated from the sinus by a thin layer of bone. Occasionally, the maxillary sinus will extend forward far enough to overlie the premolars also. It is not uncommon to find the bone covering the alveoli of some of the posterior teeth extending above the floor of the cavity of the maxillary sinus, forming small hillocks.

Regardless of the irregularity and the extension of the alveoli into the maxillary sinus, there is always a layer of bone separating the roots of the teeth and the floor of the sinus in the absence of pathologic conditions. There is always, also, a layer of sinus mucosa between the root tips and the sinus cavity.

Maxillary Articulation

The maxilla articulates with the nasal, frontal, lacrimal, and ethmoid bones, above, and laterally with the zygomatic bone and occasionally with the sphenoid bone. Posteriorly and medially, it articulates with the palatal bone. Medially, it supports the inferior turbinate and the vomer, and articulates with the opposite maxilla.

The Mandible

The mandible (Figs. 14–11 through 14–22) is horseshoe-shaped and supports the teeth of the lower dental arch. This bone is movable and has no bony articulation with the skull. It is the heaviest and strongest bone of the head and serves as a framework for the floor of the mouth. It is situated immediately below the maxillary and zygomatic bone, and its *condyles* rest in the *mandibular fossa* of the temporal bone. This articulation is the temporomandibular joint, or TMJ.

The mandible has a horizontal portion, or *body,* and two vertical portions, or *rami*. The rami join the body at an obtuse angle.

The body consists of two lateral halves, which are joined at the median line shortly after birth. The line of fusion, usually marked by a slight ridge, is called the *symphysis*. The body of the mandible has two surfaces, one external and one internal, and two borders, one superior and one inferior.

To the right and left of the symphysis, near the lower border of the mandible, are two

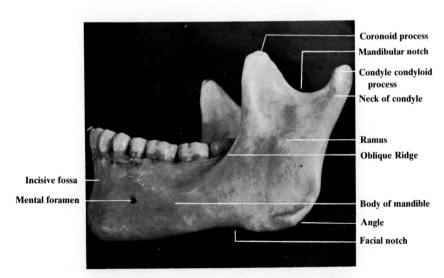

Coronoid process
Mandibular notch
Condyle condyloid process
Neck of condyle
Ramus
Oblique Ridge
Body of mandible
Angle
Facial notch
Incisive fossa
Mental foramen

Figure 14–11. Lateral view of outer surface of mandible.

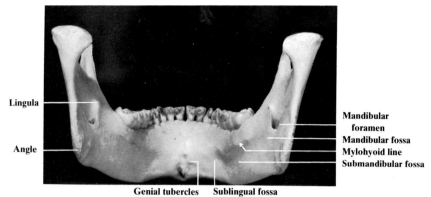

Lingula

Angle

Mandibular foramen
Mandibular fossa
Mylohyoid line
Submandibular fossa

Genial tubercles   Sublingual fossa

Figure 14–12. Posterior view of mandible.

prominences called *mental tubercles*. A prominent triangle surface made by the symphysis and these two tubercles is called the *mental protuberance* (Fig. 14–15).

Immediately posterior to the symphysis and immediately above the mental protuberance is a shallow depression called the *incisive fossa*. The fossa is immediately below the alveolar border of the central and lateral incisors and anterior to the canines. The alveolar portion of the mandible overlying the root of the canine is prominent and is called the *canine eminence* of the mandible. However, this eminence does not extend down very far toward the lower border of the mandible before it is lost in the prominence of the mental protuberance and the lower border of the mandible.

The external surface of the mandible from a lateral viewpoint presents a number of important areas for examination.

The *oblique ridge* (oblique line) extends obliquely across the external surface of the mandible from the mental tubercle to the anterior border of the ramus, with which it is continuous. It lies below the mental foramen. It is usually not prominent except in the molar area (Fig. 14–11).

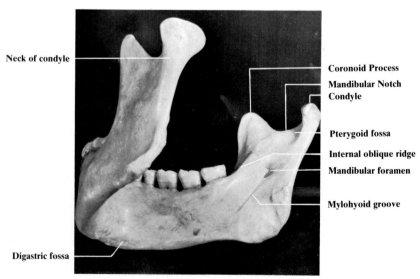

Neck of condyle

Digastric fossa

Coronoid Process
Mandibular Notch
Condyle

Pterygoid fossa

Internal oblique ridge

Mandibular foramen

Mylohyoid groove

Figure 14–13. Posterolateral view of medial surface of mandible.

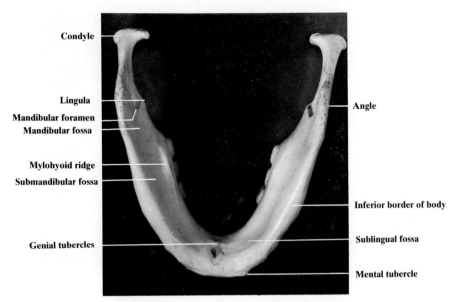

Figure 14–14. View of mandible from below.

This ridge thins out as it progresses upward and becomes the anterior border of the ramus and ends at the tip of the *coronoid process.* The coronoid process is one of two processes making up the superior border of the ramus. It is a pointed, flattened, smooth projection and is roughened toward the tip to give attachment for a part of the temporal muscle.

The *condyle,* or *condyloid process,* on the posterior border of the ramus, is variable in form. It is divided into a superior or articular portion and an inferior portion, or *neck.* Although the articular portion, the condyle, appears as a rounded knob when we view the mandible from a lateral aspect, from a *posterior* aspect the condyle is much wider and is oblong in outline (compare Figs. 14–11 and 14–12).

The condyle is convex above, fitting into the mandibular fossa of the temporal bone

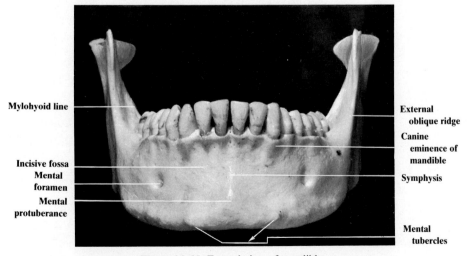

Figure 14–15. Frontal view of mandible.

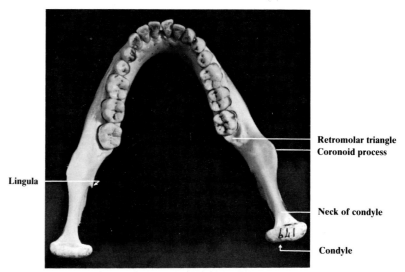

Lingula

Retromolar triangle
Coronoid process

Neck of condyle

Condyle

Figure 14–16. View of mandible from above.

when the mandible is articulated to the skull, and forms, with the interarticular cartilage which lies between the two surfaces and with the tissue attachment, the *temporomandibular joint*.

The neck of the condyle is a constricted portion immediately below the articular surface. It is flattened in front and presents a concave pit medially—the *pterygoid fovea*. A smooth semicircular notch, the *mandibular notch,* forms the sharp upper border of the ramus between the condyle and coronoid process (Fig. 14–13).

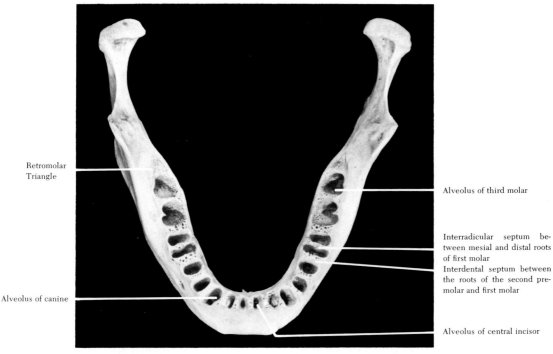

Retromolar
Triangle

Alveolus of canine

Alveolus of third molar

Interradicular septum between mesial and distal roots of first molar
Interdental septum between the roots of the second premolar and first molar

Alveolus of central incisor

Figure 14–17. The alveolar process of the mandible showing alveoli.

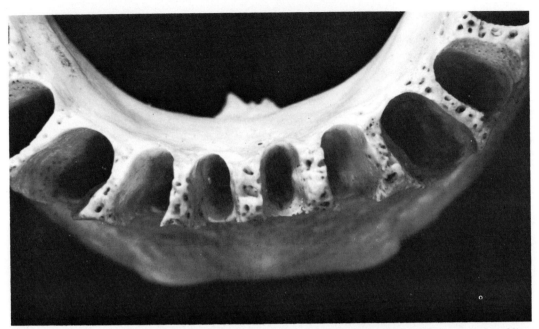

Figure 14–18. Close-up views of three separate divisions of mandibular alveoli (Figs. 14–18, 14–19, and 14–20). This picture indicates the relative sizes and shapes of the incisors for comparison with other mandibular teeth.

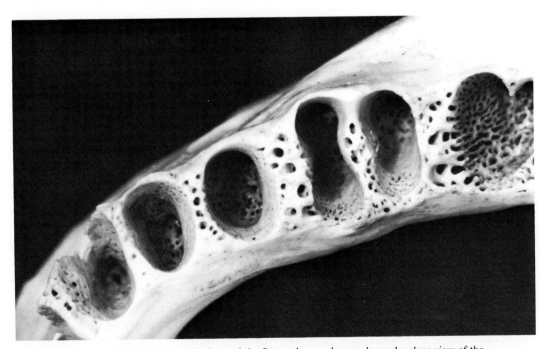

Figure 14–19. This view includes the canine and the first and second premolar and a clear view of the mandibular first molar alveoli. Note the excellent design for the anchorage of first molar roots. Apparently, the blood supply for the interseptal bone lessens as anterior teeth are approached. The apical portion of the canine alveolus displays the single opening in the bone for the blood and nerve supply to the tooth pulp.

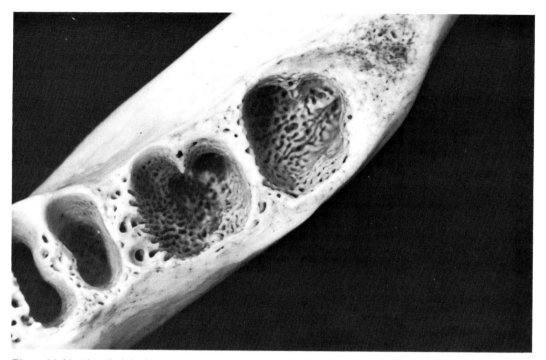

Figure 14–20. Alveoli of the first, second and third molars. Items for special attention: the thin and perforated surface of the retromolar triangular space distal to the third molar alveolus and the cancellous formation in the alveoli proper and also in the interdental septa, which would allow a rich blood supply.

The distal border of the ramus is smooth and rounded and presents a concave outline from the neck of the condyle to the angle of the jaw, where the posterior border of the ramus and the inferior border of the body of the mandible join. The border of this angle is rough, being the attachment of the masseter muscle and the stylomandibular ligament.

An important landmark on the lateral aspect of the mandible is the *mental foramen*. It should be noted that this opening of the anterior end of the mandibular canal is directed upward and backward as well as laterally. The foramen is usually located midway between the superior and inferior border of the body of the mandible when the teeth are in position, and most often it is below the second premolar tooth, a little below the apex of the root. The position of this foramen is not constant, and it may be between the first premolar and the second premolar tooth. After the teeth are lost and resorption of alveolar bone has taken place, the mental foramen may appear near the crest of the alveolar border. In childhood, before the first permanent molar has come into position, this foramen is usually immediately below the first primary molar and nearer the lower border.

It is interesting to note, when we observe the mandible from a point directly opposite the first molar, that most of the distal half of the third molar is hidden by the anterior border of the ramus. When the mandible is viewed from in front, directly opposite the median line, the second and third molars are located 5 to 7 mm lingually to the anterior border of the ramus (compare Figs. 14–11 and 14–15).

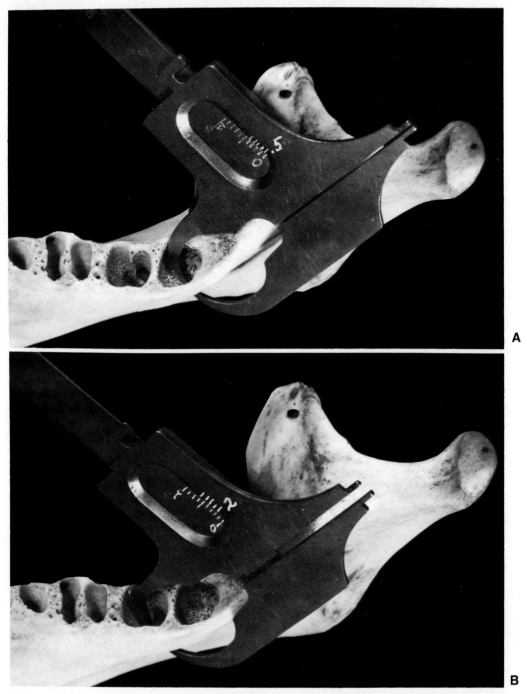

Figure 14–21. Illustration of the relative thickness of bone covering lingual mandibular second and third molar roots. *A,* Measurement of the thickness of bony cover lingual to the apex of the third mandibular molar immediately below the mylohyoid ridge. It measured only 0.5 mm. *B,* Repetition of measurement in the deepest portion lingually of the second molar alveolus. It measured fully 2 mm.

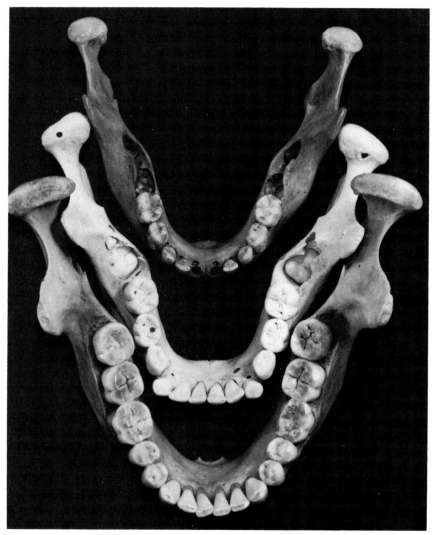

Figure 14–22. Comparison of size and shape of mandibles at various ages. *Top,* Mandible of 5-year-old. Notice the rounded bowlike form. Notice also the amount of space between the second deciduous molar and the ramus. *Middle,* Mandible of 9-year-old. Notice the angular outline with constriction at the point of second permanent molar development. *Lower,* Well-developed mandible of an individual approximately 50 years of age. The bone is regular in outline. The lingual constriction has lessened and has retreated to the third molar area.

The Internal Surface of the Mandible

Observation of the mandible from the rear shows that the median line is marked by a slight vertical depression, representing the line of union of the right and left halves of the mandible, and immediately below this, at the lower third, that the bone is roughened by eminences called the superior and inferior mental spines or *genial tubercles* (Figs. 14–14 and 14–33, *C*).

The internal surface of the body of the mandible is divided into two portions by a well-defined ridge, the *mylohyoid line*. It occupies a position closely corresponding to the lateral oblique ridge on the surface. It starts at or near the lowest part of the mental spines and passes backward and upward, increasing in prominence until the anterior portion of the ramus is reached; there it smooths out and gradually disappears (Figs. 14–13 and 14–33).

This ridge is the point of origin of the mylohyoid muscle, which forms the central portion of the floor of the mouth. Immediately posterior to the median line and above the anterior part of the mylohyoid ridge a smooth depression, the *sublingual fossa,* may be seen. The sublingual gland lies in this area.

A small oval roughened depression, the *digastric fossa,* is found on each side of the symphysis immediately below the mylohyoid line and extending onto the lower border. Toward the center of the body of the mandible, between the mylohyoid line and the lower border of the bone, a smooth oblong depression is located, called the *submandibular fossa.* It continues back on the medial surface of the ramus to the attachment of the lateral pterygoid muscle. The submandibular gland lies within this fossa.

The *mandibular foramen* is located on the medial surface of the ramus midway between the mandibular notch and the angle of the jaw and also midway between the internal oblique line and the posterior border of the ramus. The mandibular canal begins at this point, passing downward and forward horizontally.

The anterior margin of the foramen is formed by the *lingula,* or *mandibular spine,* which gives attachment to the *sphenomandibular ligament.* Coming obliquely downward from the base of the foramen beneath the lingula is a decided groove, the *mylohyoid groove.* Behind this groove toward the angle of the mandible, a roughened surface for the attachment of the medial pterygoid muscle may be seen.

The Alveolar Process

The border of this process outlines the alveoli of the teeth and is very thin at its anterior portion around the roots of the incisor teeth but thicker posteriorly where it encompasses the roots of the molars. The alveolar process, which comprises the superior border of the body of the mandible, differs from the same process in the maxillae in one very important particular: It is not as cancellous, and instead of the facial plate being thin and frail, it is equally as heavy as the lingual plate. Although the bone over the anterior teeth, including the canine, is very thin and over the cervical portion of the root may be entirely missing, the bone that does cover the root is the compact type.

The inferior border of the mandible is strong and rounded and gives to the bone the greatest portion of its strength (see Fig. 14–14).

When looking down on the mandible from a point above the alveoli of the first molars (Fig. 14–17), we may notice that although the alveolar border may be thinner anteriorly than posteriorly, the body of the bone is uniform throughout. The lines of direction of the posterior alveoli are inclined lingually to conform to the lingual inclination of the teeth when they are in position. The anterior teeth, of course, have their alveoli tipped labially; therefore, when we look down upon the mandible from above the alveolar process, more of the bone may be seen lingual to the anterior teeth than lingual to the posterior teeth. In contrast posteriorly, more of the bone may be seen buccal to the teeth than lingual. *Therefore, the outline of the arch of the teeth does not correspond to the outline of the arch of the bone.* The dental arch is narrower posteriorly than the mandibular arch.

The lingual walls of the alveoli of the second and third molars are relatively thin near the bottoms of the sockets, although the bone near the periphery is somewhat thicker and very compact. If a specimen of the mandible from which the third molar has been removed is held up to the light, the bone at the bottom of the socket is so thin that light will penetrate it. This is caused by the mandible being undercut at this point for the submaxillary fossa below the mylohyoid ridge (Figs. 14–14 and 14–21, *A* and *B,* Fig. 14–23).

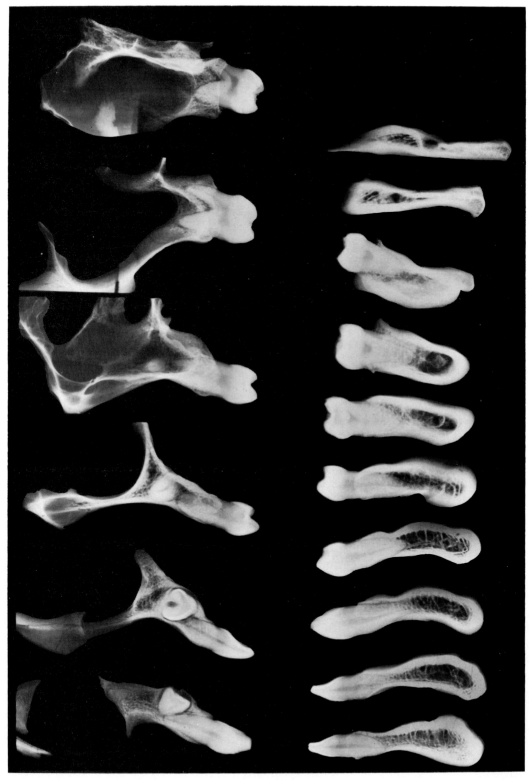

Figure 14-23. Some fine vertical sections of a skull made with radiographic problems in view. Faciolingual views of the teeth and their attachment cannot be obtained by clinical radiographic methods.

These radiographs of faciolingual sections show the extent of tooth attachment, the way in which individual teeth compare with each other, and the variances between cortical and cancellous bone in anchorage. (See also Figures 14–24 through 14–31.) The maxillary canine was impacted in this specimen. Maxillary third molars were missing. (From Updegrave, W. J.: Normal radiodontic anatomy. Dent. Radiogr. Photogr., 31:57, 1958.)

The bone buccal to the last two molars is very heavy and thick, being reinforced by the external oblique ridge. Posterior to the third molar a triangular shallow fossa is outlined; it is called the *retromolar triangle* (Fig. 14–16). The cortical plate over this fossa is not as heavy as the bone surrounding it, and it is more cancellous under the thin cortical plate covering it.

The Alveoli

The first alveolus right or left of the median line is that of the *first,* or *central, incisor.* The periphery of the alveolus often dips down lingually and labially and exposes the root for part of its length. This arrangement makes an interdental spine out of the interdental septum separating the alveoli of the mandibular central incisors. The central incisor alveolus is flattened on its mesial surface and is usually somewhat concave distally to accommodate the developmental groove on the root (Figs. 14–17 and 14–18).

The alveolus of the mandibular *second,* or *lateral, incisor* is similar to that of the central incisor. It usually has the following variations: The socket is larger and deeper to accommodate a larger and longer root; the periphery does not dip down as far on the lingual surface but may dip more on the labial aspect of the tooth, exposing more of the root of the lateral incisor. The interdental septum extends up just as high between the teeth as that between the central incisors.

The *canine alveolus* is quite large and oval and, of course, deep to accommodate the root of the mandibular canine. The lingual plate is stronger and much heavier than over the alveoli just described, although the thin labial plate may thin out at its edges and expose just as much of the canine root on the labial side. The labial outline of the alveolus is wider than the lingual outline, and the mesial and distal walls of the sockets will be irregular to accommodate developmental grooves, both mesially and distally, on the canine root (Figs. 14–17 and 14–19).

The alveoli of the *first* and *second premolars* are similar in outline. The outline is smooth and rounded, although the dimensions are greater buccolingually than mesio-distally. The alveolus of the second premolar is usually somewhat larger than that of the first premolar. The buccal plate of the alveoli is relatively thin, but the lingual plate is heavy; the interdental septum has become heavier at this point when compared with the interdental septa found between the anterior teeth. The interdental septum between the canine and first premolar is relatively thin although uniform in outline. The septum between the first premolar and second premolar is nearly twice as thick.

Progressing posteriorly (Figs. 14–17 and 14–19), we find that the interdental septum between the second premolar socket and the alveolus of the mesial root of the *first molar* is twice as thick as that found between the first and second premolars. The socket of the first molar is divided by an interroot septum which is strong and regular. The alveolus of the mesial root is kidney-shaped, much wider buccolingually than mesiodistally, and constricted in the center to accommodate developmental grooves found mesial and distal to the mesial root of the first molar. The alveolus of the distal root of the first molar is evenly oval with no constriction, conforming to the rounded shape of this root. The interdental septum between the alveoli of the mandibular first molar and the socket of the second molar is thick mesiodistally although cancellous in character.

The mandibular *second molar alveolus* may be divided into *two* alveoli, as was the case in the first molar. However, often it is found to be one compartment near the periphery of the alveolus but divides into two compartments in the deeper portions. A septal spine occurs where the developmental grooves on the root are deep enough, or an interradicular septum will appear where the roots are entirely divided. The interdental septum between the second molar sockets and the third molar sockets is not as thick mesiodistally as the two interdental septa immediately anterior.

The mandibular *third molar alveolus* is usually irregular in outline (Fig. 14–20). Usually it is much narrower toward the distal than toward the mesial aspect of the alveolus. It may have interradicular septa or septal spines to accommodate itself to the irregularity of the root.

Classical illustrations by Dr. Hugh W. MacMillan are shown in Figs. 14–24 through 14–31. The sections demonstrate the directional lines of the axes of the teeth and their alveoli. In addition, the radiographs of the sections graphically illustrate the relative

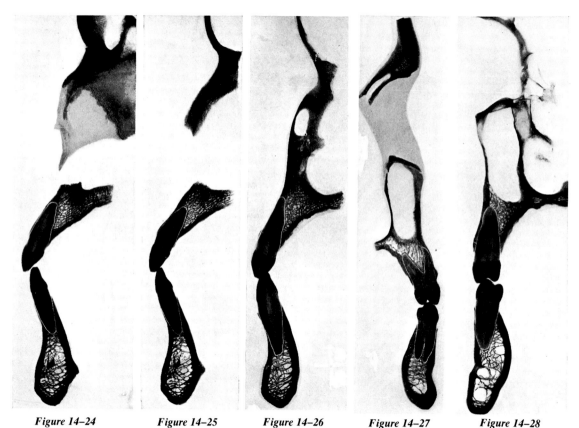

| *Figure 14–24* | *Figure 14–25* | *Figure 14–26* | *Figure 14–27* | *Figure 14–28* |

Figure 14–24 through 14–28. Note the axial relations of the superior and inferior teeth, the relative thickness of labial and lingual alveolar plates, the characteristics of the cancellous tissue, the relative densities, and the relation of the teeth to important structures. Compare the changes in the external contour and internal architecture of the adjacent sections. The sections in this series, with the exception of Fig. 14–27, were taken from the same cadaver and are from the left side. A plaster cast was made before sectioning. The sections were reassembled in the cast and held in exact relation while being x-rayed.

Figure 14–24. Central incisor regions, showing relation of superior central incisor to inferior lateral incisor.

Figure 14–25. Lateral incisor regions. Note position of apex of superior lateral incisor.

Figure 14–26. Canine regions. Note anterior extremity of maxillary antrum.

Figure 14–27. The first premolar regions.

Figure 14–28. The second premolar regions.
(From Macmillan, H. W.: The structure and function of the alveolar process. J. Am. Dent. Assoc., 11:1059, 1924.)

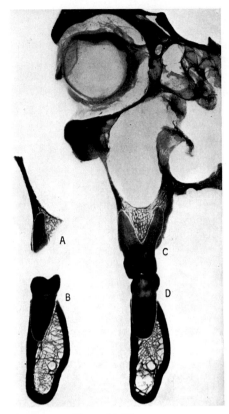

Figure 14–29

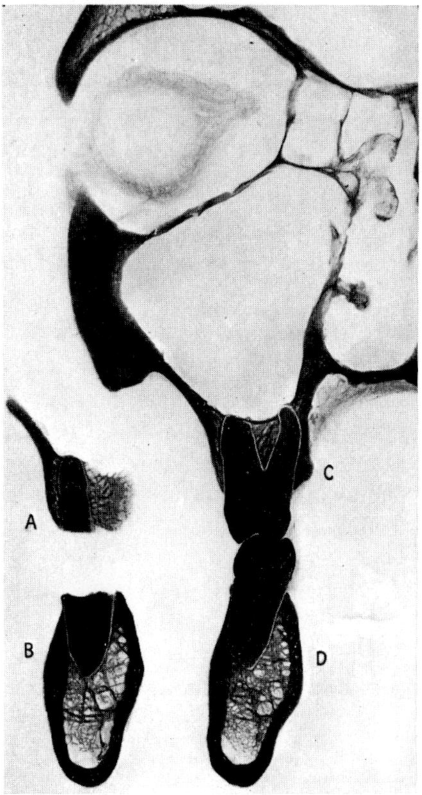

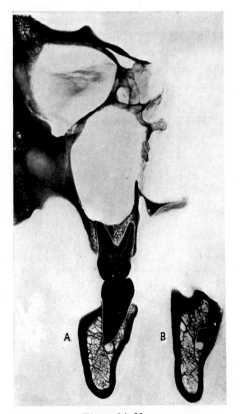

Figure 14–31

Figure 14–30

Figure 14–29. The first molar regions, showing relations of *(C)* mesiobuccal and lingual roots with *(D)* mesial half of lower molar, *(A)* distobuccal root, *(B)* distal half. (From MacMillan. H. W.: The structure and function of the alveolar process. J. Am. Dent. Assoc., 11:1059, 1924.)

Figure 14–30. The second molar regions, showing relations of *(C)* mesiobuccal and lingual roots with mesial half *(D)*, distobuccal root *(A)*, and distal root *(B)*.

Figure 14–31. The third molar regions. *(A)* Mesial root. *(B)* Apex of distal root. Note deep groove for descending palatine artery.

(From MacMillan, H. W.: The structure and function of the alveolar process. J. Am. Dent. Assoc., 11:1059, 1924.)

densities of the teeth and supporting structures and show the outline and relative thickness of the bone over the various teeth at the site of each section.

Figures 14–32, I and II, illustrate the appearance of some of the bony landmarks of the maxilla and mandible as visualized in intraoral periapical radiography. Surface as well as dento-osseous structures are often important to recognize in relation to diagnostic and treatment aspects (Fig. 14–33).

Arterial Supply to the Teeth

The arteries and nerve branches to the teeth are mere terminals of the central systems. This book must confine itself to dental anatomy and the parts immediately associated, and references will therefore be made only to those terminals that supply the teeth and the supporting structures.

Internal Maxillary Artery (Fig. 14–34)

The arterial supply to the jaw bones and the teeth comes from the *maxillary artery,* which is a branch of the *external carotid artery.* The *branches* of the maxillary artery which feed the teeth directly are the *inferior alveolar artery* and the *superior alveolar arteries.*

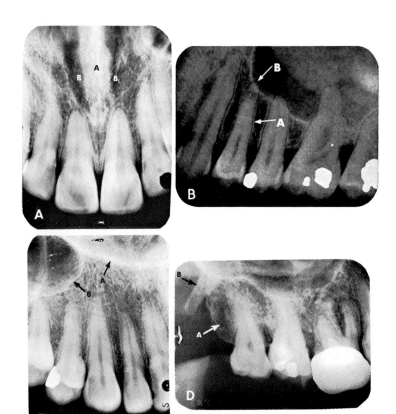

Figure 14–32, I. A, Radiograph of central incisor region visualizes the nasal septum *(A)* and fossae *(B). B,* Radiograph demonstrates the normal appearance of the lamina dura *(A)* and the periodontal membrane *(B). C,* Radiograph depicts the Y (inverted) formed by the junction of the lateral wall *(A)* of the nasal fossa and the antemedial wall *(B)* of the maxillary sinus. *D,* Radiograph visualizes the tuberosity of the maxilla *(A)* and the hamular process of the sphenoid bone *(B).* (From McCauley, H. B.: Anatomic characteristics important in radontic interpretation. Dent. Radiogr. Photogr., 18:1, 1945.

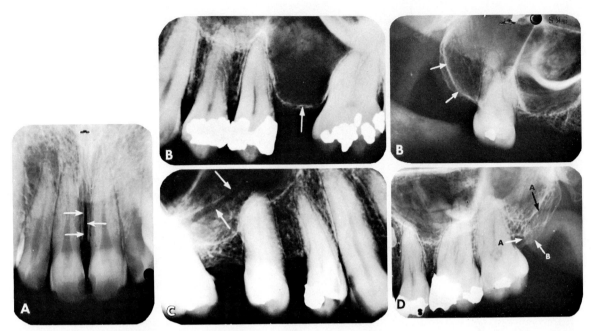

Figure 14-32, II. A, Radiograph of the medial palatine suture, the appearance of which might be interpreted as a fracture. *B,* Radiographs visualize various extensions of the maxillary sinus; left, alveolar extension; right, tuberosity extension. *C,* Radiograph in which the canal for a superior alveolar artery is seen. *D,* Radiograph showing typical superimposition of the coronoid process: *(A)* of the mandible on the tuberosity, *(B)* of the maxilla. (From McCauley, H. B.: Anatomic characteristics important in radontic interpretation. Dent. Radiogr. Photogr., 18:1, 1945.)

Inferior Alveolar Artery

The *inferior alveolar artery* branches from the maxillary artery medial to the ramus of the mandible. Protected by the sphenomandibular ligament, it gives off the *mylohyoid branch,* which rests in the mylohyoid groove of the mandible and continues along on the medial side under the mylohyoid line. After giving off the mylohyoid branch, it immediately enters the mandibular foramen and continues downward and forward through the mandibular canal, giving off branches to the premolar and molar teeth. In the vicinity of the mental foramen, it divides into a *mental* and an *incisive branch.* The mental branch passes through the mental foramen to supply the tissues of the chin and to anastomose with the *inferior labial* and *submental arteries.* The incisive branch continues forward in the bone to supply the anterior teeth and bone and to form anastomoses with its fellows of the opposite side.

The anastomoses of the mental and incisive branches furnish a good collateral blood supply for the mandible and teeth.

In their canals, the inferior alveolar and incisive arteries give off *dental* branches to the individual tooth roots for the supply of the pulp and of the periodontal membrane at the root apex. Other branches enter the interdental septa, supply bone and adjacent periodontal membrane and terminating in the gingivae. Numerous small anastomoses connect these vessels with those supplying the neighboring alveolar mucosa.

Superior Alveolar Arteries

The *posterior superior alveolar artery* branches from the maxillary artery superior to the maxillary tuberosity to enter the alveolar canals along with the posterior superior alveolar nerves and supplies the maxillary teeth, alveolar bone, and membrane of the sinus. A

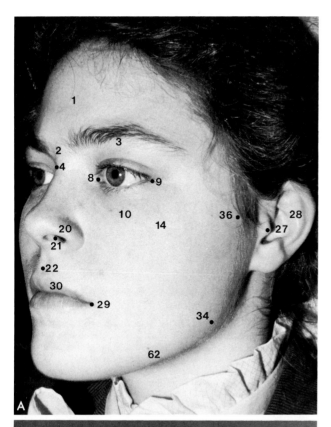

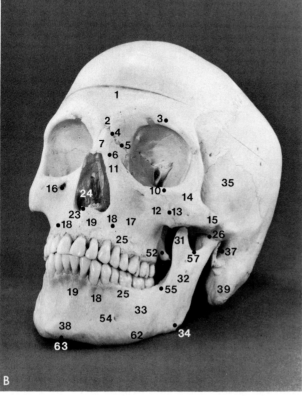

Figure 14–33. Surface landmarks

Various dental structures in the patient's face can be quickly located by means of surface landmarks. Surface landmarks are identified in A. The photograph of the bony skull *(B)* was made from the same angle of view. Features of both are numbered and identified in the legend. The medial aspect of the mandible *(C)* shows anatomic details not clearly seen in the other illustrations. The maxilla and zygoma are shown in *D*. The bony anatomy of the hard palate and its adjoining structures is shown in *E*. Structures are identified by numbers in the legend.

1 Frontal bone—forehead
2 Glabella
3 Supraorbital ridge—superciliary ridge
4 Frontonasal suture—bridge of nose
5 Maxillofrontal suture
6 Maxillonasal suture
7 Nasal bone
8 Medial canthus
9 Lateral canthus
10 Infraorbital ridge
11 Frontal process of maxilla
12 Zygomatic process of maxilla
13 Zygomaticomaxillary suture
14 Zygomatic bone—cheekbone
15 Zygomatic arch
16 Infraorbital foramen
17 Canine fossa
18 Canine eminence
19 Incisive fossa
20 Nasal ala
21 Nares
22 Philtrum
23 Anterior nasal spine
24 Inferior nasal concha

Illustration continued on opposite page.

*Figure 14–33 Continued. **Surface landmarks.***

25 Alveolar process
26 Temporomandibular articulation
27 Tragus of ear
28 Auricula
29 Labial commissure
30 Vermilion border of lip
31 Coronoid process of mandible
32 Ramus of mandible
33 Body of mandible
34 Gonial angle of mandible
35 Infratemporal fossa
36 Condyle
37 External acoustic meatus
38 Mental protuberance
39 Mastoid process of temporal bone
40 Maxillary tuberosity
41 Posterior nasal spine
42 Articular eminence
43 Styloid process of temporal bone
44 Mandibular fossa
45 Vomer
46 Greater palatine foramen
47 Lesser palatine foramen
48 Palatine bone
49 Palatine process of maxilla
50 Midpalatal suture
51 Incisive foramen
52 Lateral pterygoid plate of sphenoid bone
53 Inferior orbital fissure
54 Mental foramen
55 Oblique line
56 Mandibular foramen
57 Mandibular notch
58 Internal oblique ridge
59 Submandibular fossa
60 Sublingual fossa
61 Genial tubercle
62 Inferior border of mandible
63 Symphysis
64 Mylohyoid line
65 Hamular process of sphenoid bone
66 Zygomaticotemporal suture
67 Greater wing of sphenoid bone
68 Lacrimal bone
69 Maxillolacrimal suture
70 Lacrimal fossa

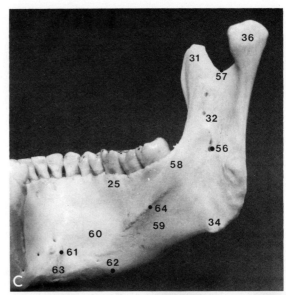

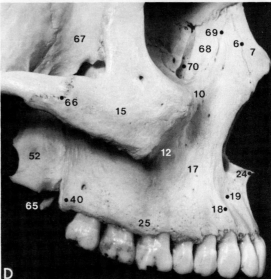

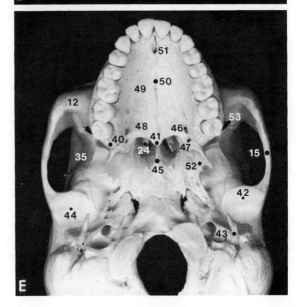

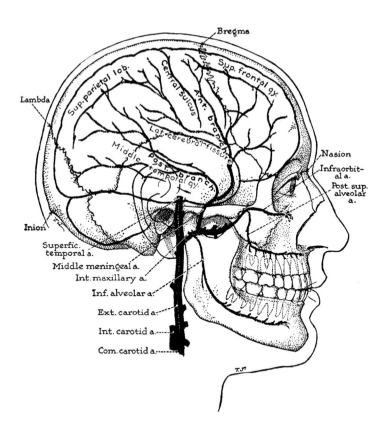

Figure 14–34. Projection of maxillary artery and its branches in relation to brain, skull, and mandible, including the teeth. (From Jones, T. S., and Shepard, W. C.: *A Manual of Surgical Anatomy*. Philadelphia, W. B. Saunders Company, 1945.)

branch of variable size runs forward on the periosteum at the junction of the alveolar process and maxillary body supplying the gingiva, alveolar mucosa, and cheek. When it is large, it may supplant in part the buccal artery.

A *middle superior alveolar branch* is usually given off by the infraorbital continuation of the maxillary artery somewhere along the infraorbital groove or canal. It runs downward between the sinus mucosa and bone or in canals in the bone and joins the *posterior* and *anterior alveolar vessels*. Its main distribution is to the maxillary premolar teeth.

Anterior superior alveolar branches arise from the infraorbital artery just before this vessel leaves its foramen. They course down the anterior aspect of the maxilla in bony canals to supply the maxillary anterior teeth and their supporting tissues and to join the *middle* and *posterior superior alveolar branches* in completing an anastomotic plexus.

Branches to the teeth, periodontal ligament, and bone are derived from the superior alveolar in the same manner as described for the inferior alveolar artery.

Descending Palatine and Sphenopalatine Arteries

The palatal blood supply comes from two sources but chiefly from the *descending palatine* artery, which descends from its origin from the maxillary through the greater canal. Its *greater palatine* branch enters the palate through the greater palatine foramen and runs forward with its accompanying vein and nerve in a groove at the junction of the palatine and alveolar processes. It is distributed to the bone, glands, and mucosa of the hard palate and to the bone and mucosa of the alveolar process, in which it forms anastomoses with fine branches of the superior alveolars. Minor branches of the descending palatine artery pass to the soft palate through lesser palatine foramina in the palatine bone.

The *nasopalatine* branch of the *sphenopalatine artery* courses obliquely forward and downward on the septum and enters the palate through the incisive canal. It has a limited distribution to the incisive papilla and adjacent palate and forms an anastomosis with the greater palatine.

Nerve Supply

The sensory nerve supply to the jaws and teeth is derived from the *maxillary* and *mandibular* branches of the *fifth cranial*, or *trigeminal*, nerve, whose ganglion, the *trigeminal*, is located at the apex of the petrous portion of the temporal bone.

Maxillary Nerve (Fig. 14–35)

The *maxillary* nerve courses forward through the wall of the cavernous sinus and leaves the skull through the foramen rotundum. It crosses the pterygopalatine fossa, where it gives branches to the pterygopalatine ganglion, a parasympathetic ganglion. This ganglion gives off several branches, now containing visceral motor as well as sensory fibers, to the mucous membrane of the mouth, nose, and pharynx.

The branches of clinical significance include: a *greater palatine* branch that enters the hard palate through the greater palatine foramen and is distributed to the hard palate and palatal gingivae as far forward as the canine tooth; a *lesser* palatine branch from the ganglion that enters the soft palate through the lesser palatine foramina; and a *nasopalatine* branch of the posterior or superior lateral nasal branch of the ganglion that runs downward

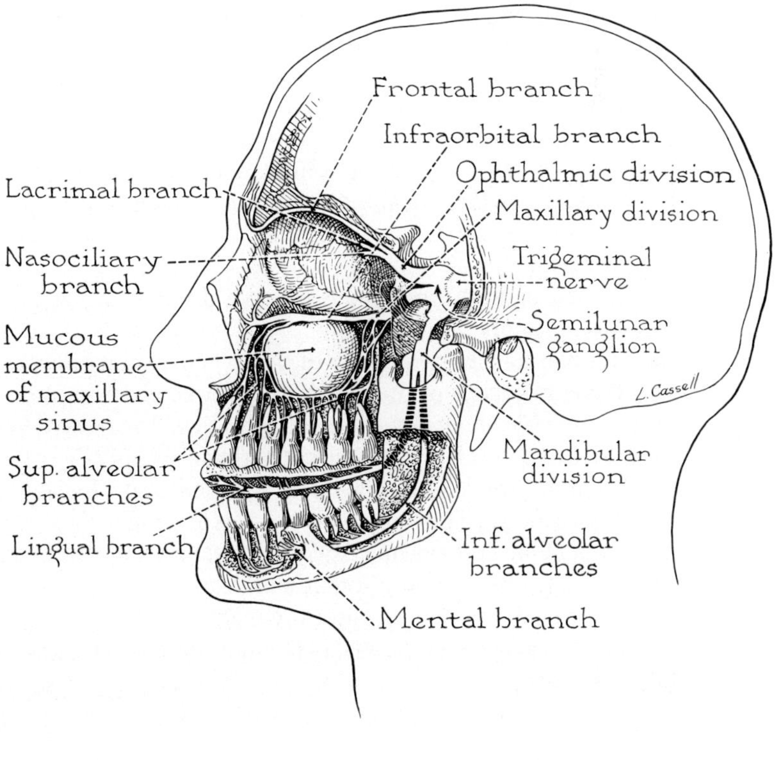

Figure 14–35. Diagram showing distribution of the trigeminal nerve. (From King, B. G., and Showers, M. T.: *Human Anatomy and Physiology*, 6th ed. Philadelphia, W. B. Saunders Company, 1969.)

and forward on the nasal septum. Entering the palate through the incisive canal, it is distributed to the incisive papilla and to the palate anterior to the anterior palatine nerve.

The maxillary nerve also has a *posterior superior alveolar* branch from its pterygo-palatine portion. This nerve enters the alveolar canals on the infratemporal surface of the maxilla and, forming a plexus, is distributed to the molar teeth and the supporting tissues.

The maxillary nerve enters the orbit and, as the *infraorbital nerve,* runs forward in its floor first in the infraorbital groove and then in the infraorbital canal. It terminates at the infraorbital foramen in branches distributed to the upper face. At a variable distance after it enters the orbit, a *middle superior alveolar* branch arises from the infraorbital nerve and runs through the lateral wall of the maxillary sinus. It is distributed to the premolar teeth and surrounding tissues and joins the alveolar plexus. The middle superior alveolar nerve may be associated closely with the posterior superior alveolar nerve as its origin but frequently branches near the infraorbital foramen.

An anterior superior alveolar branch leaves the infraorbital nerve just inside the infraorbital foramen and is distributed through bony canals to the incisor and canine teeth. All three superior alveolar nerves join in a plexus above the process. From the plexus, *dental branches* are given off to each tooth root and *interdental branches* to the bone, periodontal membrane and gingivae, the distribution being similar to that described for the arteries.

Mandibular Nerve (Fig. 14–35)

The *mandibular nerve* leaves the skull through the foramen ovale and almost immediately breaks up into its several branches. The chief branch to the lower jaw is the *inferior alveolar* nerve, which at first runs directly downward across the medial surface of the lateral pterygoid, at the lower border of which it is directed laterally and downward across the outer surface of the medial pterygoid muscle to reach the mandibular foramen. Just before entering the foramen, it releases the mylohyoid branch, which is a motor branch to the mylohyoid muscle and anterior belly of the digastric muscle.

The inferior alveolar nerve continues forward through the mandibular canal beneath the roots of the molar teeth to the level of the mental foramen. During this part of its course, it gives off branches to the molar and premolar teeth and their supporting bone and soft tissues. The nerve to the teeth does not arise as individual branches but as two or three larger branches that form a plexus from which *inferior dental* branches enter individual tooth roots and *interdental* branches supply alveolar bone, periodontal membrane, and gingivae.

At the mental foramen, the nerve divides and a smaller incisive branch continues forward to supply the anterior teeth and bone—and a larger mental branch emerges through the foramen to supply the skin of the lower lip and chin.

Other branches of the mandibular nerve contribute in some degree to the innervation of the mandible and its investing membranes. The *buccal nerve,* while chiefly distributed to the mucosa of the cheek, has a branch that is usually distributed to a small area of the buccal gingiva in the first molar area, but in some cases its distribution may extend from the canine to the third molar. The *lingual nerve,* as it enters the floor of the mouth, lies against the body of the mandible and has mucosal branches to a variable area of lingual mucosa and gingiva. The *mylohyoid nerve* may sometimes continue its course forward on the lower surface of the mylohyoid muscle and enter the mandible through small foramina on either side of the midline. It has been implicated in the innervation of central incisor teeth and their periodontal ligaments.

References

Brash, J. C., and Jamieson, E. B. (eds.) (1940). *Cunningham's Manual of Practical Anatomy,* 10th ed. *Volume 3: Head and Neck: Brain.* New York: Oxford University Press.

Callander, C. L. (1939). *Surgical Anatomy,* 2nd ed. Philadelphia: Saunders.

Deaver, J. B. (1926). *Surgical Anatomy of the Human Body,* 2nd ed. Philadelphia: Blakiston's.

Jones, T. S., and Shepard, W. C. (1945). *A Manual of Surgical Anatomy.* Philadelphia: Saunders.

King, B. G., and Showers, M. J. (1969). *Human Anatomy and Physiology,* 6th ed. Philadelphia: Saunders.

McCauley, H. B. (1945). Anatomic characteristics important in radiodontic interpretation. Dent. Radiogr. Photogr. 18:1.

Morris, H. (1942). *Human Anatomy,* 10th ed. Philadelphia: Blakiston's.

Pernkopf, E. (1963). *Atlas of Topographical and Applied Human Anatomy, vol. 1: Head and Neck,* edited by H. Ferner and translated by H. Monsen. Philadelphia: Saunders.

Rohen, J. W., and Yokochi, C. (1988). *Color Atlas of Anatomy: A Photographic Study of the Human Body,* 2nd ed. New York: Igaku-Shoin Medical.

Updegrave, W. J. (1958). Normal radiodontic anatomy. Dent. Radiogr. Photogr. 31:57.

15 The Temporomandibular Joints, Muscles, and Teeth, and their Functions

The Temporomandibular Articulation

The temporomandibular joint is an example of diarthrosis, and its movements are a combination of gliding movements and a loose hinge movement. The osseous portions of the joint are the anterior portion of the *mandibular (glenoid) fossa* and *articular eminence* of the temporal bone and the *condyloid process* of the mandible (Fig. 15–1). The functional surfaces of both the condyle and the eminence and the anterior aspects of the condyle are the functional articular surfaces, not the mandibular fossa. Interposed between the condyle and temporal bone is the *articular disc*. It consists of dense collagenous connective tissue which, in the central area, is relatively avascular, hyalinized, and devoid of nerves (Fig. 15–7). The disc is not seen on radiographs, but the bony structures in one plane can be viewed by a transcranial projection (Fig. 15–2).

The Mandibular Fossa

The mandibular fossa is an oval or oblong depression in the temporal bone just anterior to the auditory canal (Fig. 15–3). It is bounded anteriorly by the *eminentia articularis* (articular eminence), externally by the middle root of the zygoma and the auditory process, and posteriorly by the tympanic plate of the petrous portion of this bone. The shape of the mandibular fossa conforms to some extent, though not exactly, to the posterior and superior surfaces of the condyloid process of the mandible.

The Condyloid Process

The condyloid process of the mandible is convex on all bearing surfaces, although somewhat flattened posteriorly, and its knoblike form is wider lateromedially than anteroposteriorly (Fig. 15–4). It is perhaps two and one half times as wide in one direction as in the

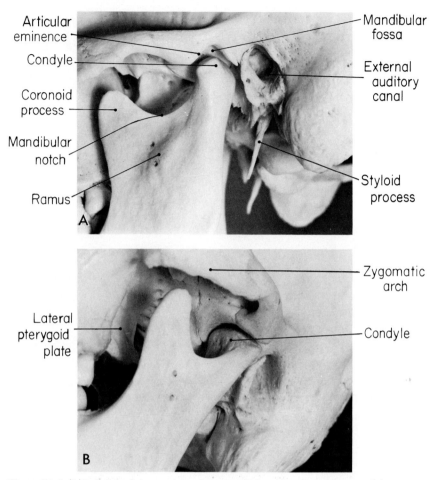

Figure 15–1. *A,* Relation of the condyle of the mandible to the glenoid fossa and the articular eminence of the temporal bone with the teeth in the intercuspal position *B,* View of mandibular fossa and infratemporal fossa.

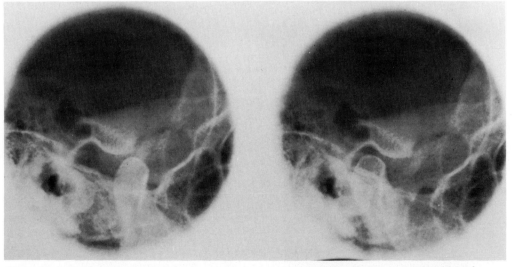

Figure 15–2. Radiograph showing temporamandibular joint in open (*left*) and closed (*right*) position of mandible.

STYLOID PROCESS   ANGULAR SPINE OF SPHENOID

MASTOID
PROCESS

FORAMEN
OVALE

MEDIAL
GLENOID
LIP

AUDITORY
MEATUS

ZYGOMA

POST-
GLENOID
PROCESS

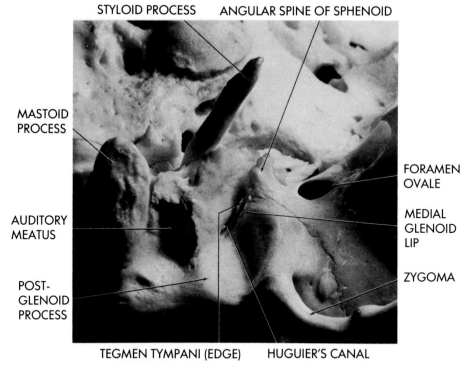

TEGMEN TYMPANI (EDGE)   HUGUIER'S CANAL

Figure 15–3. Exterior of base of skull showing the mandibular fossa in the inferior surface of the squamous part of the temporal bone at the base of the zygomatic process. It is divided into two halves by the petrotympanic fissure. The anterior half is included in the temporomandibular articulation.

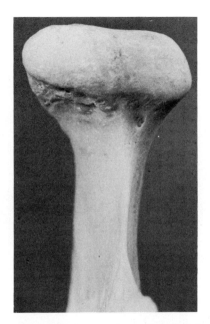

Figure 15–4. Condyloid process viewed from front (left side).

other. Although the development of the condyle differs in individuals, the functional design remains the same. The long axes of the condyles are in a lateral plane, and at first sight they seem to be out of alignment, since the long axes, if the lines were prolonged, would meet at a point anterior to the foramen magnum at an angle of approximately 135°. The condyle is perpendicular to the ascending ramus of the mandible (Fig. 15–4).

Joint Capsule

The temporomandibular joint is enclosed in a capsule (Fig. 15–5) that is attached at the borders of the articulating surfaces of the mandibular fossa and eminence of the temporal bone and to the neck of the mandible. The anterolateral side of the capsule may be thickened to form a band referred to as the "temporomandibular ligament." It is not always so thickened but, when clearly distinguishable as a ligament, it appears to originate on the zygomatic arch and to pass backward to attach on the lateral and/or distal surfaces of the neck of the mandible.

The capsule consists of an internal synovial layer and an outer fibrous layer containing veins, nerves, and collagen fibers. The innervation for the capsule arises from the trigeminal nerve and several kinds of receptors have been described. The vascular supply arises from the maxillary, temporal, and masseteric arteries.

Mandibular Ligaments

Accessory ligaments are considered a part of the masticatory apparatus, including the stylomandibular and sphenomandibular ligaments (Fig. 15–6). These ligaments do not have a direct relationship with mandibular articulation, although they may stabilize the articular system during jaw movements.

The sphenomandibular ligament arises from the angular spine of the sphenoid bone and from the petrotympanic fissures and ends broadly at the lingula of the mandible. In some instances there is a continuation of ligament fibers through the petrotympanic fissure via Huguier's canal (Fig. 15–3) to the middle ear, where they attach to the malleus.

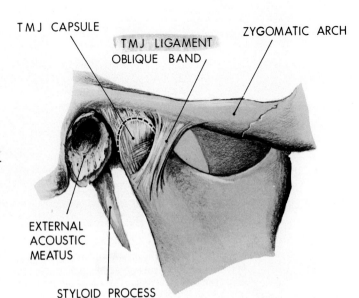

Figure 15–5. TMJ capsule and TMJ ligament.

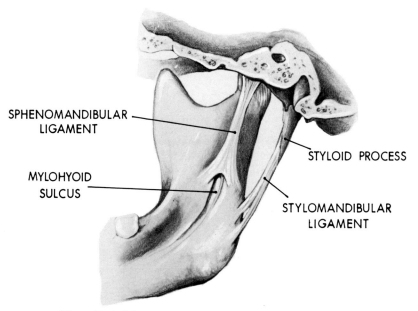

Figure 15–6. Sphenomandibular and stylomandibular ligaments.

There are otomandibular ligaments which connect the middle ear and the temporomandibular joint. These small ligaments, e.g., discomalleolar and tympanomandibular (sphenomandibular), have been described as connecting the malleus to the TMJ disk and to the sphenomandibular ligaments (Figs. 15–7 and 15–8). The role of these ligaments as causal factors in the TMJ mediated auditory symptoms remains to be substantiated (Ash and Pinto, 1991).

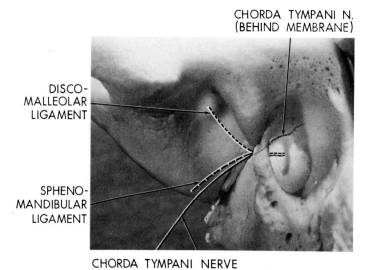

Figure 15–7. Ligaments attached to the malleus. (From Ash et al. Current Concepts of the Relationship and Management of Temporomandibular Disorders and Auditory Symptoms. J. Mich. Dent. Assoc. 72:550, 1990.)

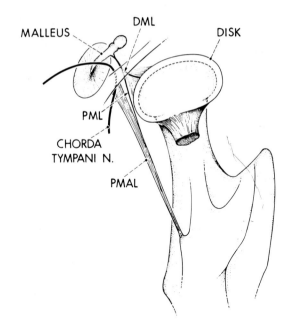

Figure 15–8. Ligaments attached to malleus: PML, fibers from sphenomandibular ligament; DML, discomalleolar ligament fibers. (Ash and Pinto, 1991)

Articular Disk

The interarticular disk (Fig. 15–9) consists of fibrous tissue shaped to accommodate the shape of the condyle and concavity of the mandibular fossa. There are thicker anterior and posterior bands and a thin central zone (Fig. 15–10). The superior and inferior heads of the lateral pterygoid muscle both insert into the pterygoid fovea of the mandible with a part of the superior head inserting into the disk and capsule. The disk divides the articulating surfaces into upper and lower compartments that provide for smooth gliding function. As the jaw opens and moves forward, the intermediate zone of the disk is interposed between the anterior slope of the articular eminence and the condyle and the bilaminar region of the disk fills in the mandibular fossa (Fig. 15–11). The relationship of the disk to the eminence is stabilized by the upper head of the lateral pterygoid muscle, which does not appear to be

Figure 15–9. Schematic representation of temporomandibular joint. The well-defined division of the lateral pterygoid muscle is for illustrative purposes only. A significant number of fibers of the upper part of the lateral pterygoid muscle attach to the neck of the condyle along with the inferior head of the lateral pterygoid muscle.

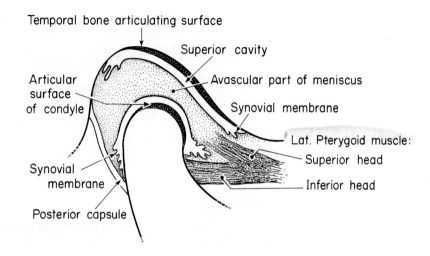

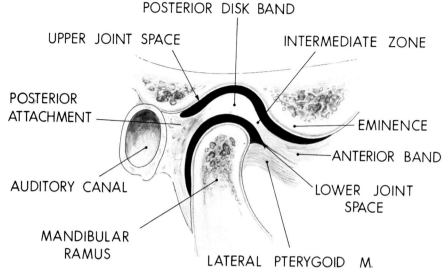

Figure 15–10. Articular disk and associated structures (From Dolwick, M. F. and Sanders, B.: *TMJ Internal Derangement and Arthrosis*, St. Louis, CV Mosby, 1985.)

active during mandibular opening movement. Anterior displacement of the disk (Fig. 15–12) with the posterior band in an anterior position with the jaw closed can prevent the jaw from opening normally ("locking"). The cause of this disk derangement is multifactorial, but may include acute and chronic truma with ischemic necrosis.

Mandibular Positions

Basic jaw positions are usually described as centric occlusion (CO) or the intercuspal (IC) position, centric relation (CR), or the retruded contact position, and rest position of the mandible. *Centric occlusion* is defined as maximum intercuspation of the teeth. *Centric*

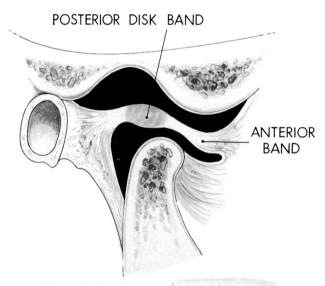

Figure 15–11. Articular disk: jaw in open position.

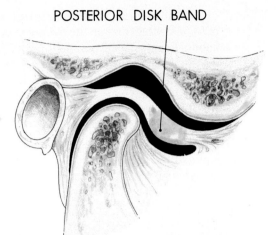

POSTERIOR DISK BAND

Figure 15–12. Articular disk, anterior displacement: jaw in closed position.

relation is a position (or path of opening and closing without translation of the condyles) of the mandible in which the condyles are in their uppermost, midmost positions in the mandibular fossae and related anteriorly to the distal slope of the articular eminence. Because the mandible appears to rotate around a transverse axis through the condyle in centric relation movement, guidance of the jaw by the clinician in opening and closing movements that do not have translation is referred to as *hinge axis movement* (Fig. 15–13). In this position, the condyles are considered to be in the terminal hinge position. Under physiologic conditions of the masticatory system, centric relation is used to transfer the position of the mandible (in relation to the maxilla) to an articulator.

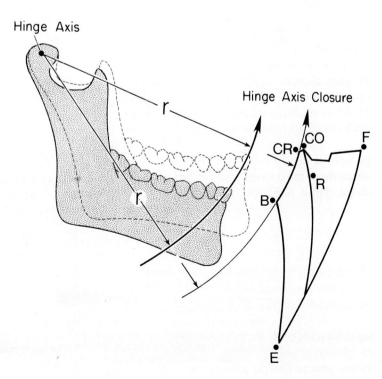

Hinge Axis

Hinge Axis Closure

Figure 15–13. Schematic representation of mandibular movement envelope in sagittal plane. *CR*, Centric relation; *CO*, centric occlusion; *F*, maximum protrusion; *R*, rest position; *E*, maximum opening; *B to CR*, opening and closing on hinge axis with no change in radius (r).

In the natural dentition, centric occlusion is, in a majority of people, anterior to centric relation contact and on the average approximately 1 mm. Centric occlusion (or acquired or habitual centric as it is sometimes called) is a tooth-determined position, whereas centric relation is a jaw-to-jaw relation determined by the condyles in the fossae.

Rest position is a postural position of the mandible determined largely by neuromuscular activity and to a lesser degree by the viscoelastic properties of the muscles. Thus, tonicity of muscles may be influenced by the central nervous system as a result of such factors as emotional stress and by local peripheral factors such as a sore tooth. The interocclusal space with the mandible in rest position, head in upright position, is about 1 to 3 mm at the incisors but has considerable normal variance even up to 8 to 10 mm without evidence of dysfunction.

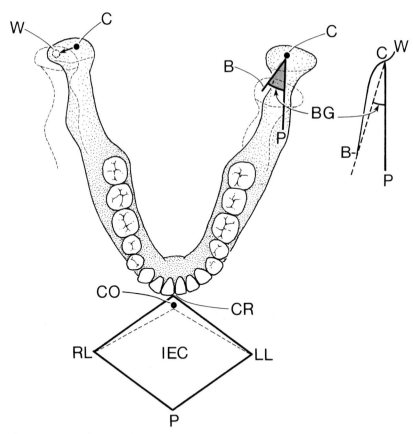

Figure 15–14. Right mandibular movement with schematic representation of movement at incisal point in horizontal plane *(CR, LL, P, RL)* and at the condyle *(W, C, B, P)* made by a pantograph. Teeth are not in occlusion. *CR,* Centric relation; *LL,* left lateral; *P,* protrusive; *RL,* left lateral; *CO,* centric occlusion. On the right side, condyle moves from *C* (centric) to right working *(W).* On the balancing side, left condyle moves from *C* along line *B* and makes an angle *BG,* called Bennett angle. *C to P,* Straight protrusive movement.

Mandibular Movements

In lateral movements (Fig. 15–14), the condyle appears to rotate with a slight lateral shift in the direction of the movement. This movement is called Bennett movement and may have immediate as well as progressive components. By the use of recording equipment (such as a pantograph or kinesiograph) it is possible to record mandibular movements in relation to a particular plane of reference (e.g., sagittal, horizontal, or frontal planes). If a point (the incisive point) located between the incisal edges of the two mandibular central incisors is tracked during maximal lateral and protrusive movements, in retrusive movement, and wide opening movement, such movements take place within a border or envelope of movements (Posselt, 1952). Functional and parafunctional movements take place within these borders. However, most functional movements, such as those associated with mastication, occur chiefly around centric. Border movements in the horizontal plane are shown in Figure 15–14.

The maximum opening movement is 50 to 60 mm, depending on the age and size of the individual. An arbitrary lower limit for normal of 40 mm may be in error inasmuch as some individuals may have no difficulty incising a large apple and have no history of TMJ muscle dysfunction. The maximum lateral movement in the absence of TMJ muscle dysfunction, including pain, is about 10 to 12 mm. The maximum protrusive movement is approximately 8 to 11 mm, again depending on size of the subject and skull morphology. The retrusive range for adults and children is about 1 mm, although 2 to 3 mm may be observed infrequently. The retrusive range, as measured from centric occlusion to centric range, is referred to as a discrepancy between CO and CR. Border movements in the sagittal plane are shown in Figure 15–13.

All values for border movements must be related to function; i.e., a maximum lateral movement of 7 to 8 mm to the right (10 to 12 mm to the left) must be related to the occlusion and to whether or not there is translation of the left condyle, which may be "fixed" because of dysfunction or pain. Such values should also be related to other functions such as incising, chewing, swallowing, and speaking. However, if such values are made a part of every patient's dental record, any change can be evaluated in terms of dysfunction.

Muscles

Masticatory functions, as well as speaking and swallowing, involve reflex contraction and relaxation of the muscles of mastication whose activity is initiated voluntarily. It is impossible to determine clinically if a particular muscle is participating in a particular movement solely from its origin and insertion. Patterns of muscle contraction are complex and even in the same different areas may have different functions.

The complex movements of the temporomandibular joint suggest that muscles of mastication exhibit differential regional action as well as regional differences in their histochemical profiles. Thus, to consider a "muscle" as a contracting entity is an oversimplification. In reality, each muscle is a collection of motor units with different properties located in different parts of a single muscle and exhibiting different activities. However, for obvious reasons, the action of the various muscles will be given as a contracting entity.

The masticatory muscles concerned with mandibular movements include the lateral pterygoid, digastric, masseter, medial pterygoid, and temporalis muscles. Also, the mylohyoid and geniohyoid muscles are involved in masticatory functions (Figs. 15–15 through 15–19).

Several muscles associated with the ear, throat, and neck are of interest to the dentist,

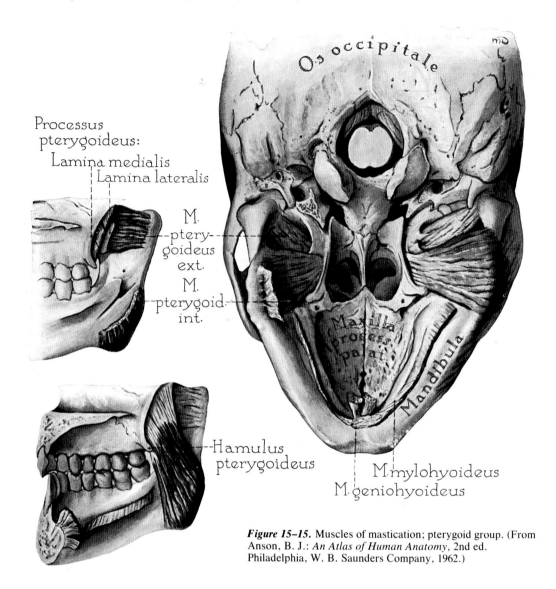

Os occipitale

Processus
pterygoideus:
    Lamina medialis
        Lamina lateralis

M.
pterygoideus
ext.
M.
pterygoid
int.

Maxilla
process
palat

Mandibula

Hamulus
pterygoideus

M.mylohyoideus
M.geniohyoideus

Figure 15–15. Muscles of mastication; pterygoid group. (From
Anson, B. J.: *An Atlas of Human Anatomy,* 2nd ed.
Philadelphia, W. B. Saunders Company, 1962.)

including tensors tympani and palatini, because they may relate to subjective hearing
disorders.

Lateral Pterygoid Muscle

The lateral pterygoid muscle has two origins: One head originates on the outer surface of
the lateral pterygoid plate, and an upper or superior head originates on the greater sphenoid
wing (Figs. 15–15 and 15–16). The insertion is on the anterior surface of the neck of the
condyle. In addition, there is an insertion of some fibers to the capsule of the joint and to the
anterior aspect of the articular disc.

The superior head is active during various jaw-closing movements only, whereas the
inferior head is active during jaw-opening movements and protrusion only. The lateral
pterygoid is anatomically suited for protraction, depression, and contralateral abduction. It

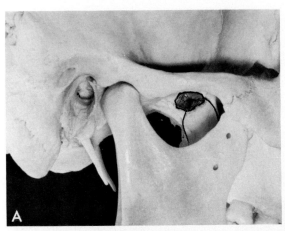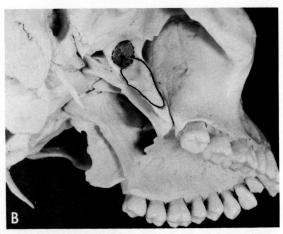

Figure 15–16. Origin of the lateral pterygoid muscle. *A,* Upper head arises from the infratemporal surface of the greater wing of the sphenoid (dark area). Lower head arises from the lateral surface of the lateral pterygoid plate. *B,* Same as in *A* with mandible removed. The lower part ends in the pterygoid fovea of the neck of the mandible. The upper head inserts into the articular disc of the joint and into the upper part of the condyle.

may also be active during other movements for joint stabilization. The superior head is active during such closing movements as chewing and clenching of the teeth and during swallowing. Presumably, the superior head positions or stabilizes the condylar head and disc against the articular eminence during mandibular closing. The inferior head assists in the translation of the condyle downward, anteriorly, and contralaterally during jaw opening. The lateral pterygoid is innervated by nerve V.

Masseter Muscle

The masseter muscle extends from the zygomatic arch to the ramus and body of the mandible. The insertion of this muscle is broad, extending from the region of the second molar on the lateral surface of the mandible to the posterior lateral surface of the ramus (Figs. 15–17 and 15–20). The masseter muscle is covered partly by the platysma muscle (Fig. 15–19) and by the risorius muscle (Fig. 15–19). The platysma is activated during firm clenching in some individuals and, having some insertion in the orbicular muscle (orbicularis oris), is sometimes active in facial expression. The risorius is affected by emotion and is active in facial expression.

The superficial part of the masseter muscle is separated distinctly only from the deeper layer of the muscle at the posterior upper part of the muscle. The masseter muscle is covered partly and to a variable degree with the parotid gland tissue. The center of the lower third of the masseter muscle is about 2 to 3 cm from the anterior border of the sternocleidomastoid muscle, which contracts during clenching in some individuals. The masseter muscle is active during forceful jaw closing and may assist in protrusion of the mandible. The masseter muscle is innervated by the fifth nerve (masseter nerve). The *zygomaticomandibular muscle* inserts at the coronoid process and originates on the inner surface of the zygomatic arch. It may be an antagonist to the posterior temporalis and a synergist for the lateral pterygoid muscle.

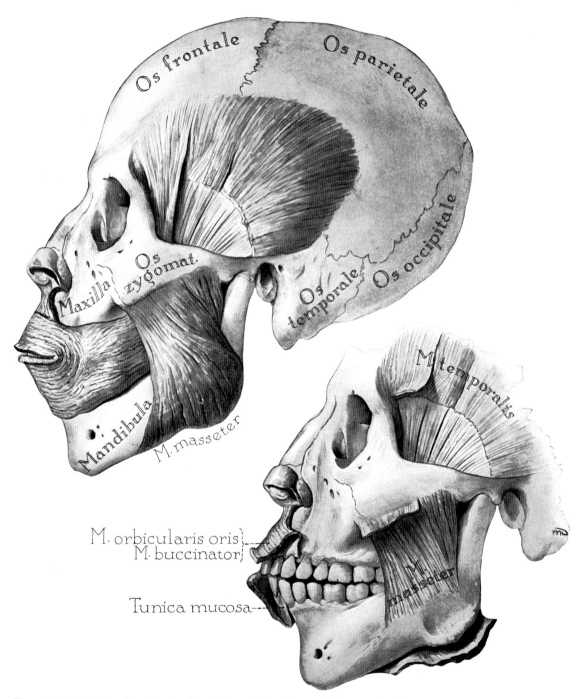

Figure 15–17. Muscles of mastication, lateral views. (From Anson, J. B.: *An Atlas of Human Anatomy*, 2nd ed. Philadelphia, W. B. Saunders Company, 1962.)

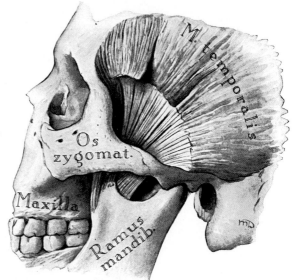

Figure 15–18. Muscles of mastication, lateral view. (From Anson, B. J.: *An Atlas of Human Anatomy,* 2nd ed. Philadelphia, W. B. Saunders Company, 1962.)

Medial Pterygoid Muscle

The medial pterygoid muscle arises from the medial surface of the lateral pterygoid plate and from the palatine bone (Fig. 15–15). It inserts on the medial surface of the angle of the mandible and on the ramus up to the mandibular foramen. The principal functions of the medial pterygoid muscle are elevation and lateral positioning of the mandible. It is active during protrusion. The innervation is a branch of the mandibular division of the fifth nerve.

Temporalis Muscle

The temporalis muscle is fan-shaped and originates in the temporal fossa (Figs. 15–17 and 15–18). On passing to the zygomatic arch, it forms a tendon that inserts into the anterior border and mesial surface of the coronoid process of the mandible and along the anterior border of the ascending ramus of the mandible. The anterior fibers extend along the anterior border of the ramus almost to the third molar. The muscle has three component parts and appears to behave as if it consisted of three distinct parts. The temporal muscle is the principal positioner of the mandible during elevation. The posterior part is active in retruding the mandible and the anterior part is active in clenching. The anterior part may act as a synergist with the masseter in clenching, whereas the posterior part acts as an antagonist to the masseter in retruding the jaw. The temporalis muscle is innervated by temporal branches of the mandibular division of the fifth nerve.

Digastric Muscle

The attachment of the anterior digastric muscle is at or near the lower border of the mandible and near the midline. There is a tendon between the anterior and posterior digastric muscles that is attached by a looplike strip of fascia to the hyoid bone. The anterior digastric muscle is covered by the platysma muscle, and beneath lie the mylohyoid

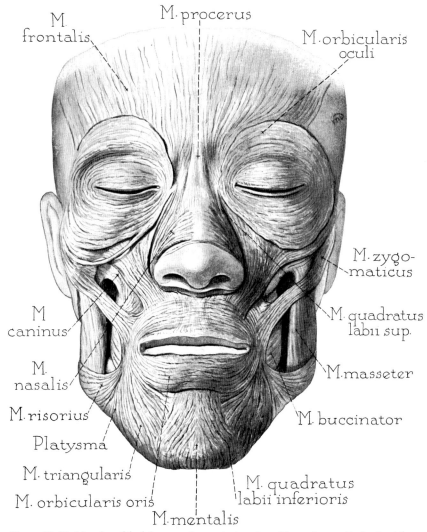

M.
frontalis

M. procerus

M. orbicularis
oculi

M. zygo-
maticus

M
caninus

M. quadratus
labii sup.

M.
nasalis

M. masseter

M. risorius

M. buccinator

Platysma

M. triangularis

M. quadratus
labii inferioris

M. orbicularis oris

M. mentalis

Figure 15–19. Muscles of facial expression, anterior view. (From Anson, B. J.: *An Atlas of Human Anatomy*, 2nd ed. Philadelphia, W. B. Saunders Company, 1962.)

and the geniohyoid muscles. All of these muscles are considered to be active during various phases of jaw opening. A mylohyoid branch of the mandibular division of the fifth nerve innervates the anterior digastric muscle; the digastric branch of the facial nerve innervates the posterior digastric muscle.

Geniohyoid Muscles

The geniohyoid muscle lies superior to the mylohyoid muscle and adjacent to the midline. It arises from the mental spine on the posterior aspect of the symphysis menti of the mandible. It inserts on the anterior surface of the hyoid bone. When the mandible is fixed, the hyoid bone is drawn forward and upward; when the hyoid bone is fixed, the lower jaw is depressed. Innervation is C_1, C_2, and possibly the hypoglossal nerve.

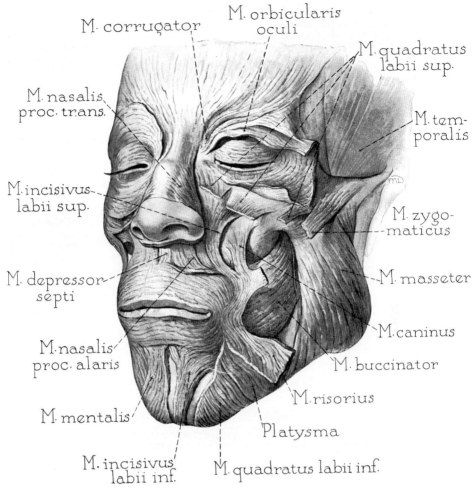

Figure 15–20. Muscles of facial expression, anterolateral view. (From Anson, B. J.: *An Atlas of Human Anatomy,* 2nd ed. Philadelphia, W. B. Saunders Company, 1962.)

Tensor Tympani and Palatini Muscles

The tensor tympani (Fig. 15–21) and tensor veli palatini muscles (Fig. 15–22) are innervated by the trigeminal nerve and therefore may respond to similar kinds of ascending information from joints, skin and muscles, as well as from descending inputs from higher centers that converge on interneurons and the trigeminal motor nucleus (Fig. 15–24). Disturbances of active auditory tube opening during swallowing that occur frequently with TMJ and muscle disorders (TMD) are consistent with restricted function and anatomy of the tensor palatini and levator veli palatini muscles.

Restricted jaw opening and prevention of yawning seen in TMJ and muscle disorders can lead to otologic symptoms such as subjective hearing loss and "stuffy" sensations in the ear. Thus pain in and around the joints and muscles may influence the otomandibular muscles via interneurons in the intertrigeminal area and be responsible for a few cases of tinnitus, and restricted jaw opening due to TMJ and muscle disorders may be responsible for the subjective hearing loss.

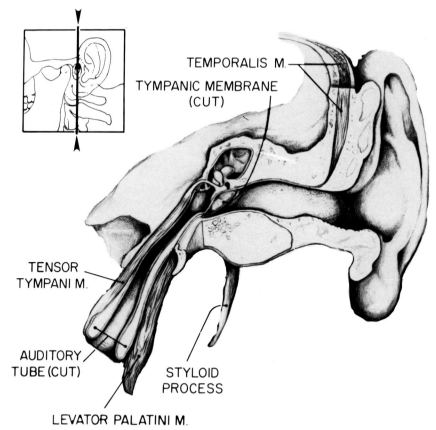

Figure 15–21. Section through ear showing inner ear structures and tensor tympani muscle which is active in stretching the tympanic membrane.

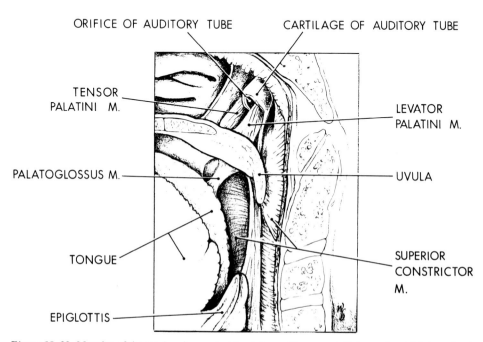

Figure 15–22. Muscles of throat showing eustachian tube and tensor palatini muscle which is active in opening the auditory tube.

Head and Neck Muscles

The muscles of the head and neck have been of interest to the dentist because of a potential relationship among the occlusion, temporomandibular joints, and pain in these muscles and/or muscle contraction headache. The possible role of the *epicranius muscles* in tension headache has yet to be clarified. The *sternocleidomastoid muscle* (Fig. 15–23) is often affected in patients with temporomandibular joint muscle dysfunction and often co-contracts with jaw clenching. The functions of the *orbicularis oris* and the *buccinator* muscles (Fig. 15–19) appear to have a significant role for optimal function of complete dentures. The muscles of facial expression are all innervated by the seventh nerve.

Other muscles that are of interest to the dentist because of TMJ and muscle disorders are the scalenus, splenius, iliocostalis cervicis, and omohyoideus. A number of problems in oral motor function, such as lip posture in the aged, may be related to a generalized deterioration in performance or to a specific motor function rather than the dental state or prescription medication. Most reports on motor disorders and aging have focused on disturbances in control originating in the nervous system.

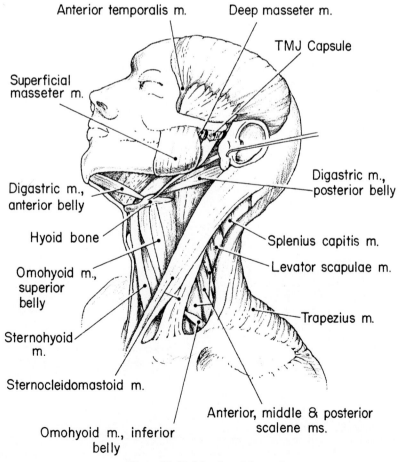

Figure 15–23. Muscles of the neck.

Mandibular Movements and Muscle Activity

Mandibular movement during normal function and during parafunction (e.g., bruxism) involve complex neuromuscular patterns originating in part in a pattern generator in the brain stem and modified by influences from higher centers (Fig. 15–24) (namely, the cerebral cortex and basal ganglia) and from peripheral influences (e.g., the periodontium, muscles, and so on). However, a detailed discussion of such movements is beyond the scope of this text. Rather, the discussion will be related to muscle activity as seen in electromyography for jaw opening and closing, protrusion, retrusion, and lateral movements.

Mandibular Opening

The digastric, mylohyoid, and geniohyoid muscles are active during jaw opening, either slowly or maximally against resistance. No activity occurs in the temporalis and masseter muscles while the mouth is opened slowly and when the jaw is opened maximally, although some activity may occur in the medial pterygoid muscle. When the jaw is opened against resistance, the temporalis muscle remains silent. During opening movements, the lateral pterygoid muscles show initial and sustained activity. In forced depression, the digastric muscle is activated almost as soon as the lateral pterygoid muscle is. Generally, the activity of the anterior digastic muscle follows that of the lateral pterygoid muscle.

Mandibular Closing

While the mandible is being elevated slowly, without contact of the teeth, there is no activity in any portion of the temporalis muscle. Elevation without contact or resistance is brought about by contraction of the masseter and medial pterygoid muscle. Elevation against resistance is affected by the temporalis, masseter, and medial pterygoid muscles. The suprahyoid muscles act as an antagonist of the elevator muscles. Closure into maximal intercuspation (centric occlusion) may involve contraction of facial and neck muscles.

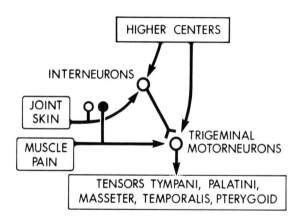

Figure 15–24. Information from joints, skin, muscles, and higher centers converge on the interneurons and trigeminal motor nucleus.

Retrusion

Voluntary mandibular retrusion with the mouth closed is brought about by contraction of the posterior fibers of the temporalis muscle and by the suprahyoid and infrahyoid muscles. Retraction of the mandible from protrusion and without occlusal contact is effected by the contraction of the posterior and middle fibers of the temporalis muscles. Slight activity of the suprahyoid may be due to slight jaw opening to allow the teeth to glide over each other from centric occlusion to centric relation.

Protrusion

Protrusion of the mandible without occlusal contact results from contraction of the lateral and medial pterygoid muscles and from contraction of the masseter muscles. Protraction against resistance is brought about by contraction of the lateral and medial pterygoid muscles and of the masseter and suprahyoid muscle group. Protrusion with the teeth in occlusion is achieved by contraction of the pterygoid and masseter muscles. Only slight activity occurs in the suprahyoid muscles. In combined protraction and opening, there is activity in the medial and lateral pterygoid muscles, the masseter muscles, and sometimes the anterior fibers of the temporalis muscles.

Lateral Movements

Lateral movement of the mandible to the right side (without occlusal contact) is achieved by ipsilateral contraction of primarily the posterior fibers of the temporalis muscle. The suprahyoid muscles are active in maintaining the jaw slightly depressed and protruded. Movement to the left side without occlusal contact is brought about by the contralateral contraction of the medial pterygoid and masseter muscles. Lateral movement to the right side against resistance is achieved by the ipsilateral contraction of the temporalis muscle and by some activity in the ipsilateral masseter and medial pterygoid muscles. Movement to the left side against resistance is achieved by the contralateral contraction of the medial pterygoid and masseter muscles. Lateral movement of the right with occlusal contact is achieved by ipsilateral contraction of the temporalis muscle. Movement to the left with occlusal contact is brought about by contralateral contraction of the medial pterygoid and masseter muscles. Both lateral pterygoid muscles initiate depression of the mandible, and the contralateral muscle initiates a lateral transversion. Lateral movements of the jaw are achieved by ipsilateral contraction of the posterior and middle fibers of the temporalis muscle and by contralateral contraction of the lateral and medial pterygoid muscles and the anterior fibers of the temporalis muscle. Parts of the temporal and masseter muscles may act as antagonists or synergists during horizontal movements and minimum separation of the teeth.

Chewing

Chewing is highly complex and oral motor behavior usually seen in the frontal plane in simple form (Fig. 15–25). There is no archetypal chewing cycle. The means of the vertical dimension of the chewing cycle are between 16 and 20 mm and between 3 and 5 mm for lateral movements. The duration of the cycle varies between 0.6 to 1 second depending on the type of food. The speed of masticatory movement varies within each cycle, according to

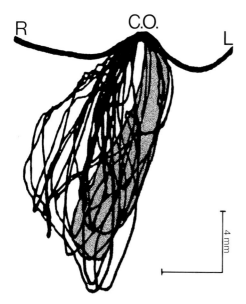

R   C.O.   L

4 mm

Figure 15–25. Mandibular movements during the process of chewing naturally. Incisor point movement seen in frontal plane.

types of foods, and among individuals. Speed, duration, and form of the chewing cycle vary with the type of occlusion, kind of food, and presence of dysfunction.

Occlusal contacts occur in centric occlusion in at least 80 to 90 percent of all chewing cycles, especially near complete trituration of the bolus. With closing and opening movements, there is contact gliding. In the closing phase, the contact glide depends on the type of occlusion and type of food. Where tough food is the normal diet (e.g., as with Australian aborigines), with corresponding occlusal wear, the chewing movement shows a long contact glide ($\overline{X}$ = 2.8 ± 0.35; Beyron, 1964) compared with the short contact glide ($\overline{X}$ = 0.90 mm ± 0.36) of Europeans living on a modern diet of easily titurated food (Ahlgren, 1976). The chewing force reaches a maximum in centric occlusion and lasts for 40 to 170 msec, and the peak electromyographic activity of the temporal and masseter muscles lasts for a mean value of 41 ± 26 msec. Some chewing force is maintained for gliding tooth contact on the opening phase. In the intercuspal position, the jaw is stationary or it pauses for approximately 100 msec before the next cycle begins.

Swallowing

Swallowing involves most of the tongue muscles and buccal musculature. In the initial stage of swallowing, the bolus moves from the mouth to the fauces (Fig. 15–26). The bolus is then moved from the fauces to the esophagus and finally through the esophagus to the stomach. When saliva is swallowed, there is total participation of the suprahyoid muscles, with marked activity of the digastric and mylohyoid muscles, followed by moderate activity in the geniohyoid muscles. The medial pterygoid muscle is frequently active; less frequently, the temporalis and masseter muscles are active with occlusal contact.

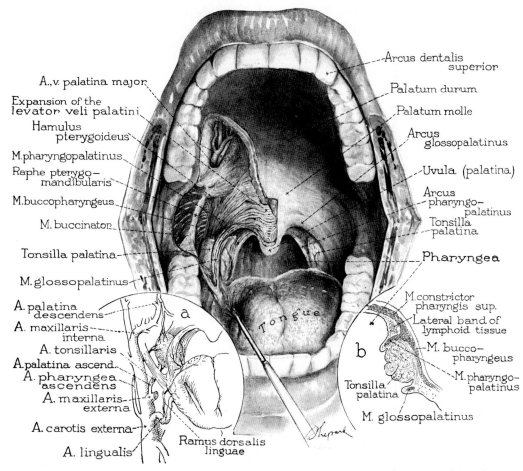

A.,v. palatina major

Expansion of the
levator veli palatini

Hamulus
pterygoideus

M.pharyngopalatinus

Raphe pterygo-
mandibularis

M.buccopharyngeus

M. buccinator

Tonsilla palatina

M.glossopalatinus

A. palatina
descendens

A. maxillaris
interna

A. tonsillaris

A.palatina ascend.

A. pharyngea
ascendens

A. maxillaris-
externa

A. carotis externa

A. lingualis

Arcus dentalis
superior

Palatum durum

Palatum molle

Arcus
glossopalatinus

Uvula (palatina)

Arcus
pharyngo-
palatinus

Tonsilla
palatina

Pharyngea

M.constrictor
pharyngis sup.

Lateral band of
lymphoid tissue

M. bucco-
pharyngeus

M.pharyngo-
palatinus

M. glossopalatinus

Tonsilla
palatina

Tongue

a

b

Ramus dorsalis
linguae

Figure 15–26. Oral pharynx, with special reference to the palatine tonsil and the musculature of the palate. (From Anson, J. B.: *An Atlas of Human Anatomy,* 2nd ed. Philadelphia, W. B. Saunders Company, 1962.)

Oral Motor Behavior

Oral motor behavior refers to function and parafunction of the mouth and associated structures. More generally, behavior includes observable actions ranging from simple movements such as retrusion or protrusion to more complex movements such as chewing. To accomplish complex behavior, sensory-motor systems consisting of muscles and neural processes are required for the initiation, programming, and execution of motor functions. Chewing movements depend on complex integrative neural processes of the central nervous system that may be initiated by either internal or external influences, including innate drives, emotional states, and instructions to patients. During chewing, a large amount of proprioceptive (i.e., muscle "sense") and exteroceptive (i.e., tactile "sense") information is fed to the central nervous system (e.g., cerebral cortex, brain stem, basal ganglia, spinal cord). Rhythmic movements such as chewing are largely programmed or preprogrammed involving learning, which reduces the need for peripheral sensory input. However, inputs from muscle joint, tendon, and periodontal receptors still have important functions, especially in relation to learning, new experiences, and protective reflexes. Neuronal mechanisms must be present to provide for modification of reflexes and continued updating of masticatory movements by information about such factors as occlusal forces and the state and location of the bolus.

Mastication (An Overview)

The act of mastication begins with "setting the system" by sight, tactile sense, and smell to receive the food. The tactile sense may relate to picking up the food to grasping the food with the incisor teeth. When the food is taken into the mouth, the lips, tongue, and periodontium function to estimate size, hardness, and other characteristics that must be compared with previous behavior required for chewing. This information sets the chewing program in the pattern generator, including subsequences that relate to central and peripheral influences already in progress. Orofacial receptors, such as periodontal mechanoreceptors, may monitor occlusal forces and control the jaw-closing muscles. The chewing program may be altered according to stages of chewing or by information from receptors in specific areas such as the palatal mucosa and tongue. The chewing rhythm may be stopped because of noxious stimuli. It is probable that rhythmic and repetitive chewing behavior is disturbed by dysfunctional states of the occlusion and/or the temporomandibular joints whereby the bolus is shifted and the jaw moved to another position for the next forceful tooth-food contact. Thus chewing cycles may occur without the development of an actual power stroke in dysfunction states.

References

Aarstad, T. (1954). *The Capsular Ligament of the Temporomandibular Joint and Retrusion Facets of the Dentition in Relation to Mandibular Movements.* Translated by Helga Christie. Oslo: Acad. Forlag.

Ahlgren, J. (1966). Mechanisms of mastication. Acta. Odont. Scand. 24(Suppl.) 44:1.

Ahlgren, J. (1976). Masticatory movements in man. In Anderson, D. J., and Matthews, B. (eds.), *Mastication.* Bristol, England: John Wright and Sons.

Ash, C. M., and Pinto, O. F. (1991). The TMJ and the middle ear: Structural and functional correlates for aural symptoms associated with temporomandibular joint dysfunction. Int. J. Prosthodont. 4:51.

Ash, M. M., et al. (1990). Current concepts of the relationship and management of temporomandibular disorders and auditory symptoms. J. Michigan Dent. Assoc. 72:550.

Beyron, H. (1964). Occlusal relations and mastication in Australian aborigines. *Acta Odont. Scand.* 22:597.

Buxbaum, J. D., et al. (1982). A comparison of centric relation with maximum intercuspation based upon quantitative electromyography. J. Oral Rehabil. 9:45.

Callander, C. L. (1939). *Surgical Anatomy,* 2nd ed. Philadelphia: Saunders.

Carlsoo, S. (1952). Nervous coordination and mechanical function of the mandibular elevators. Acta. Odont. Scand. 10(Suppl.) 11:1.

Deaver, J. B. (1926). *Surgical Anatomy of the Human Body,* 2nd ed. Philadelphia: Blakiston's.

Dolwick, M. F., and Sanders, B. (1985). *TMJ Internal Derangement and Arthrosis.* St. Louis, Mo.: Mosby.

Duthie, N., and Yemm, R. (1982). Muscles involved in voluntary mandibular retrusion in man. J. Oral Rehabil. 9:155.

Eagle, W. W. (1949). Asymptomatic styloid process. Arch. Otolaryngol. 49:490.

Eriksson, P.-O., et al. (1981). Special histochemical muscle-fibre characteristics of the human lateral pterygoid muscle. Arch. Oral Biol. 26:495.

Gandevia, S. C., and Mahutte, C. K. (1980). Joint mechanics as a determinant of motor unit organization in man. Med. Hypotheses 6:527.

Gibbs, C. H., et al. (1971). Functional movements of the mandible. J. Prosthet. Dent. 26:604.

Gosen, A. J. (1974). Mandibular leverage and occlusion. J. Prosthet. Dent. 31:369.

Grant, P. G. (1973). Lateral pterygoid: Two muscles? Am. J. Anat. 138:1.

Hansson, T., et al. (1977). Thickness of the soft tissue layers and the articular disk in the temporomandibular joint. Acta. Odont. Scand. 35:77.

Hickey, J. C. (1963). Mandibular movements in three dimensions. J. Prosthet. Dent. 13:72.

Hjortsjo, C. H. (1953). The mechanism in the temporomandibular joint. Acta. Odont. Scand. 11:5.

Hylander, W. L. (1975). The human mandible: Lever or link? Am. J. Phys. Anthrop. 43:227.

Kawumura, Y., and Nobuhara, M. (1957). Studies on masticatory function. II. The swallowing threshold of persons with normal occlusion and malocclusion. Med. J. Osaka Univ. 8:241.

Lehr, R. P., and Owens, S. E. (1980). An electromyographic study of the human lateral pterygoid muscles. Anat. Rec. 196:441.

McNamara, J. A. (1973). The independent functions of the two heads of the lateral pterygoid muscle. Am. J. Anat. 138:197.

Moller, E. (1966). The chewing apparatus. Acta. Physiol. Scand. 69(Suppl.) 280:1.

Owall, B., and Moller, E. (1974). Tactile sensibility during chewing and biting. Odontol. Revy 25:327.

Posselt, U. (1952). Studies in the mobility of the human mandible. Acta. Odont. Scand. 10(Suppl.):3.

Ramfjord, S. P., and Ash, M. M. (1983). *Occlusion,* 3rd ed. Philadelphia: Saunders.

Rees, L. A. (1954). The structure and function of the mandibular joint. J. Brit. Dent. A. 96:125.

Smith, R. J. (1978). Mandibular biomechanics and temporomandibular joint function in primates. Am. J. Phys. Anthrop. 49:341.

Stohler, C. S., and Ash, M. M. (1982). Mandibular displacement in complete chewing sequence (abstract). J. Dent. Res. 61:273.

Stores, A. T. (1981). Joint and tooth articulation in disorders of jaw movement. In Kawamura, Y., and Dubner, R. (eds.), *Oral-Facial Sensory and Motor Function.* Tokyo: Quintessence Publishing.

Takahashi, T., et al. (1983). The role of oral kinesthesia in the determination of the swallowing threshold. J. Dent. Res. 62:327.

Thilander, B. (1961). Innervation of the temporomandibular joint capsule in man. Trans. Ray. Sci. Dent. 7:9.

Toller, P. A. (1961). The synovial apparatus and temporomandibular joint function. Br. Dent. J. 111:355.

Vitti, M., and Basmajian, J. V. (1977). Integrated actions of masticatory muscles: Simultaneous EMG from eight intramuscular electrodes. Anat. Rec. 187:173.

Wompler, H. W., et al. (1980). Scanning electron microscopic and radiographic correlation of articular surfaces and supporting bone in the mandibular condyle. J. Dent. Res. 59:754.

Wyke, B. D. (1974). Neuromuscular mechanisms influencing mandibular posture: A neurologist's view of current concepts. J. Dent. 2:111.

Yurkstas, A. A. (1965). The masticatory act. J. Prosthet. Dent. 15:248.

16 *Occlusion*

The term "occlusion" as used in dentistry may mean the contact relationship of the teeth in function or parafunction. However, the term refers not only to contact of the arches at an occlusal interface but also to all those factors concerned with the development and stability of the masticatory system and with the use of the teeth in oral motor behavior. Because definitions of occlusion are too brief to be useful as a basis for dental practice, more complete explanations evolve into concepts of occlusion that reflect prevailing interests and clinical convenience. Thus a modern concept of occlusion must include the idea of an integrated system of functional units involving teeth, joints, and muscles of the head and neck. The solutions to such problems as orthodontic relapse, denture instability, and periodontal trauma require concepts of occlusion that extend well beyond the arrangement of teeth, occlusal contacts, and jaw position.

Concepts of Occlusion

Concepts of occlusion vary with almost every specialty of dentistry. Common to some are definitions based on a static view of the dentition in which descriptions of the occlusion emphasize the fit of particular parts of individual maxillary teeth with specified parts of mandibular teeth. Until recently, only a few concepts of occlusion have included functional criteria. And because the dentofacial complex is highly mobile, ideas of occlusal stability and homeostasis are often misunderstood and seldom mentioned as a part of a concept of occlusion.

Early ideas regarding occlusion were often based on complete dentures. And because of the problems of instability of denture bases, the concept of "balanced occlusion" was developed. It considers that bilateral contacts in all functional excursions prevent tipping of the denture bases. Although such concepts have been advocated by some clinicians for the natural dentition, acceptance has been limited and unsupported by research evidence. Even so, some of the concepts related to condylar guidance, cusp height, incisal guidance, curve of Spee, and plane of occlusion have been useful in the restoration of natural teeth.

Several concepts of an "ideal" or optimal occlusion of the natural dentition have been suggested by Angle (1887), Beyron (1954), D'Amico (1958), Friel (1954), Hellman (1941), Lucia (1962), Ramfjord and Ash (1983), and Stallard and Stuart (1963). These concepts stress to varying degrees static (see Fig. 16–23) and/or functional characteristics of an occlusion considered to be theoretical or practical goals for diagnosis and treatment of the occlusion. Some of the ideas have developed principally in relation to orthodontics and

414

others for full mouth rehabilitation. None are completely applicable to the natural dentition; some provide for specific occlusal relations and joint positions, and few concepts of occlusion consider in principle or practical ways the muscle and oromotor functions. Thus, the idea of a functional rather than simply a static relationship of occlusal surfaces has become increasingly important because of the recognition that functional disturbances of the masticatory system can be related to malocclusion, occlusal dysfunction, and disturbances of oral motor behavior, including bruxism.

An Outline of Items Suggested for the Study of Occlusion

The following topics are suggestions for the study of occlusion. Important areas such as the development of the neuromuscular system have not been included, but it is recommended that the interested reader consult some of the references included in this chapter.

1. Development of occlusion
2. Dental arch form
3. Compensating curvatures of the dental arches (curved occlusal planes)
4. Angulation of individual teeth in relation to various planes (including root form)
5. Functional form of the teeth at their incisal and occlusal thirds
6. Facial and lingual relations of each tooth in one arch to its antagonist or antagonists in the opposing arch in centric occlusion
7. Occlusal contact and intercusp relations of all the teeth of one arch with those in the opposing arch in centric occlusion
8. Occlusal contact and intercusp relations of all the teeth during the various functional mandibular movements
9. Neurobehavioral aspects of occlusion

Development of Occlusion

Primary Dentition

Any consideration of the development of occlusion should begin with the occlusion of the deciduous teeth (Fig. 16–1). It is during this period in the development of the oral-facial complex that oral motor behavior reflects learning related to the advent of the teeth. Human oral functions that are acquired or modified during the natural progression from neonate, through infancy to adulthood are in part related to the development of occlusion, both of the deciduous and permanent teeth, i.e., occlusion in its broadest meaning. Perhaps many of the reflex mechanisms of the oral-facial area and sensory and higher center influences are important for the acquisition of masticatory skills, just one of the many motor behaviors that come under the phrase oral motor function. Thus of particular importance is the novel sensory apparatus of the teeth that makes their appearance with the deciduous teeth at an important time in the maturation of the nervous system and its interface with the environment. The development of the muscle matrix and the active growth of the facial skeleton occurs at a very strategic time for the maturation of the nervous system and the development of oral motor functions involving the teeth and chewing. It is also at this time that jaw positions and posturing of the mandible in relationship to the teeth takes place.

The timing of eruption of the teeth is due in large part to heredity and only somewhat to environmental factors (Table 16–1). Development and eruption of the primary dentition are quite independent of the development and maturation of the child as a whole (Falkner,

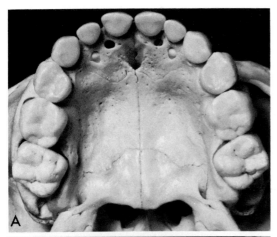

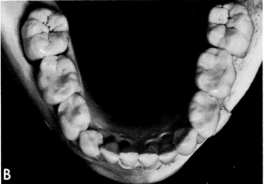

Figure 16–1. *A, B,* Occlusal surfaces of deciduous dentition with permanent first molars present.

1957). The significance of local environmental factors on the development of occlusion considered in its broadest sense is relatively unknown. Thus learning of mastication may be highly dependent on the stage of development (type and number of teeth present) of the occlusion, maturation of the neuromuscular system, and such factors as diet.

The primary arch form is oval and by the age of 9 months the width of the arch has been established largely for both the deciduous and permanent dentitions (Richardson and Castaldi, 1967). This observation may seem untrue in view of the apparent difference in facial appearance between the child of this age and a young adult with a permanent dentition. What does change substantially, of course, is the increased anterior-posterior dimension of the jaws, which is necessary for the incorporation of the permanent molars into the occlusion.

Table 16–1. **Sequence and Age at Eruption of Primary Teeth**

Teeth	*Age*	*Mean Number Teeth Present*	*Distribution in Number of Teeth*
$\overline{A}$	6 months	—	1–3, 33%
$\underline{A}$	9 months	3	1–6, 80%
$\underline{B}$	12 months	6	4–8, 50%
$\dfrac{D}{\overline{B}, \overline{D}}$	18 months	12	9–16, 85%
$\dfrac{C}{\overline{C}}$	24 months	16	15–18, 60%
$\overline{E}, \underline{E}$	30 months	19	20, 70%

The position of the deciduous teeth in the arches demonstrates generally some degree of interdental spacing, which tends to decrease slightly with age. The contact relations of the teeth tend to vary with the degree of bruxism present in the child. A number of factors appear to be related to the development of contact relations at the time of eruption of the teeth, including the position of the tooth germ, presence of permanent teeth, development of the condyles, cuspal inclines, and neuromuscular influences. Generally, little attention has been paid to the cusp-fossa and temporomandibular joint relationships, and usually only tooth-to-tooth observations have been made, namely, the mesiolingual cusp of the maxillary molar occludes in the central fossa of the deciduous mandibular molar. Jaw-to-jaw relations in regard to the position of the condyle have received little attention. Perhaps discrepancies between condylar position and tooth position have little meaning in a relatively plastic, rapidly growing and changing system, including the nervous system.

Of particular interest to the orthodontist is the fact that the mandibular second deciduous molar has a greater mesiodistal diameter than the maxillary second molar. This difference in dimensions of the two teeth results in the distal surfaces of these two molars being in the same plane, i.e., there is a flush terminal plane at the end of the deciduous dentition. If a "step" (deviation of the flush terminal plane) occurs because of carious lesions or other disturbances, it has been suggested that there is a tendency to interfere with the development of normal occlusal relations of the permanent first molars. Also it has been suggested that wearing away naturally of the cusps in the deciduous dentition allows the mandible to assume a more forward position during a period of time when the mandible is growing more rapidly than the maxilla. In the absence of cuspal interferences, there is some evidence that the permanent incisors erupt with less vertical overlap and the permanent molars erupt into a more favorable occlusion. Several orthodontic techniques have been directed toward the functional protraction of the mandible during growth in patients with anterior-posterior jaw discrepancies.

Permanent Dentition

The sequence of eruption of the permanent dentition is more variable than that of the primary dentition and does not follow the same anterior-posterior pattern. In addition, there are significant differences in the eruption sequences between the maxillary arch and the mandibular arch that do not appear in the eruption of the primary dentition.

The most common sequences of eruption in the maxilla are 6-1-2-4-3-5-7-8 and 6-1-2-4-5-3-7-8. The most common sequences for the mandibular arch are (6-1)-2-3-4-5-7-8 and (6-1)-2-4-3-5-7-8 (Knott and Meredith, 1966). These are also the most favorable sequences for the prevention of malocclusion (Fig. 16–2). Should the second molars erupt before the premolars are fully erupted, significant shortening of the arch perimeter resulting in malocclusion is likely to occur, even if the alveolar bone arch dimensions are adequate for the size of the permanent dentition (Lo and Moyers, 1953).

The eruption of permanent teeth also follows the tendency for the mandibular tooth of one type to erupt before the maxillary tooth erupts. This tendency is reversed in the premolar eruption sequence. This is due to the difference in eruption timing of the canine in the two arches. In the mandibular arch, the canine erupts before the premolar, whereas in the maxillary arch the canine generally erupts after the premolar.

The timing of eruption of the permanent dentition is not critical as long as the eruption times are not too far from the normal values. The sequence of eruption varies somewhat, with the dentition in girls erupting on an average of 5 months earlier than that in boys. However, sexual differences are less significant than the tendency exhibited by the individual in eruption times of previously erupted teeth. If any tooth has erupted early or late, succeeding teeth will also be early or late in their eruption.

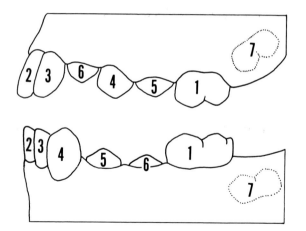

Figure 16–2. Favorable eruption sequence of permanent teeth.

An important portion of the dental arch in the development of occlusion of the permanent dentition is the premolar segment. In this section, the erupting premolars are significantly smaller in mesiodistal dimension than the primary molars which they replace. The dynamics of this change in arch dimensions, particularly in the mandibular arch, is important to a proper understanding of the development of occlusion and malocclusion.

An often confusing point in the analysis of the mixed dentition is the actual *decrease* in arch perimeter during the growth of the mandible. The arch perimeter of the permanent dentition, as measured from the mesials of the mandibular first molars, decreases an average of about 4 mm (Moorrees, 1959). This occurs at the same time during which the mandible and basal bone are experiencing significant growth posteriorly. Because this change is found to a greater extent in the mandible than in the maxilla and because of the pronounced tendency for the lower molars to drift mesially, occlusal relationships are in a flux during the later stages of the mixed dentition.

Some of the space made available by the "leeway space" (the difference in sizes between the premolars and primary molars) must be utilized for alignment of the lower incisors as these teeth erupt with an average of 1.6 mm of crowding (Moorrees, 1965). The remainder of the space will be utilized by the mandibular molar. This movement of the mandibular molar may correct an end-to-end molar relationship (normal for the mixed dentition) into a normal molar relationship in the permanent dentition; i.e., the mesial lingual cusp of the maxillary first molar occludes in the central fossa of the mandibular first molar and the mesial buccal cusp of the maxillary first molar occludes between the mesial and distal buccal cusps of the mandibular first molar (Angle Class I Molar Relationship). These relationships are discussed under item 7, occlusal contact and intercusp relations.

Dental Arch Form

The basic pattern of tooth position is the arch. The arch has long been known architecturally (as the word architecture itself implies) to be a strong, stable arrangement. Forces transmitted normal to the apex of a catenary arch are transmitted entirely to the base units of the arch. If the two base units are stabilized against lateral thrusts, the remainder of the arch units experience only compressive forces and therefore do not move relative to each other.

The maxillary teeth are positioned on the maxilla, as are the mandibular teeth on the mandible, in such a way as to produce a curved "arch" when viewed from the occlusal surface (Fig. 16–3). This form is in large part determined by the shape of the underlying basal bone. Malpositioning of individual teeth does not alter the arch form. However, when multiple teeth are misplaced, then irregularities or asymmetries may develop in arch form.

The shape of the arch form of the facial surfaces of the teeth has been found by Currier (1969) to be a segment of an ellipse. The arch form as defined by the centroids (center of the occlusal form) of the teeth is a parabolic curve.

Variations of arch form from the elliptical have been described variously as "U"-shaped (or square arch form) and tapered. The tapered arch form generally occurs in the maxillary arch and quite often as the result of a pathological narrowing of the anterior maxilla left palate and less commonly a severe thumb-sucking habit may result in arch narrowing of the anterior maxilla.

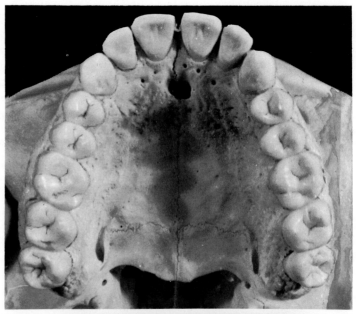

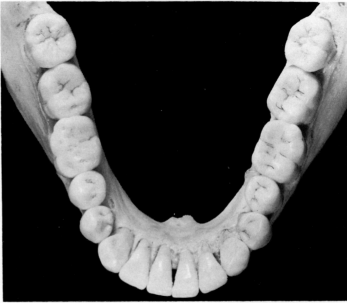

Figure 16–3. Anatomic specimen showing normal alignment of teeth. Although the mandibular arch gives the impression that it is longer from the median line to the distal of the third molars, this is an optical illusion. Because the teeth adapt themselves to compensating occlusal curvature, the mandibular arch is spoken of as being "concave." This comes close to putting the axis of each posterior tooth in the line of vision; this also puts each occlusal surface of a posterior mandibular tooth in "perfect profile," which registers mesiodistal measurements completely. Because the maxillary curvature is the reverse of the mandibular and "convex" rather than "concave," the mesiodistal measurement of maxillary posterior teeth is foreshortened in the camera lens, creating the misconception.

Changes in arch form, within anatomic limits, do not have any significant effect on occlusion unless the change is in only one of the two dental arches. Discrepancies in arch form between the maxillary and mandibular arches generally result in poor occlusal relationships. Arch form distortion in only one arch can be advantageous when the basal bone structure is incorrectly positioned as in severe mandibular retrognathism or prognathism. In such cases, the arch form distortion in one arch allows a better occlusion on the posterior aspect than is otherwise possible.

Changes in the sizes of the arches, within anatomic limits, do not have a large effect on occlusion. The arch form of the maxilla tends to be larger than that of the mandible. This results in the maxillary teeth "overhanging" the mandibular teeth when the teeth are in centric occlusion (the position of maximal intercuspation). The lateral or anterior-posterior aspect of this overhang is called "overjet."

This arch relation has a useful feature: During opening and closing movements of the jaws, the cheeks, lips, and tongue are less likely to be caught. Since the facial occlusal margins of the maxillary teeth extend beyond the facial occlusal margins of the mandibular teeth, and since the linguo-occlusal margins of the mandibular teeth extend lingually in relation to the linguo-occlusal margins of the maxillary teeth, the soft tissues are displaced during the act of closure until the teeth have had an opportunity to come together in occlusal contact.

Although the overall shape of the arch may be elliptical, the facial surfaces are not all on the curve of the ellipse. Certain teeth, because of their shape and/or size are generally positioned somewhat to the labial or lingual aspect of the ideal ellipse (or "U" or tapered form). These are the maxillary lateral incisors, maxillary and mandibular cuspids, and maxillary first molars.

The maxillary lateral incisors are positioned so that their lingual surfaces, along with the lingual surfaces of the maxillary central incisors and cuspids, describe a smooth curve. Because of the lesser buccolingual thickness of the lateral incisors, the buccal surface of the lateral incisors are more lingually placed. The greater buccolingual dimension of the cuspid places its buccal surface more buccally with respect to an ideal ellipse than either incisor.

The buccal surface of the maxillary first molar is positioned (Fig. 16–4) to the buccal aspect of the ideal elliptical pattern owing to the buccolingual width of this tooth. This surface is also substantially angled, with the distal buccal surface more lingual than the mesiobuccal, allowing the distobuccal cusp to occlude properly with the lower first molar.

The stability of the occlusion and the maintenance of tooth position are dependent upon all of the forces that act upon the teeth. Occlusal forces, eruptive forces, lip and cheek pressure, and tongue pressure are all involved in maintaining the position of the teeth. As long as all of these forces are balanced, the teeth and the occlusion will remain stable. Should one or more of the influences change in magnitude, duration, or frequency, stability is lost and the teeth will shift, disrupting a previously stable occlusion.

Compensating Curvatures of the Dental Arches (Curved Occlusal Planes)

The occlusal surfaces of the dental arches do not generally conform to a flat plane. The mandibular arch conforms generally to one or more curved planes, which appear concave, and the opposing maxillary arch, the curvature of which appears convex. Although Bonwill (1899) was the first to describe the mandible and mandibular arch as adapting itself in part to an equilateral triangle (Fig. 16–5), such measurements cannot be established arbitrarily. There is no scientific evidence that an approximation of the curvature of the arches to a 4-inch equilateral triangle has any direct application to function or dysfunction.

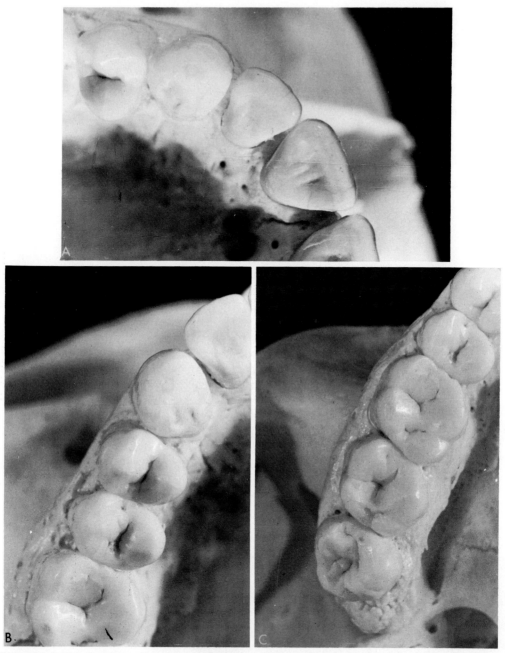

Figure 16–4. Close-up views of sections of a dental arch. These pictures were taken of the same specimens shown in Figure 16–3. They show the variations in the design of individual units in the arch, contact form, occlusal form, group alignment, and so forth. The photographs of the teeth of one half of the arch were taken by means of three different angulations of camera focus. Even by this means, it is impossible to get more than one or possibly two teeth in direct profile. A more perfect approach would require a view of each of the teeth in direct alignment with individual axes. Later in the chapter, the variance in axial alignment will be discussed.

    A., This section includes maxillary central incisor, lateral incisor, canine, and first premolar. The focus was made in line with the long axis of the canine.

    B, A view of the maxillary lateral incisor, canine, and first and second premolars. The angle was in line generally with the first premolar.

    C, This section includes the maxillary second premolar and all three of the molars. The camera was focused on the first molar, putting it in profile.

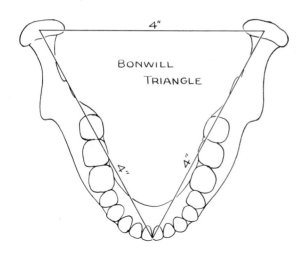

Figure 16–5. The Bonwill equilateral triangle.

von Spee noted that the cusps and incisal ridges of the teeth tended to display a curved alignment when the arches were observed from a point opposite the first molars. This alignment is spoken of still as the *curve of Spee* (Fig. 16–6). This curvature is within the sagittal planes only.

Monson (1920), at a later date, connected the curve of Spee, or curvature in sagittal planes, with related compensating curvatures in vertical planes and suggested that the mandibular arch adapted itself to the curved segment of a sphere of a 4-inch radius (see Fig. 4–8). Although these ideas of curvature have not been accepted as a goal of treatment, the importance of curved occlusal planes to clinical dentistry is demonstrated in prosthetics and orthodontics. It is probable that the curvatures represent the vector of a number of factors within the orofacial structures, including the neuromuscular system, concerned with stability.

The significance of compensating curvatures in clinical dentistry is perhaps more related to clinical convenience than knowledge of what its precise degree should be for anyone. Whatever the force vector, it cannot be determined at this time with any precision; and the degree of curvature is usually based upon several clinical ideas such as the

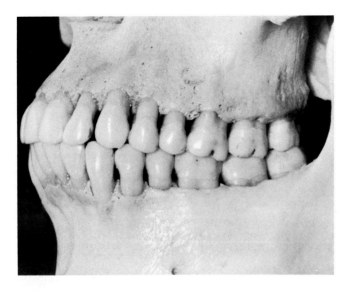

Figure 16–6. View of specimen with normal occlusion from the right side in line with first molars. This picture serves as a good example of facial relationships of maxillary and mandibular teeth.

following. There should be no posterior contacts in protrusive movements. According to Thielemann's formula for balanced occlusion (where CG refers to condylar guidance, IG to incisal guidance, CS to the curve of Spee, CH to cusp height, and PO to plane of occlusion), incisal guidance or cuspid guidance must be increased in proportion to the severity of the curve of Spee (cusp height and plane of occlusion remaining the same):

$$\text{Balance} = \frac{\text{CG} \cdot \text{IG}}{\text{CS} \cdot \text{CH} \cdot \text{PO}}$$

Although such a formula is helpful in visualizing the relationship of these five factors for "balanced" occlusion in complete dentures, its significance to the natural dentition is less apparent. From a restorative standpoint only, a limited number of these factors can be changed in the natural dentition. In relation to orthodontics, the goal is to have no more than a slight arc; flatness has been suggested to be desirable because of relapse tendencies. Also the difficulty of obtaining increased cuspid guidance for disclusion of posterior teeth is lessened by having less curvature. Also, it is possible to decrease the amount of vertical overlap of the maxillary incisors if the curve of Spee has only a slight arc. Attempts to establish a specific curve (i.e., the deepest curve as 1.5 mm) as the border between normal and abnormal have not had widespread acceptance.

Angulation of the Individual Teeth in Relation to Various Planes; Root Form

The relationship of axes of maxillary and mandibular teeth to each other varies with each tooth group, i.e., incisors, canines, premolars, and molars (Figs. 16–7 through 16–11).

Sections through the jaws with the teeth in centric occlusion, made to show the mesial aspect of each tooth in either arch, are shown in MacMillan's illustrations (see Figs. 14–24 to 14–31). In this specimen it may be noted that the incisors are placed with their axes at about 60 degrees to the horizontal plane at the occlusal contact, the axis of the maxillary tooth being placed at an acute angle to the axis of the mandibular tooth. The canines are placed so that the axes form angles less acute, followed by the first premolars, which resemble the canines in their placement.

The second premolars and the first molars differ from the teeth anterior to them in their axial relations to each other and in their angulations to a horizontal plane. The axes of these maxillary and mandibular teeth are nearly parallel. From a study of Figure 14–29, it may be seen that there is a possibility of error here. More than likely, the second premolar mandibular and first molar maxillary should have been related as pictured in Figure 14–30, which depicts the second molar region correctly.

The second and third mandibular molars have their axes at angles somewhat more acute in relation to the horizontal than the first molar axis. Prolongations of the lines bisecting the mandibular second and third molars tend to bisect the lingual roots of the maxillary second and third molars. The axis line of the mandibular first molar, when prolonged, would tend to pass between the buccal and lingual roots of the maxillary first molar.

No absolute rules may be assumed when describing the axial relations of maxillary and mandibular teeth in centric occlusion. Nevertheless, even though skulls and specimens show some variations in the degree of angulations, normally developed specimens show angulations of crowns and roots similar to the generalizations just described (Figs. 16–12 and 16–13).

Each tooth must be placed at the angle that best withstands the lines of forces brought

1   2

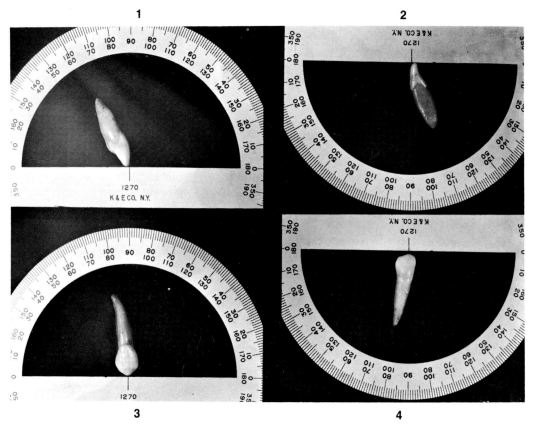

3   4

Figure 16–7. Individual teeth placed within a protractor to show their axial inclinations. The placement of the roots in relation to occlusal levels of the crowns governs the association of occlusal levels in the dental arch. The combination of occlusal levels exhibits curvature, which in turn assists in arriving at occlusal compensation during jaw movements. *1,* Maxillary central incisor. *2,* Mandibular central incisor. *3,* Maxillary canine. *4,* Mandibular canine.

against it during function. The angle at which it is placed depends upon the function the tooth has to perform. If the tooth is placed at a disadvantage, its functional efficiency is limited.

The anterior teeth, as shown in Figures 14–24 through 14–26, seem to be placed at a disadvantage when we view them from mesial or distal aspects. The lines of force during mastication, or when the jaws are merely opened or closed, are tangent generally to the long axes of these teeth (Fig. 14–24). It must be remembered that they are designed for momentary *biting* and *shearing* only, and not for the assumption of the full force of the jaws. Neuromuscular control mechanisms are highly developed for the control of such transient forces.

The mesiodistal and faciolingual axial inclinations of the teeth are usually described in terms of angles between the long axis of a tooth and a line drawn perpendicular to a horizontal plane or to the median plane. Photographs of teeth placed within a protractor show the axial inclination of the teeth and roots (Figs. 16–7 through 16–11). Although such measurements are somewhat arbitrary, they follow closely those suggested by Dempster (1963) and Kraus (1969) and their colleagues for the teeth and by Andrews (1976) for crowns. A summary is shown in Table 16–2.

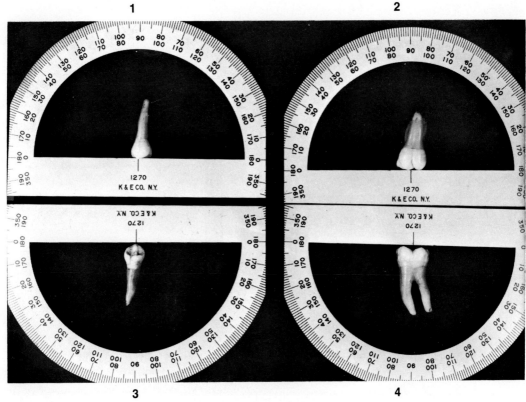

Figure 16–8. Individual teeth placed within a protractor to show their axial inclinations. *1*, Maxillary first premolar. *2*, Maxillary first molar. *3*, Mandibular first premolar. *4*, Mandibular first molar.

Functional Form of the Teeth at Their Incisal and Occlusal Thirds

The incisal and occlusal thirds of the tooth crowns present convex or concave surfaces at all contacting occlusal areas (Fig. 16–14). When the teeth of one jaw come into occlusal contact with their antagonists in the opposite jaw during various mandibular movements, curved surfaces come into contact with curved surfaces. These curved surfaces may be convex or concave. A convex surface, representing a segment of the occlusal third of one tooth, may come into contact with a convex or a concave segment of another tooth; always, however, curved segments contact curved segments, large or small (Fig. 16–15).

Lingual surfaces of maxillary incisors present some concave surfaces where convex portions of the incisal ridges of mandibular incisors come into occlusal contact.

The posterior teeth show depressions in the depth of sulci and developmental grooves; nevertheless, the enamel sides of the sulci are formed by convexities that point into the developmental grooves. Cusps that are rather pointed will contact the rolls of hard enamel that make up marginal ridges on posterior teeth. Until the cusps are worn flat, the deeper portions of the sulci and grooves act as escapements for food, since the convex surfaces of opposing teeth are prevented from fitting into them perfectly by the curved sides of the sulci (Fig. 16–16).

Although the teeth when in centric occlusion seem to intercuspate rather closely, on examination it is found that escapements have been provided. These escapement spaces are needed for efficient occlusion during mastication. When occluding surfaces come

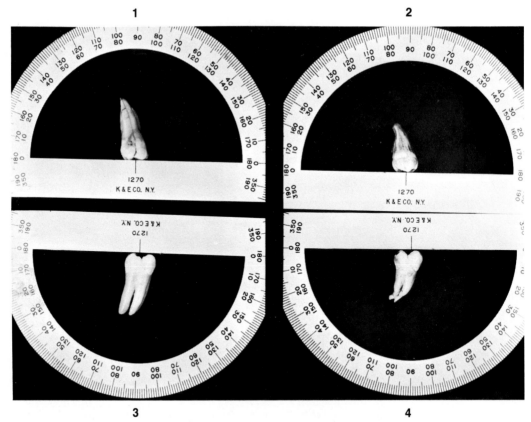

Figure 16–9. Individual teeth placed within a protractor to show their axial inclination. *1*, Maxillary second molar. *2*, Maxillary third molar. *3*, Mandibular second molar. *4*, Mandibular third molar.

together, some escapement spaces are so slight that light is scarcely admitted through them; they vary in degree of opening from such small ones to generous ones of a millimeter or more at the widest points of embrasure.

Escapement space is provided in the teeth by the form of the cusps and ridges, the sulci and developmental grooves, and the interdental spaces or embrasures when teeth come together in occlusion.

The significance of the incisal and occlusal thirds of the teeth has been an area of controversy because there is so little objective information on the influence of flat or convex surfaces on function. The use of anatomic and nonanatomic occlusal surfaces of denture teeth has only heightened interest in the role of cuspal form, "escapements" for food, and "cutting" surfaces in mastication. An examination of contemporary Eskimo or aboriginal dentitions shows that by the age of 20 most of the teeth are flattened and it has been suggested (Poole, 1976) that the only advantage of cusps on the teeth in humans is the establishment of the teeth in their correct position during the development of occlusion. Although such ideas have little acceptance, some clinicians grind the posterior teeth flat under the impression that dental caries may be reduced as well as some forms of TMJ muscle dysfunction and perhaps periodontal disease. Although the evaluation of mastica-

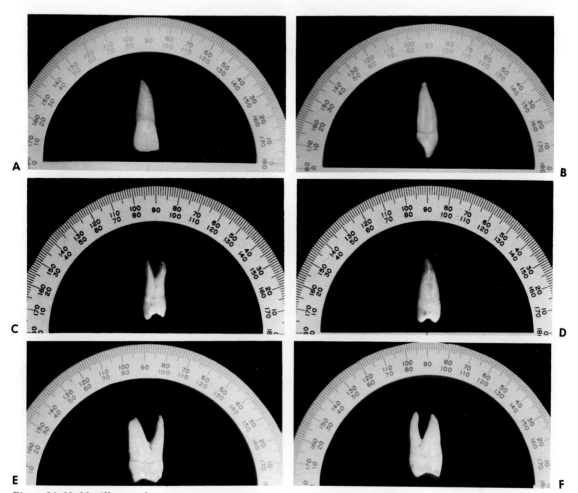

Figure 16–10. Maxillary teeth.

Photos depicting further experimentation in the study of the angulation of axes, which, it is realized, could have an effect upon lines of force in occlusion. Here the approach was from different aspects (mesial and distal), placing the teeth in their approximate alignment with occlusal levels. The crown portions of the teeth, along with the cervical third of the roots, seem to be straight with the horizontal line (see Figs. 14–30 and 14–31). However, close scrutiny of the roots will suggest varied curvatures.

A, Central incisor.
B, Canine.
C, First premolar.
D, Second premolar.
E, First molar.
F, Another maxillary first molar showing some differentiation in form when compared with *E.*

tion is an interesting subject, and even though the persistence of cusps into early middle age has occurred only in Western man for the last 200 to 300 years (Butler, 1974; Mills, 1976), it must be accepted that cusp form and function at this time have to be consistent with the dentition of modern man. Although a number of concepts of occlusal morphology have been suggested for restorations, none has been demonstrated to increase the health and comfort of patients more than another.

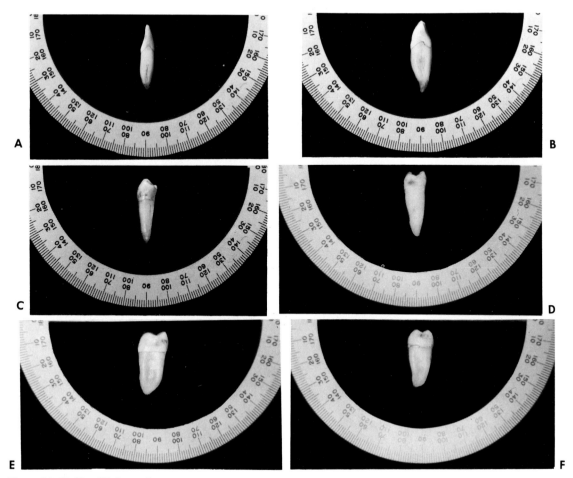

Figure 16–11. Mandibular teeth.

    Generally speaking, the mandibular teeth will show angulation similar to that of the maxillary when viewed from mesial or distal aspects. However, the root forms must conform to the manner in which the teeth are anchored, so the teeth in the two jaws differ; the mandibular has no spreading roots from mesial or distal aspects. The developmental grooves and depressions in many roots of mandibular teeth furnish anchorage akin to fused roots; the somewhat kidney-shaped roots (on cross section) resist movement when imbedded in bone. Also, close scrutiny here will demonstrate some curvature from the cervical third of the root to the apex *(E)* when the crest of contour is followed on each side of the developmental depression, as if following the direction of fused roots.

    A, Central incisor.
    B, Canine.
    C, First premolar.
    D, Second premolar.
    E, First molar.
    F, Another first molar, smaller and differing somewhat from *E.*

Facial and Lingual Relations of Each Tooth in One Arch to its Antagonists in the Opposing Arch in Centric Occlusion

    In centric occlusion, facial views of the normal denture show each tooth of one arch in occlusal with portions of two others in the opposing arch (Fig. 16–17) with the exception of the mandibular central incisors and the maxillary third molars. Each of the exceptions named has one antagonist only in the opposing jaw (Fig. 4–22).

    Since each tooth has two antagonists, the loss of one still leaves one antagonist

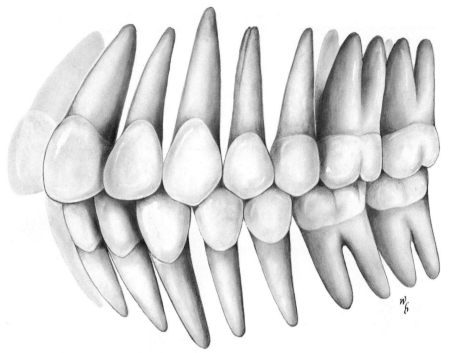

Figure 16–12. Orientation of crowns and roots of the teeth (lateral view).

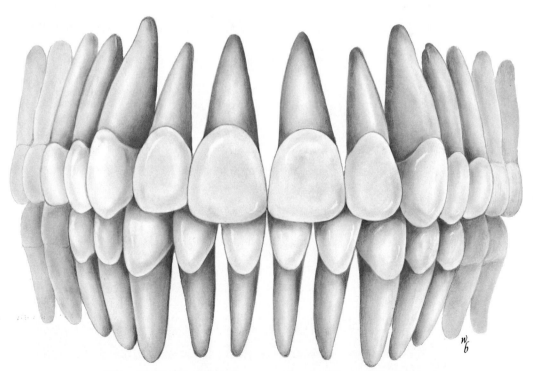

Figure 16–13. Orientation of crowns and roots of the teeth (frontal view).

Table 16–2. **Angulation/inclination of teeth**

Mesiodistal													Faciolingual
7⌋	6⌋	5⌋	4⌋	3⌋	2⌋	1⌋	⌊1	⌊2	⌊3	⌊4	⌊5	⌊6	⌊7
8°	10°	5°	9°	17°	7°	2°	28°	26°	16°	5°	6°	8°	10°
14°	10°	9°	6°	6°	0°	2°	22°	23°	12°	9°	9°	20°	20°
7⌉	6⌉	5⌉	4⌉	3⌉	2⌉	1⌉	⌈1	⌈2	⌈3	⌈4	⌈5	⌈6	⌈7

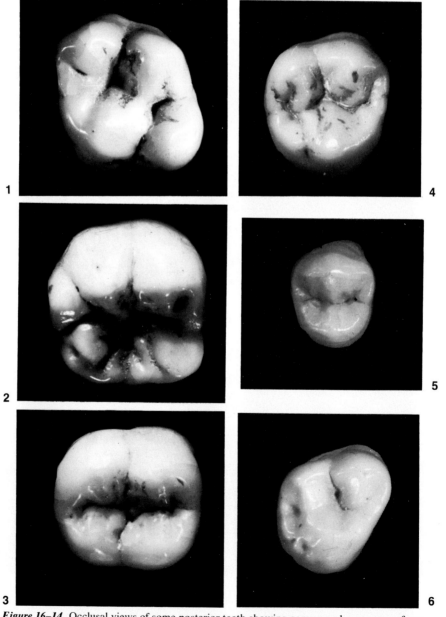

Figure 16–14. Occlusal views of some posterior teeth showing convex and concave surfaces and no vestige of flat planes or sharp angles. *1,* Maxillary first molar. *2,* Mandibular first molar. *3,* Mandibular second molar. *4,* Maxillary second molar. *5,* Maxillary first premolar. *6,* Maxillary third molar.

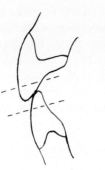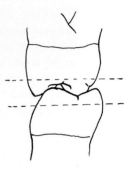

Figure 16–15. The incisal or occlusal thirds of the tooth crowns present convex or concave surfaces at all contacting occlusal areas.

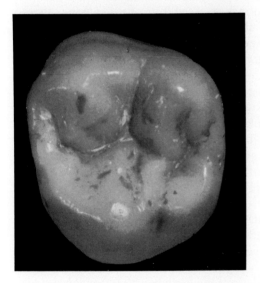

Figure 16–16. Natural occlusal third surface of maxillary second molar. The occlusal surface contour illustrated here is a good example of the irregular contour of cusps and ridges to be found on all maxillary molars. Note rounded cusp tips and cusp ridges; also note the rounded and turned "triangular" ridges folding into the generous central fossa and into the smaller mesial and distal fossae as well.

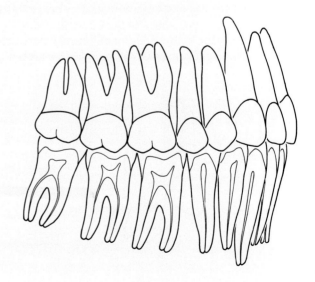

Figure 16–17. Schematic drawing showing the facial relations of teeth in opposing arches in an idealized occlusion.

remaining, which will keep the tooth in occlusal contact with the opposing arch and keep it in its own arch relation at the same time by preventing elongation and displacement through the lack of antagonism. The permanency of the arch forms depends on the mutual support of the teeth in contact with each other. When a tooth is lost, the adjoining teeth in the same arch may, depending on occlusal forces, migrate in an effort to fill the void. The migration of adjoining teeth disturbs the contact relationships in that vicinity. In the meantime, tooth movement changes occlusal relations with antagonists in opposing dental arches. The common result is hypereruption of the tooth opposing the space left by the lost tooth (Fig. 16–18).

If one of the maxillary central incisors is lost, the mandibular central incisor on the same side is left without an opposing tooth. The same situation exists regarding the maxillary third molar if the mandibular third molar is lost.

The dental arches are composed throughout by teeth in pairs, starting at the median line, one right, one left. Each pair is made up of two teeth alike in form and dimension, but since one is right and the other left, the outline form is reversed from one side to the other to accommodate the situation. Central incisors only are in contact with each other at the median line; other pairs are divided distal to the centrals and each member of each pair will be to the left or to the right and will be in contact on both of its sides with other members of other pairs (Fig. 16–19). To repeat: The right and left central incisors are together at the median line; right and left lateral incisors are placed distal to them. The lateral incisors will contact central incisors as well as canines. Right and left canines are distal to lateral incisors, contacting them, as well as first premolars, and so forth.

The mandibular arch is narrower when calibrated at the buccal surfaces of posterior teeth than is the maxillary arch. This relation is brought about by the differences in mesiodistal width between mandibular and maxillary anterior teeth (particularly the incisors) and by the lingual projection of mandibular posterior tooth crowns, an arrangement that brings about proper intercuspation.

Horizontal overlap (overjet) is that characteristic of the teeth in which the incisal ridges or buccal cusp ridges of the maxillary teeth extend labially or buccally to the incisal ridges or buccal cusp ridges of the mandibular teeth, when the teeth are in centric occlusal relation (Fig. 16–20).

Vertical overlap (overbite) is that characteristic of the teeth in which the incisal ridges of the maxillary anterior teeth extend below the incisal ridges of the mandibular anterior teeth when the teeth are placed in centric occlusal relation (Fig. 16–21). The presence of horizontal overlap in the molars prevents cheek biting.

Lingual views of the occlusal relations with the teeth in centric occlusion (Fig. 16–22) show the intercuspation of lingual cusps and how far the maxillary teeth occlude laterally to the lingual cusps of the mandibular arch.

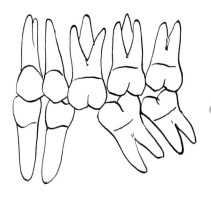

Figure 16–18. This illustration demonstrates possible migration and improper contact and occlusal relation resulting from the loss of a mandibular first molar.

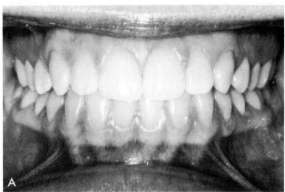

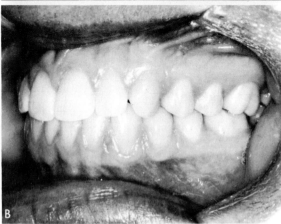

Figure 16–19. *A,* Alignment of incisors, frontal view. Note slight deviation of midline. *B,* Same patient from lateral facial view.

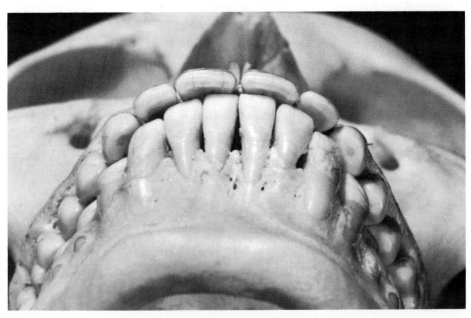

Figure 16–20. Demonstration of horizontal overlap.

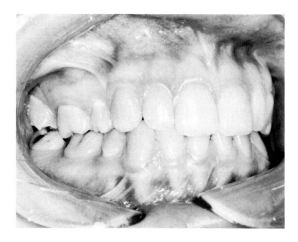

Figure 16–21. Vertical overlap in patient with teeth in centric occlusion.

The significance of vertical and horizontal overlap has to be related to the type of diet and jaw movement possible in humans. Excessive vertical overlap of the anterior teeth may result in tissue impingement and is referred to as an *impinging overbite*. The degree of vertical and horizontal overlap should be sufficient to allow jaw movement in function without interference. There should be sufficient vertical overlap (with cuspid providing the primary guidance) to enable the disclusion of the posterior teeth. Such movement in masticatory function is controlled by neuromuscular mechanisms developed out of past learning in relation to physical contact of the teeth. When protective reflexes are bypassed in parafunction, trauma from occlusion involving the teeth, supporting structures, and the temporomandibular joints may occur. However, aside from cheek biting due to insufficient horizontal overlap of the molars and trauma to the gingiva from an impinging overbite, there is no convincing evidence that a certain degree of overbite or overjet is optimal for effective mastication or stability of the occlusion. However, a vertical and/or horizontal overlap may be excessive and lead to dysfunction.

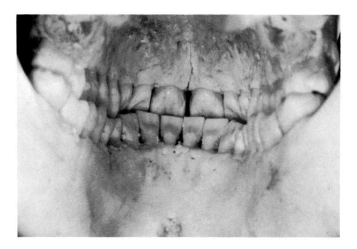

Figure 16–22. Lingual views of the teeth in centric occlusion.

Occlusal Contact and Intercusp Relations of All the Teeth of One Arch with Those in the Opposing Arch in Centric Occlusion

Occlusal contact and intercusp relations are the most difficult to study and also the most difficult to illustrate. However, it must be kept in mind that the knowledge acquired in the study of this item has practical application in any phase of daily practice. It might be said that a working knowledge of occlusal contact and intercusp relations of both dental arches in centric occlusion is necessary for any discussion of occlusal relations, whether for the natural dentition or a proposed restoration of the dentition. Thus the dentist should know for discussion purposes where a particular *supporting cusp* makes contact with a *centric stop* on the opposing tooth. For example, the lingual cusps of the maxillary posterior teeth and the buccal cusps of the posterior mandibular teeth are the supporting cusps. Centric stops are areas of contact that a supporting cusp makes with opposing teeth. Thus the mesial lingual cusp of the maxillary first molar (a supporting cusp) makes contact with the central fossa (central stop) of the mandibular first molar (Figs. 16–23 and 16–25). An idealized schematic representation of all centric stops is shown in Fig. 16–24.

Centric occlusion is frequently the position of the jaw for bracing during swallowing and the terminal position of the masticatory stroke. When the teeth of both jaws come together in centric occlusion, forces should be equalized so that the teeth are stabilized by all the forces acting on them.

Following suggestions made many years ago by Friel (1927), the technique of description will be borrowed from Hellman (1941) as told in reports on comparative anatomy and paleontology.

Their plan in describing occlusion of the teeth was to list the prospective occluding surfaces into the following divisions:

1. Surface contact
2. Cusp and fossa contact
3. Ridge and embrasure contact
4. Ridge and groove contact

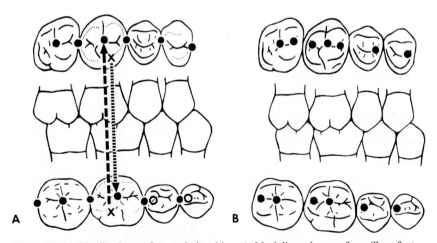

Figure 16–23. Idealized cusp-fossa relationships. *A*, Mesiolingual cusp of maxillary first molar occluding in central fossa of lower first molar. Distal buccal cusp of mandibular first molar occludes in central fossa of maxillary first molar. *B*, Occlusal concept, in which all supporting cusps occlude in fossae.

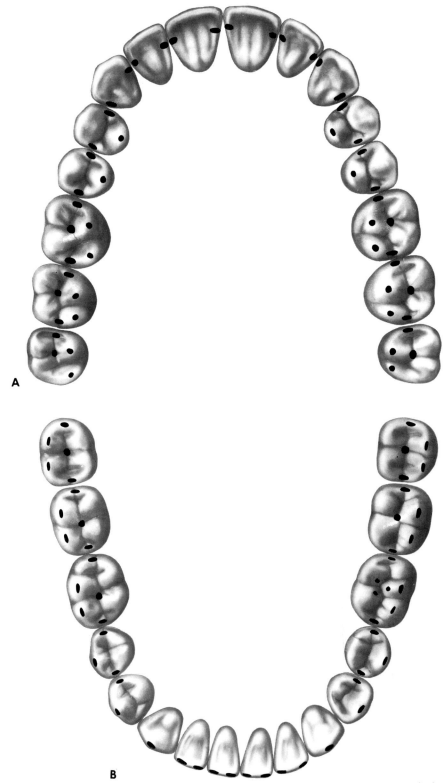

Figure 16–24. Idealized scheme for all contacts of supporting cusps with fossae and marginal ridges of opposing teeth. Such contact relations on all teeth are seldom found in the natural dentition. *A*, Maxillary arch. *B*, Mandibular arch.

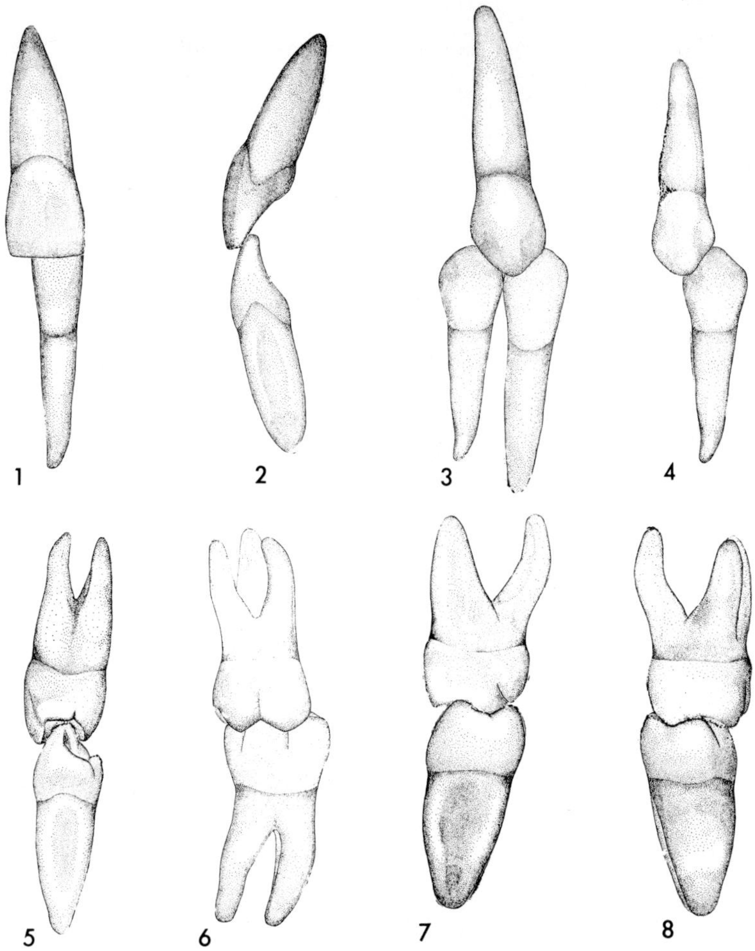

Figure 16–25. Normal intercuspation of maxillary and mandibular teeth.

1, Central incisors, labial aspect.

2, Central incisors, mesial aspect.

3, Maxillary canine, in contact with mandibular canine and first premolar, facial aspect.

4, Maxillary first premolar and mandibular first premolar, buccal aspect.

5, Maxillary first premolar and mandibular first premolar, mesial aspect.

6, First molars, buccal aspect.

7, First molars, mesial aspect.

8, First molars, distal aspect.

It must be remembered that when this listing was made, the investigators were interested primarily in descriptions of functional form and development and not in the detail required for dental treatment or restoration. In order to focus on the latter activities some minor changes in nomenclature that are intended to be of assistance in understanding the detailed descriptions have been added.

The list, as it was changed for the purpose at hand, is as follows:

1. Interocclusal offset relationship of opposing teeth
2. Surface contact
3. Cusp and fossa apposition
4. Cusp and embrasure apposition
5. Ridge and sulcus apposition (includes ridge and developmental groove apposition)

Figures and legends featuring landmarks on teeth are to be repeated for use in ready reference during the reading (Fig. 16–26 through 16–29). Illustrations for reference include close-up photographs of specimen teeth in occlusion (Figs. 16–30 through 16–33). It would be well to emphasize again the unyielding, hard, rounded surfaces to be seen everywhere on the occlusal ''working surfaces'' of the teeth (Fig. 16–34).

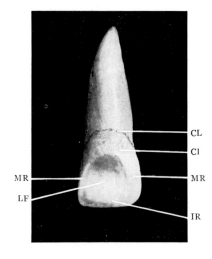

Figure 16–26. Maxillary right central incisor (lingual aspect). *CL*, Cervical line; *CI*, cingulum; *MR*, marginal ridge; *IR*, incisal ridge; *LF*, lingual fossa.

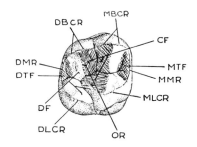

Figure 16–27. Maxillary right first molar, occlusal landmarks. *MBCR*, Mesiobuccal cusp ridge; *CF*, central fossa (shaded area); *MTF*, mesial triangular fossa (shaded area); *MMR*, mesial marginal ridge; *MLCR*, mesiolingual cusp ridge; *OR*, oblique ridge; *DLCR*, distolingual cusp ridge; *DF*, distal fossa; *DTF*, distal triangular fossa (shaded area); *DMR*, distal marginal ridge; *DBCR*, distobuccal cusp ridge.

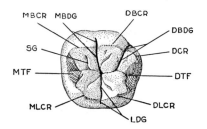

Figure 16–28. Mandibular right first molar, occlusal aspect. *DBCR*, Distobuccal cusp ridge; *DBDG*, distobuccal developmental groove; *DCR*, distal cusp ridge; *DTF*, distal triangular fossa (shaded area); *DLCR*, distolingual cusp ridge; *LDG*, lingual developmental groove; *MLCR*, mesiolingual cusp ridge; *MTF*, mesial triangular fossa (shaded area); *SG*, a supplemental groove; *MBCR*, mesiobuccal cusp ridge; *MBDG*, mesiobuccal developmental groove.

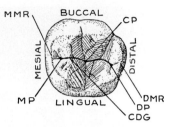

Figure 16–29. Mandibular right first molar, occlusal aspect. Shaded area—central fossa. *CP*, Central pit; *DMT*, distal marginal ridge; *DP*, distal pit; *CDG*, central developmental groove; *MP*, mesial pit; *MMR*, mesial marginal ridge.

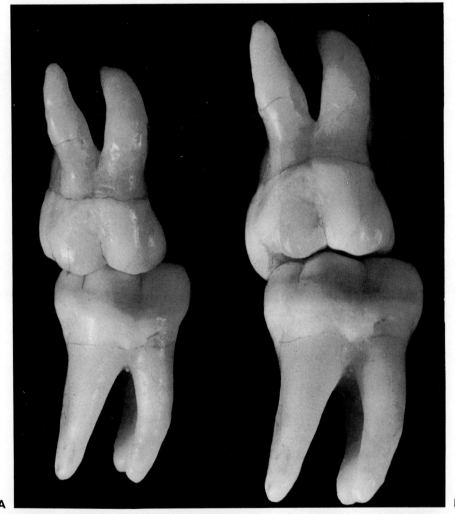

A   B

Figure 16–30. First molars in centric occlusion, facial view. Because the first molars are instrumental in establishing occlusal relations anterior to them—and posterior to them as well—their study should receive special attention in order to facilitate understanding of the fundamentals of occlusion generally.

A, This view is at right angles to facial portions about level with occlusal surfaces. This is the classic view, giving the impression (held by most observers) of the mesiobuccal cusp of the maxillary molar fitting snugly into the sulcus of the mesiobuccal groove of the mandibular first molar.

B, The combination has been tipped so that one is able to peer under the buccal cusps of the maxillary molar. It is apparent that the triangular ridge of the mesiobuccal cusp is slightly distal to the groove mentioned previously.

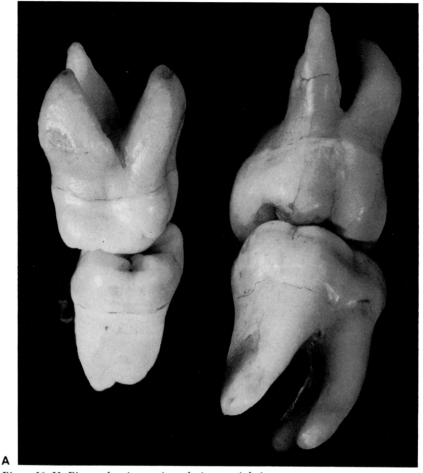

A   B

Figure 16–31. First molars in centric occlusion, mesial view.

  A, This view is directly mesial to the combination and considerably above the level of the occlusal surface of the mandibular molar. Note the escapement provided by the tooth form of the crowns when in centric relation.

  B, A perspective view from an odd angle that portrays the efficiency of the occlusal form of the molars.

  The rounded folds of ridges and cusp forms contact opposing teeth without rigid interlocking. This formation permits some adjustment in alignment without trauma. Yet the cusp-fossa and ridge-sulcus arrangement still fits well enough to promote stability.

Interocclusal Offset Relationship of Opposing Teeth

This subject was discussed at length under facial and lingual relations. To summarize: Each premolar or molar tooth is in contact mainly with its namesake in the opposite jaw (e.g., the first molar to first molar; see Fig. 16–17).

Surface Contact

These contacting occlusal surfaces are found at *incisal portions of mandibular anteriors,* which become functional when they come into contact with the *lingual surfaces of maxillary anterior teeth.* However, even these contacting areas exhibit some curvature.

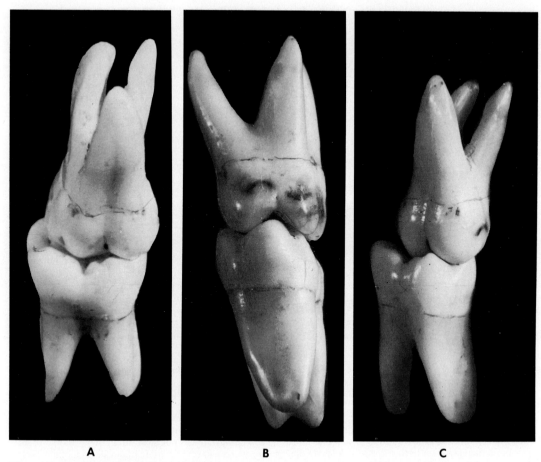

A   **B**   **C**

Figure 16–32. First molars in centric occlusion.

A, Above and lingual to occlusal surface of mandibular first molar. Relation of the two teeth showing considerable escapement mesially—close adaptation distally near the distal marginal ridge of the maxillary molar.

B, Articulation of the first molars distally. Note the close adaptation of the distolingual cusp of the maxillary molar to the distolingual and distal cusps of the mandibular molar. Also note the lack of contact of the distobuccal cusp of the upper molar, creating escapement space. Lateral relation of the jaw would put the upper molar triangular ridge of the distobuccal cusp in contact.

C, Distolingual view of first molars in centric occlusion. Compare this aspect with *A.* Note the spacing which has opened up mesially and the close adaptation of the distolingual cusp of the upper molar with the distal marginal ridge and the distal cusp of the lower molar. The distolingual cusp of the mandibular molar opposes the lingual sulcus of the lingual developmental groove.

Cusp and Fossa Apposition

Examples under this heading are the cusp-fossa relationships of premolars and molars (Figs. 16–35 through 16–36). Of particular importance is the massive and pointed mesiolingual cusp portions of the maxillary molars that fit into the major fossae of lower molars in centric occlusion. This occlusal design is not only useful in the act of chewing; it is most effective as a stabilizer of alignment because of the way the cusps "key into" the fossae. The manner in which these parts fit together in centric occlusion is more important than the relationship of buccal cusps of maxillary molars to buccal grooves of mandibular molars. The molar relationship is often referred to as the key to occlusion.

The distolingual cusps of maxillary molars are in apposition to the distal triangular

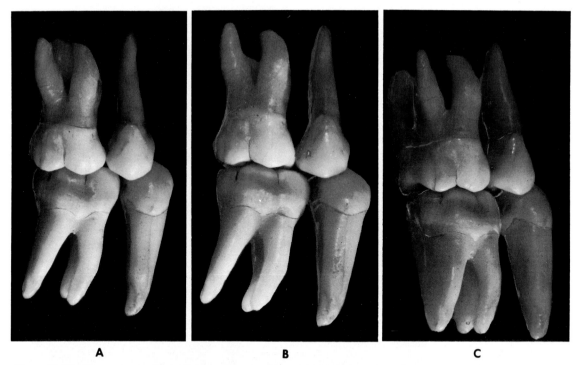

A   **B**   **C**

Figure 16–33. The specimens shown in occlusal contact in centric relation are second premolars and first molars, maxillary and mandibular. They were photographed from the buccal aspect.

A, The sighting of the aspect is about 90°, with the buccal surfaces of the molars approximately level with the tips of the buccal cusps of the mandibular teeth.

B, Without changing occlusal relations, the specimens were tipped so the view was directed somewhat under the maxillary teeth occlusally. Note the actual distal relationship of cusp tips and triangular ridges of the maxillary molar to the buccal developmental grooves of the mandibular molar. This relationship was not apparent in A.

C, From the viewpoint farther distally, the cusp tips and grooves seem to be more in line with each other. Note the lack of occlusal contact in some areas that promotes escapement by creating free space even in centric relation.

fossae (Fig. 16–38) and marginal ridge (Fig. 16–39) of mandibular molars and often to the mesial marginal ridge of the molar distal to their namesakes (e.g., maxillary first molar distolingual cusp to mesial of mandibular second molar).

Another *cusp-fossa* relationship to be noted is the contact of relatively sharp lingual cusps of *maxillary premolars* with triangular fossae of *mandibular premolars*.

The *cusp-fossa* apposition, including the *buccal cusps* of *mandibular posterior teeth*, follows:

The *mesiobuccal* cusps of *mandibular molars* are in apposition to the distal fossa, or the marginal ridge bordering it, of the tooth above, mesial to its namesake (e.g., first molar mandibular to distal of second maxillary premolar).

The *distobuccal cusps* of *mandibular molars* are accommodated by the central fossae of their namesakes in the opposite jaw.

The *buccal cusp tip* of the *second mandibular premolar* approaches the *mesial occlusal fossa* of the *opposing second premolar*, while the *first mandibular premolar* occludes partly with the *first premolar* above and partly with the *maxillary canine* (Fig. 16–37, A, B, and C).

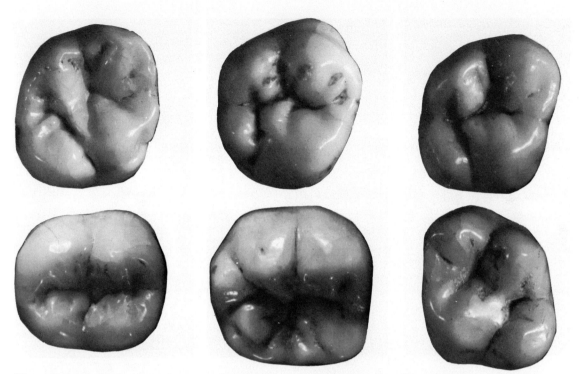

Figure 16–34. Occlusal aspects of several fine specimens of molars. These teeth suggest the possibility that during development, the smooth contoured enamel was "folded" into the developmental grooves.

It is quite apparent that rounded contours and cusp formations of similar design will strike opposing teeth with like surfaces in points and constricted areas only.

No flat surfaces are to be found on occlusal third portions of posterior teeth unless they are caused by wear or accident.

The normal limits on occluding surfaces are illustrated. The registration of all occlusal contacts, including centric relation, should be held within these limitations in order to establish physiological activity.

Cusp and Embrasure Apposition

Under this heading, some description is made that is often omitted when defining normal occlusion in centric occlusion. Some *cusp* tips are actually *opposed* to *embrasure spaces.* Other cusps are in partial contact with marginal and cusp ridges, in addition to straddling the embrasure spaces created by the ridges (Fig. 16–39).

Ridge and Sulcus Apposition

A short reminder of the parts under discussion: *"triangular ridges,* a continuation of prominently formed enamel that extends from cusp tips toward the center of occlusal surfaces, usually ending in fossae or developmental grooves (Figs. 16–27 through 16–29).

Sulci are linear depressions between these enamel ridges with developmental grooves at the bottom of the enamel valleys; the grooves extend at times on to buccal and lingual surfaces.

The main ridge and sulcus occlusion that dominates discussion is that of the triangular ridges of the buccal cusps of maxillary molars as they are accommodated into buccal grooves with their sulci in mandibular molars (Figs. 16–27 and 16–31).

Another important combination is that of the triangular ridge of the distolingual cusp of

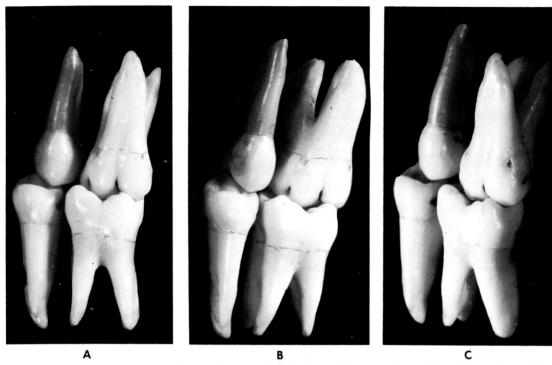

| | | |
| A | B | C |

Figure 16–35. The specimens shown in occlusal contact include the maxillary second premolar and first molar and the mandibular second premolar and first molar.

A, The teeth were posed so that the view was almost directly opposite the lingual surface of the maxillary molar. The occlusal relationship of first molars here is interesting, as it is assisted by the inclusion of second premolars.

B, Compare *B* with *A* and notice how a slight change in angle clarifies the study. The view is now almost from directly opposite the mandibular premolar and from slightly above its occlusal surface. Note particularly the cusp-fossa relationship.

C, This is a distolingual view with the occlusal relationship comparable to *B*. Note how escapement spacing varies and cusp relations are clarified when the teeth are studied from more than one aspect.

the mandibular first molar as it fits into the lingual groove sulcus of the maxillary first molar (Fig. 16–32, *C*).

The ridge and sulcus contact of significant note in lateral occlusal movements, as well as in centric relation, is the *oblique transverse ridge* of the *maxillary first molar,* a triangular ridge extending obliquely from the distobuccal cusp to the mesiolingual cusp. This ridge fits into the sulcus formed on the occlusal surface of the mandibular first molar, marked by the junction of distobuccal, central, and lingual developmental grooves.

Taking these most important ridge-sulcus listings as starting points, it is possible to formulate many other combinations if a complete and ideal picture of occlusion is desired.

Hellman (1941) listed 138 points of possible occlusal contacts to be observed and tabulated in a complete description of occlusion. The tabulation included 32 teeth. The list of points (total, 138) is as follows:

1. Lingual surfaces of upper incisors and canines, 6
2. Labial surface of lower incisors and canines, 6
3. Triangular ridges of upper buccal cusps of premolars and molars, 16
4. Triangular ridges of lingual cusps of lower premolars and molars, 16
5. Buccal embrasure of lower premolars and molars, 8

A

B

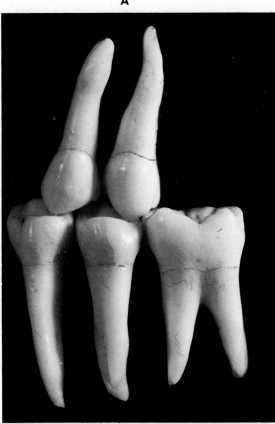

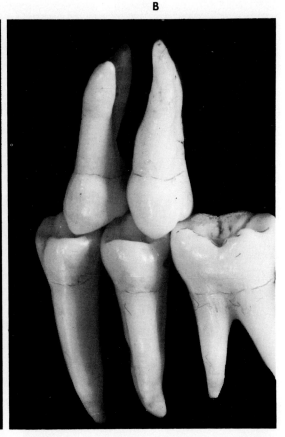

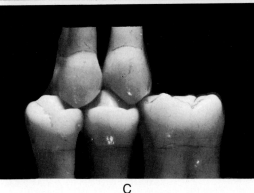

C

Figure 16–36. These photos of specimen teeth are made
from four separate angulations lingually. The specimen
teeth show the occlusal relations of maxillary premolars in
contact with mandibular premolars and first molar.

A, Viewed from directly opposite the lingual surface
of the mandibular second premolar; the viewer is to make
an independent analysis.

B, A view of the occlusal relations taken
distolingually above the occlusal surfaces of the
mandibular teeth. Note particularly the occlusal contact
of the lingual cusps of the maxillary premolars.

C, This picture of the crowns exclusively may be
compared with *A;* there is a slight variation in angle and
lighting.

    6. Lingual embrasures of upper premolars and molars (including the canine and first
       premolar embrasure accommodating the lower premolar), 10
    7. Lingual cusp points of upper premolars and molars, 16
    8. Buccal cusp points of lower premolars and molars, 16
    9. Distal fossae of premolars, 8
  10. Central fossae of the molars, 12
  11. Mesial fossae of the lower molars, 6
  12. Distal fossae of the upper molars, 6

A

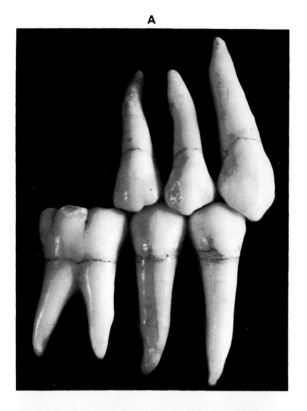

B

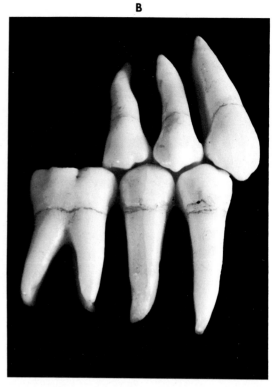

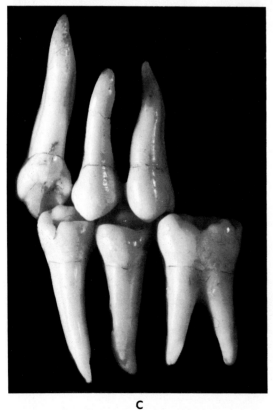

C

Figure 16–37. Natural tooth specimens set up to show occlusal relations. The teeth displayed include the maxillary canine, the maxillary first canine, and the second premolars; the mandibular first and second premolars; and the first molar.

A, View at right angles to facial surfaces. This is the typical aspect made in occlusal studies that gives the impression of surfaces fitting rather tightly together with little apparent open relief.

B, The arrangement was tipped so that the camera was allowed to see under the facial cusps of maxillary teeth. Note the point contact effect in occlusion of lowers with marginal ridge areas of uppers and the creation of escapement spaces.

C, A distolingual view of the same arrangement of teeth as seen in *A* and *B*. This view is often neglected in studies of occlusion. It illustrates occlusal contact and emphasizes the additional escapement space created by the tooth form lingually.

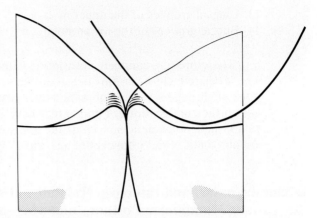

Figure 16–38. Schematic representation of the possible relationship of supporting cusps to distal fossae (premolars and molars).

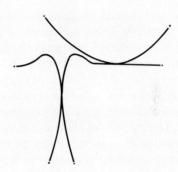

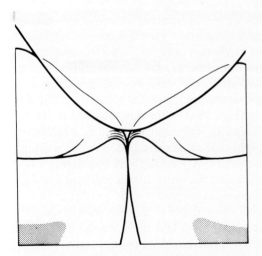

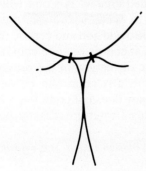

Figure 16–39. Relationship of supporting cusps to marginal ridges.

13. Lingual grooves of the upper molars, 6
14. Buccal grooves of the lower molars, 6*

Therefore, if a complete description without the omission of any detail of ideal occlusion is desired, close scrutiny of a good skull or cast showing 32 teeth would make possible a list of all ridge-sulcus combinations, all cusp embrasure combinations, and so on. Usually, if the combinations of points that have been mentioned in the last few pages can be established, some details, such as the approximate location of hard contact in occlusion, are automatic. Friel's concept of an ''ideal'' occlusion is illustrated in Figure 16–40.

Occlusal Contact and Intercusp Relations of All the Teeth During the Various Mandibular Positions and Movements

Occlusal contact relations away from centric occlusion involve all possible movements of the mandible within the envelope of border movements shown in Figures 15–8 and 15–10. These movements are generally referred to as lateral, lateral protrusive, protrusive, and retrusive movements. Lateral and lateral protrusive movements may be either to the right or to the left. Expressions of lateral movement often also do not include lateral protrusive movements and basic movements reduced to right and left lateral movement, protrusive movement, and retrusive movement.

During the *right lateral movement,* the mandible is depressed and the dental arches are separated, the jaw moves to the right and brings the teeth together at points to the right of centric occlusion in right working (Fig. 16–41, *A*). On the left side, called the balancing or nonworking side, the teeth may or may not make contact (Fig. 16–41, *C*).

Concepts of occlusion often describe idealized contact relations in lateral movements as shown in Figure 16–42. However, in the natural dentition, a variety of contact relations may be found, including group function, cuspid disclusion only, or some combination of cuspid, premolar, and molar contacts in lateral movements. *Group function* refers to multiple contacts (Fig. 16–43) in such movements rather than simply cuspid guidance (Fig. 16–44). Thus working side contacts may be single or multiple in lateral excursion. There is general agreement that balancing side contacts (Fig. 16–45) are not required in lateral movement, and that such contacts are not considered an occlusal interference. A balancing side interference is a contact on the balancing side that causes disclusion of the working side or that interferes with smooth gliding movements. A working side interference is a contact on the working side that causes working side disclusion or displacement of a mobile tooth on the working side.

During the *protrusive movement,* the mandible is depressed, then moves directly forward, bringing the anterior teeth together at points most favorable for the incision of food. Protrusive movement is followed by a retrusive movement to centric occlusion.

Retrusive movement from centric occlusion to retruded contact position where the condyles are in the rearmost, uppermost position seems to occur in bruxism but infrequently in mastication and swallowing, except where centric occlusion and centric relation are coincident, i.e., where maximum intercuspation occurs at centric relation contact. The adverse neuromuscular responses to retrusion and closure of the jaw in the presence of occlusal interferences to maximum intercuspation in centric relation can be detected electromyographically and by the clinician. However, the jaw does not go to the retrusive position necessarily even after elimination of such occlusal interferences by occlusal

---

* *Hellman did not list the distobuccal groove of the lower first molar, possibly because it is normally out of occlusal contact.*

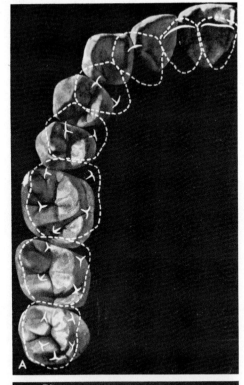

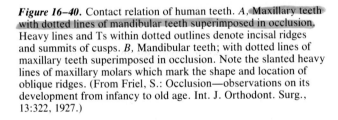

Figure 16–40. Contact relation of human teeth. *A,* Maxillary teeth with dotted lines of mandibular teeth superimposed in occlusion. Heavy lines and Ts within dotted outlines denote incisal ridges and summits of cusps. *B,* Mandibular teeth; with dotted lines of maxillary teeth superimposed in occlusion. Note the slanted heavy lines of maxillary molars which mark the shape and location of oblique ridges. (From Friel, S.: Occlusion—observations on its development from infancy to old age. Int. J. Orthodont. Surg., 13:322, 1927.)

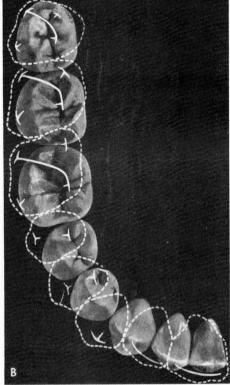

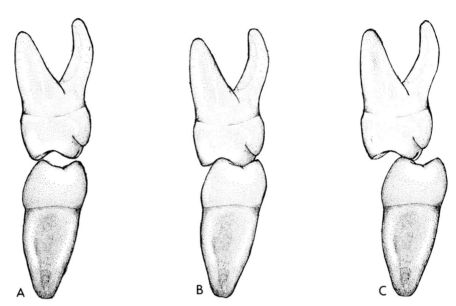

Figure 16–41. Occlusal relations of first molars during the cycle of occlusal movements (see also Fig. 16–51).

    A, Initial occlusal contact in right lateral occlusal relation.

    B, Centric occlusal relation.

    C, Final contact after leaving centric relation before the mandible drops away to begin another cycle. This is also the balancing contact for the left lateral occlusal relation.

adjustment, and although the occlusion may be reconstructed to guide the mandible into the retruded position and maximum intercuspation, a "slide in centric" (Fig. 16–46) may develop again but the significance of the return of a small "slide" has not been determined (Celenza, 1973).

Lateral Occlusal Relations of the Teeth

When the mandibular teeth make their initial contact with the maxillary teeth in right or left lateral occlusal relation, they bear a right or left lateral relation to centric occlusion. The canines, premolars, and molars of one side of the *mandible* make their occlusal contact facial (labial or buccal) to their facial cusp ridges at some portion of their occlusal thirds (Fig. 16–42). Those points on the mandibular teeth make contact with *maxillary* teeth at points just lingual to their facial cusp ridges. The central and lateral incisors of the working side are not usually in contact at the same time; if they are, the labioincisal portions of the mandibular teeth of that side are in contact with the linguoincisal portions of the maxillary teeth.

During the sliding contact action, from the most facial contact points to centric occlusion, the teeth intercuspate and slide over each other in a *directional line approximately parallel with the oblique ridge of the upper first molar*. The oblique ridge of the maxillary first molar relates occlusally to the combined sulci of the distobuccal and developmental grooves of the occlusal surface of the mandibular first molar.

As the teeth of one side move from lateral relation to centric occlusion, the cusps and ridges bear a certain relationship to each other; the cusps and ridges (including marginal ridges) of the canines and posterior teeth of the *mandibular* arch have an intercusping relationship to the cusps and ridges of the teeth of the *maxillary* arch (Fig. 16–47). The crowns of the teeth are formed in such a way that cusps and ridges may slide over each

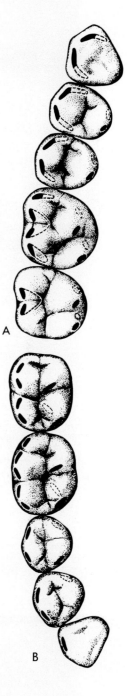

Figure 16–42. Lateral occlusal contacts from centric occlusion. *A*, Contacts in right lateral movement on the maxillary teeth. *B*, Contacts on the mandibular teeth by the maxillary teeth in right lateral movement.

other without mutual interference. In addition, the crowns of the teeth are "turned" on the root bases to accommodate the angled movement across their opponents (Fig. 16–48).

The cusp tip of the mandibular canine moves through the linguoincisal embrasure of the maxillary lateral incisor and canine. The cusp tip is often in contact with one of the marginal ridges making up the lingual embrasure above it. Its mesial cusp ridge is usually out of contact during the lateral movement. Its distal ridge contacts the mesial cusp ridge of the maxillary canine.

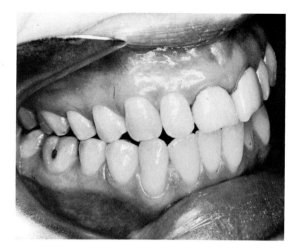

Figure 16–43. Group function. Multiple working side contacts.

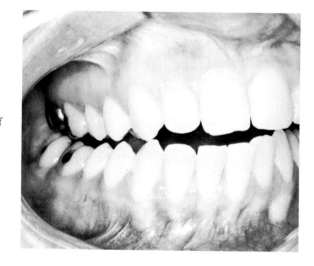

Figure 16–44. Cuspid guidance. There are no contacts of molars or premolars in right lateral movement.

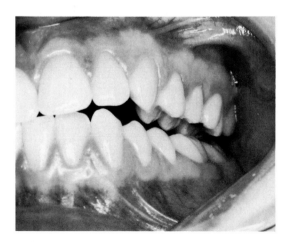

Figure 16–45. Balancing side contacts. In this case, these contacts did not cause disclusion of the teeth on the working side at any point in lateral movement.

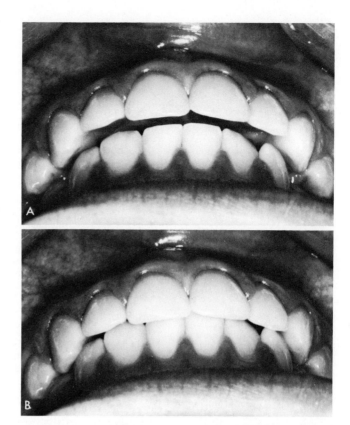

Figure 16–46. Difference in jaw position and occlusal contacts between centric occlusion and centric relation. *A,* Jaw in centric relation. *B,* Teeth in the intercuspal position (centric occlusion).

The cusp tip of the mandibular first premolar moves through the occlusal embrasure of the maxillary canine and first premolar (Figs. 16–49 and 16–50). Its mesiobuccal ridge contacts the distal cusp ridge of the maxillary canine, and its distobuccal cusp ridge contacts the mesio-occlusal slope of the buccal cusp of the maxillary first premolar.

The mandibular second premolar buccal cusp moves through the occlusal embrasure and then over the linguo-occlusal embrasure of the maxillary first and second premolars. Its mesiobuccal cusp ridge contacts the disto-occlusal slope of the buccal cusp of the maxillary first premolar, and its distobuccal cusp ridge contacts the mesio-occlusal slope of the buccal cusp of the upper second premolar.

Figure 16–47. Projected paths on maxillary *(A)* and mandibular *(B)* first molars made by supporting cusps, i.e., mesial lingual cusp of maxillary molar on mandibular molar and distal buccal cusp of mandibular molar on maxillary molar. P = Protrusive path; B = path on balancing side; W = path made during working side movement; D = distal; M = mesial.

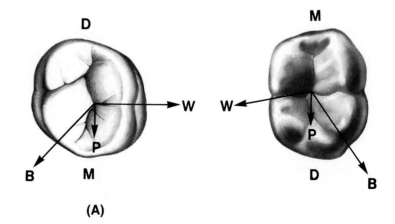

(A)

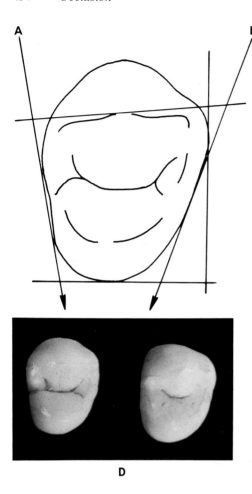

D

Figure 16–48. Outline of the occlusal aspect of the right maxillary first premolar with its distal and lingual surfaces surveyed by a right angle distolingually (see Fig. 9–14).

A, A line following the angulation of the mesial surface is not too far removed from parallelism with the vertical line of the right angle distally. This formation allows a proper contact relationship with the distal proximal surface of the maxillary canine; simultaneously it cooperates with the canine in keeping the lingual embrasure design within normal limitations.

B, Line *B* demonstrates a more extreme angulation of the distal portion of the first premolar. This form allows cusp and ridge by-pass by mandibular teeth over the distal marginal ridge surface of the maxillary tooth with normal jaw movements during lateral occlusal relations.

C, Line *C,* aligned with mesiobuccal and distobuccal line angles, demonstrates the adaptation of the form of the buccal surface of the crown to dental arch form without changing the functional position of crown and root.

D, Two natural specimens of the maxillary right first premolar that display similar characteristics compared with the accented drawing above them.

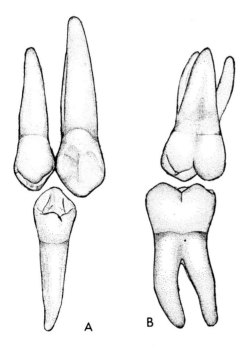

Figure 16–49. Cusps and cusp ridges, embrasures, and so forth, bear an interrelationship to each other. *A,* Mandibular first premolar relation to maxillary canine and first premolar on the verge of occlusal contact. Lingual aspect. *B,* Mandibular first molar relation to the maxillary first molar on the verge of occlusal contact. Lingual aspect.

Figure 16–50. Assembly of the maxillary canine, first and second premolars and the first molar as they appear in the maxillary arch. The arrows indicate the direction of movement of the mandibular teeth over the maxillary teeth during the masticatory cycle. The major embrasures of canines and premolars are above marginal ridges occlusally. The arrows are on a line approximately parallel to the oblique ridge of the maxillary first molar.

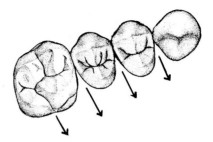

The lingual cusps of all premolars are out of contact until centric relation is attained. Then the only lingual cusps in contact are those of the maxillary premolars, with the possible addition of the distolingual cusp of a mandibular second premolar of the three-cusp type (Fig. 16–35, *B*). The molars have a more involved *lateral occlusal relation* because of their more complex design.

It has been determined previously, while describing the lateral occlusal relations of canines and premolars, that cusps, cusp ridges, sulci, and embrasures bear an interrelationship to each other. Cusps and elevations on the teeth of one arch pass between or over cusps and through embrasures or sulci. The tooth form and the alignment of the opposing teeth of both jaws make this possible. The cusps of the teeth of one jaw simply do not ride up and down the cusp slopes of the teeth in the opposing jaw. This explanation of the occlusal process has created wide misunderstanding. The cusp, ridge, fossa, and embrasure form of occlusion allow interdigitation without a "locked-in" effect. There is no clashing of cusp against cusp or any interference between parts of the occlusal surfaces if the development is proper.

A Description of the Occlusal Cycle in the Molar Areas during Right or Left Lateral Occlusal Relations

In lateral movements during mastication, the mandible drops downward and to the right or left of centric occlusion. As it continues the cycle of movement and returns toward centric occlusion, the bucco-occlusal portions of mandibular molars come into contact with the occlusal portions of the maxillary molars lingual to the summits of buccal cusps and in contact with their triangular ridges of the slopes on each side of them, continuing the sliding contact until centric occlusion is accomplished (Figs. 16–41 and 16–51).

From these first contacts the mandibular molars slide into centric occlusion with maxillary molars and then come to a momentary rest.

The movement continues with occlusal surfaces in sliding contact until the linguo-occlusal slopes of the buccal portions of the mandibular molars pass the final points of contact with the linguo-occlusal slopes of the lingual portions of the maxillary molars (Fig. 16–51). When the molars lose contact, the mandible drops away in a circular movement to begin another cycle of lateral jaw movement (Fig. 16–41).

The actual distance traveled by mandibular molars in contact across the occlusal surfaces of maxillary molars, from first contacts to final contacts at separation, is very short. When measured at the incisors, it is only 2.8 mm in Australian aborigines and only half or less of this in Europeans (Beyron, 1964). The lower molars, which are the moving antagonists, are taken out of contact before the first contact location on their buccal cusps reaches the final points of contact on the maxillary molars. (Compare *A* and *C* in Figure 16–41).

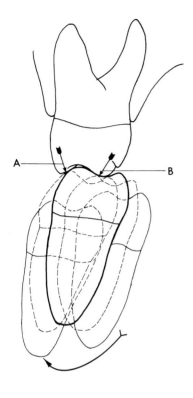

A ———

——— B

Figure 16–51. The cycle of occlusal movements, represented by a schematic drawing of first molar relations—mesial aspect. The heavy outline of the mandibular molar represents it to be in centric occlusal relation with the maxillary molar. The shadow outlines represent the mandibular molar in various relations during the cycle of mandibular movement during mastication. The two short arrows (*A* and *B*) at right angles to the occlusal surface of the maxillary molar measure the extent of movement between them over the occlusal surface from the first contact of the mandibular molar to the last contact before continuing another cycle.

Mechanism of Mastication

During the masticatory process, the individual generally chews on one side only at any one chewing stroke. Most of the work is done by shifting material from one side to the other when convenient; the shifting is confined generally to the molar and premolar regions. Occasionally, for specific reasons the shift of mastication may be directed anteriorly. Nevertheless, the posterior teeth, of right or left side, are depended upon by the host to do the major portion of the work of mastication. The posteriors are aided, of course, in various ways by the canines, but the latter do not possess the broad occlusal surfaces required for chewing efficiency overall.

The food is manipulated by the tongue, lips, and cheeks so that it is thrown between the teeth continuously during the mandibular movements which bring the teeth together in their various relations. To repeat: The major portion of the work is accomplished in the premolar and molar regions while the mandible is making right lateral and left lateral movements, bringing the teeth into right lateral and left lateral occlusal relation, terminating the strokes in centric occlusion.

The Occlusal Cycle of the Posterior Teeth with Their Canines: A Summary

The occlusal cycle of the posterior teeth, accompanied by the canines during the right and left lateral occlusal relations, may be summarized as follows:

1. There are right lateral and left lateral relations to be observed, depending on which is to be called the working side.
2. If the right side is the working side, one of two situations may be observed. Only the right side cuspids may be in contact (cuspid guidance) or the cuspid only with consecutively added posterior teeth will be in contact (group function).

3. From right lateral relation, the teeth glide into centric occlusion.
4. Left lateral occlusal relation will be a duplication of the description above for right lateral relation, except for substitution of the word "left" where the term "right" was used and vice versa.
5. From left lateral relation, the teeth return to centric occlusion.

Protrusive Occlusal Relations of the Teeth

The process of *biting* or *shearing* food material is negotiated by the *protrusive occlusal relation*.

Although the mandible may be lowered considerably in producing a wide opening of the mouth, the occlusion of the anterior teeth is not concerned with any arrangement very far removed from centric relation.

When the jaw is opened and moved straight forward to the normal protrusive relation, the mandibular arch bears a forward, or anterior, relation of only 1 or 2 mm in most cases to its centric relation with the maxillary arch.

The protrusive occlusal relation places the labioincisal areas of the incisal ridges of the mandibular incisors in contact with the linguoincisal areas of the incisal portions of the maxillary incisors. The mesiolabial portion of the mesial cusp ridge of the mandibular canine should be in contact with the maxillary lateral incisors distolinguoincisally.

From the protrusive occlusal relation the teeth glide over each other in a *retrusive* movement of the mandible, a movement that terminates in centric occlusion. During this final shearing action, the incisal ridges of the lower incisors are in continuous contact with the linguoincisal third portions of the maxillary incisors, from the position of protrusive occlusal relation to the return to centric occlusal relation.

The maxillary canines may assist by having their distal cusp ridges in contact with the mesial cusp of the mandibular first premolar. They cooperate with the incisors most of the time in one way or another. A slight movement to right or left during protrusion will bring canines together in a "biting" manner. In addition, at the end of the incisive cycle, the contact of the canines with each other in centric occlusion lends final effectiveness to the process.

Neurobehavioral Aspects of Occlusion

Up to this point in this discussion, the emphasis has been on the structural, anatomical alignment of the teeth. Chapter 15 mentioned briefly some of the aspects of mandibular positions and movements and muscle function. And although it would be impossible to do justice to the topic of neuroscience of occlusion in a brief review, it is imperative to call attention to the meaning of occlusion in its broadest sense.

Recent ideas concerning the diagnosis and treatment of disturbances, such as chronic oral-facial pain, temporomandibular disorders (TMD), craniomandibular disorders, and bruxism, and the diagnosis and treatment of malocclusion involving orthognathic surgery, require a greater knowledge of the neurobehavioral aspects of oral motor behavior than ever before in the practice of dentistry.

The neurobehavioral aspects of occlusion relate to function and parafunction of the stomatognathic system. Function includes a variety of actions or human behavior such as chewing, sucking, swallowing, speech, and respiration. Parafunction refers to action such as bruxism, e.g., clenching and grinding of the teeth. All these functions require highly developed sensory-motor mechanisms. The coordination of occlusal contacts, jaw motion, and tongue movement during mastication requires a very intricate control system involving a number of guiding influences from the teeth and their supporting structures, temporomandibular joints, masticatory muscles, and from higher centers in the central nervous system. Frequent contact of the teeth during mastication without biting the tongue, closure of the jaw to facilitate swallowing (occurring about 600 times a day), remarkable tactile sensibility in which threshold values for detecting foreign bodies between the teeth may be as little as 8 μ, and the presence of protective reflexes suggest the need for intricate mechanisms of control of jaw position and occlusal forces.

The presence of several type of teeth, powerful musculature, and a most delicate positional control system indicates that it is important to understand the strategy underlying such sensitive control mechanisms. Although the ease with which these mechanisms may be disturbed at the periphery (i.e., the teeth, joints, periodontium, peripheral neural system) and centrally (brainstem and higher centers) is not well understood, the adaptive capacity of the stomatognathic system appears to be considerable. On an individual clinical basis, however, the responses of a patient to occlusal therapy may be reflected in oral behavior outside the range of normal. Inasmuch as function and parafunction share similar anatomical, physiological, and psychological substrates, it is necessary to review briefly the neurobehavioral correlates of the activities of the stomatognathic system.

Occlusal Stability (Figs. 16–52 through 16–58)

Occlusal stability refers to the tendency of the teeth, jaws, joints, and muscles to remain in an optimal functional state. A few of the mechanisms involved include mesial migration of teeth, eruption of teeth to compensate for occlusal wear or intrusion by occlusal forces, remodeling of bone, protective reflexes and control of occlusal forces, reparative processes, and a number of others even less understood than those just listed. Although the strategy for stability related to a functional level required for survival appears obvious, orchestration of such diverse mechanisms can be couched only in such terms as "homeostasis." The influence of such factors as disease, aging, and dysfunction on occlusal stability has yet to be clarified.

From a clinical standpoint, several concepts of occlusal stability are used as goals for occlusal therapy, including stable jaw relation in centric occlusion and centric relation; occlusal forces to be directed in the long axis of a tooth; maintenance of centric stops, supporting cusps, and contact vertical dimension; replacement of lost teeth; and control of tooth mobility. These aspects of occlusal stability are more appropriately found in books on occlusal treatment.

Mesial migration is a term used to describe the migration of teeth in a mesial direction. The cause of this phenomenon has not been fully clarified, although a number of ideas have been advanced. There seems to be little doubt that mesial drift does occur, but there is no general agreement on the magnitude of movement, which teeth move, and how the movement is achieved. Suggested causes include traction of the transseptal fiber system (Picton and Moss, 1980), forces of mastication (Dewel, 1949; van Beek and Fidler, 1977), and tongue pressure (Yilmaz et al., 1980). The strategy behind the mesial migration appears to be related to closure of proximal tooth contacts. Although occlusal forces may be considered as passive and traction of transseptal fibers as active mechanisms, it is difficult to determine in what way occlusal stability is influenced. The contact relations of the teeth may promote occlusal stability, but if incorrect relations are present, opening of proximal contacts can occur (Fig. 16–52).

There is a tendency to assume that a particular arrangement of teeth is unstable (Fig. 16–53); however, such an occlusal relationship may have become stabilized, at least at a particular point in time. Whether or not an occlusion is fully stable can be observed only by periodic evaluation of that occlusion. Many factors (caries, periodontal disease, occlusal

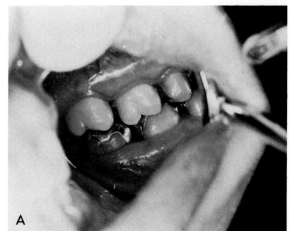

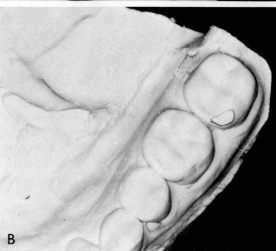

Figure 16–52. Occlusion, food impaction, and bruxism. *A,* After placement of a restoration of the lower second molar, contact between the lower first and second molar was lost, resulting in food being wedged between these teeth. Loss of contact was due to lower second molar being moved distally by an occlusal interference to protrusive movement during bruxism. *B,* Area outlined on cast to show position of occlusal interference.

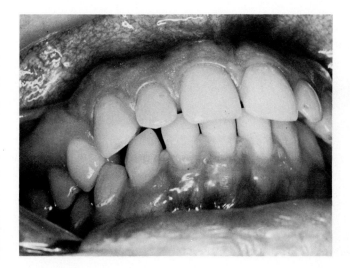

Figure 16–53 Occlusal instability cannot be determined simply on the basis of occlusal contact relations and spacing of the teeth. A change in the occlusion may reflect an adaptation to an existing disturbance in the masticatory system.

trauma, bruxism) may upset the delicate balance of an already marginally stable occlusion. An ideal occlusion has no structural, functional, or neurobehavioral characteristics that tend to interfere with occlusal stability. The response to bruxism may be increased tooth mobility and root resorption (Fig. 16–54) or decreased tooth mobility and increased density and thickness of the supporting tissues.

Guidance of Occlusion

Guidance of occlusion is discussed usually only in terms of tooth contact, anatomical or physical guidance, and more specifically in relation to cuspid and incisal guidance. Less specific is the term "anterior guidance," which may refer to tooth guidance for all or any of the anterior teeth, or to guidance involving the neuromuscular system. Yet another guidance relates to condylar guidance which, like the term "incisal guidance," may refer to so-called mechanical equivalents of guidance on an articulator. Again, like anterior guidance, the neuromuscular aspects of condylar guidance are not well understood. The paths of the condyles are not well represented in the mechanical equivalents of an articulator, especially in less than a "fully adjustable" articulator, and neuromuscular mechanisms are not represented at all.

It is of particular importance to the clinician to make certain that physical guidance of a restoration (or of the natural teeth in the treatment of dysfunction or malocclusion) is in harmony with the neuromuscular system and neurobehavioral attributes of the patient. Although some degree of compatibility may be assured on evaluation of occlusal relations and smooth gliding movements are present in various excursions, the acceptance and adaptability of the neuromuscular system may not be apparent until an unfavorable response occurs (Figs. 16–55 through 16–58).

In an ideal occlusion, there should be no need for adaptation but the criteria for it can only be guidelines, since their implementation may reflect clinical skill beyond the ordinary. Even minor occlusal discrepancies in a few individuals may result in acute TMJ muscle dysfunction. It is not uncommon to have some kind of response (structural function, and/or psychological) with the restoration of a maxillary central incisor if an interfer-

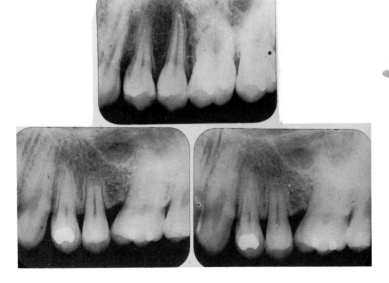

Figure 16–54. Root resorption associated with clenching habit. *Upper,* Prior to placement of restoration and clenching. *Left,* Root resorption began with placement of restoration and bruxing. Patient complained of pain in tooth. The pain subsided with the occlusal adjustment of the restoration, which was slightly "high" in centric occlusion. *Right,* Several months later, with no further evidence of resorption or pain.

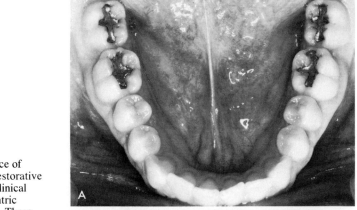

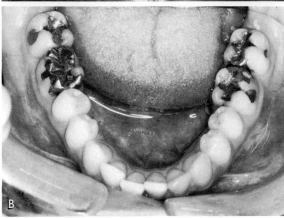

Figure 16–55. Anterior crowding. *A,* Absence of crowding. *B,* Anterior crowding following restorative treatment by only a few months. The only clinical findings were an occlusal interference in centric relation and very "tight" proximal contacts. These findings are only presumptive evidence of a cause-and-effect relationship between restorations and anterior crowding of the teeth.

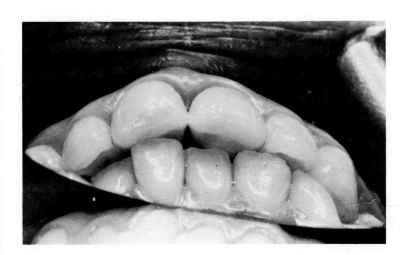

Figure 16–56. Alterations in the positions of anterior teeth following restorative treatment. Rotation reflects result of occlusal forces.

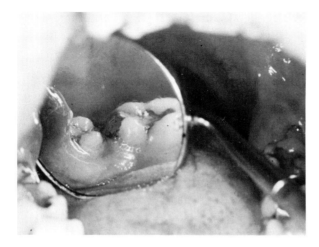

Figure 16–57. Erupting third molars may trigger clenching and grinding (bruxism). Although such parafunction may be a factor in altered occlusal relations, a direct cause-and-effect relationship between parafunction and anterior crowding, or between third molars and crowding, has not been demonstrated.

ence to complete closure in centric occlusion has been placed by mistake in the restoration. If the interferences cannot be avoided comfortably by mandibular displacement in chewing and swallowing by neuromuscular mechanisms (functional adaptation), if the tooth becomes mobile and is moved out of position (structural adaptation), and/or if the patient cannot ignore the discomfort or the "presence of change" even for a short period of time (behavioral adaptation), overt symptoms of dysfunction of the muscles, joints, periodontium or teeth (pulp) may occur. However, such adaptive response and failure of adaptation are observed only rarely and such observations do not qualify as scientific evidence. Models of research to test the validity of these clinical observations have suffered from serious flaws in design. Still, no clinician would knowingly put an occlusal interference in a restoration.

In addition to physical guidance from the teeth when the teeth are in contact during mastication or empty movements, mandibular guidance may occur prior to and during contact of the teeth from receptors in the periodontium, temporomandibular joints, and other peripheral sensory receptors as well as from higher centers in the central nervous system. It has been suggested that the anatomical relationships of the teeth and joints provide passive guidances and that active guidances involve reflexes originating in receptors in or around the teeth (Dubner et al., 1978). The question of feedback from various

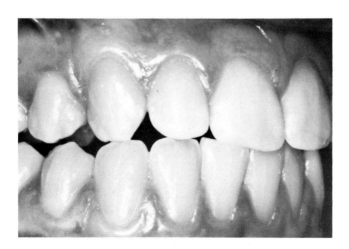

Figure 16–58. The presence of a sharply delineated pattern of wear, namely on the mandibular right central incisor, is sometimes interpreted as demonstrating the cause of a tooth being moved out of proper alignment (as this central incisor is). However, such a cause-and-effect relationship remains to be clarified.

structures influencing mandibular movements and position is a complex one and cannot at this time be clearly answered.

The tendency to equate clinical responses with reflexes elicited under laboratory conditions rather than studying responses under natural conditions has led to what may be considered contradictory findings. It is also not unusual to find it assumed that failure to observe a response (i.e., a change in chewing patterns with anesthesia, occlusal interferences, and so on) is due to the absence of a response rather than to a failure in the method of observation. Thus some responses may exist under natural conditions but have not been observed. Whether or not a changed anatomical feature of the occlusion causes an alteration of mandibular movement depends on a number of factors involving preprogramming, learning, adaptation or habituation, relationship to function and parafunction, and other central or peripheral influences.

In terms of strategy, an occlusal anatomical feature must interfere with something (function or parafunction) to cause a response (Fig. 16–59, *A,B*). Otherwise, it should not be called an occlusal interference. Thus a contact on the nonfunctional side (balancing side

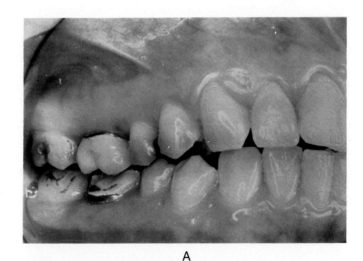

A

Figure 16–59. A, Centric occlusion relationship. *B*, Occlusal interference in right working. Note absence of canine contacts.

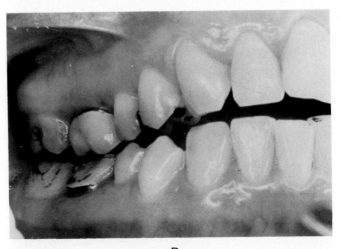

B

contact) is not an occlusal interference unless such a contact interferes with ongoing function and parafunction (i.e., prevents contact at some point on the working side). In doing an occlusal adjustment in centric relation, the clinician guides the jaw into a position of closure in a retruded contact position. In some individuals, premature occlusal contacts prevent a stable jaw relationship and during guided rapid cyclic closure by the clinician, reflex jaw movements and muscle hyperactivity may occur to prevent such closure. Training of the patient and proper manipulation of the mandible in the absence of TMJ or muscle dysfunction may eliminate the muscle hyperactivity just long enough to guide the jaw into centric relation and to mark the occlusal interference with articulating paper (Fig. 16–60). During the course of an occlusal adjustment to remove occlusal interferences to a stable occlusion in centric relation, a number of responses occur. For example, in some patients during the elimination of interferences, removal of a premature contact results in complete elimination of muscle resistance to guided jaw closure; that is, the clinician may close the jaw rapidly or slowly without any muscle response to prevent the closure. This may occur even with a slide in centric remaining, provided the contacts are bilateral and multiple and freedom to move smoothly from centric relation to centric occlusion is possible.

Another clinical observation is that before the elimination of a particular interference during the occlusal adjustment and before guiding the jaw into contact to determine whether that interference has been eliminated, all resistance and reflex muscle activity to prevent closure into the retruded contact position is gone. It should be kept in mind that during the course of an occlusal adjustment, a new but transient solitary occlusal interference may occur or an interference may have greater significance for one tooth than another. These observations agree with several studies showing that occlusal relations can lead to avoidance responses that probably serve to protect the teeth, muscles, joints, and periodontium from trauma owing to occlusion. Training the patient to a hinge axis movement in the presence of occlusal interferences requires that no contact be made or even close to contact of the occlusion be made for several up-and-down movements and that the patient relax. Relaxation involves modulation of feedback from peripheral structures (joints, teeth, muscles, periodontium) and inhibitory effects from higher centers.

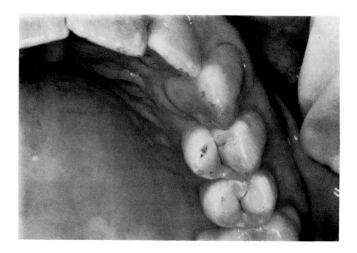

Figure 16–60. Premature contact in centric relation marked with articulating paper.

Vertical Dimension

Contact vertical dimension (occlusal vertical dimension) is the vertical component of centric occlusion. Although it would be helpful to be able to relate the contact relationship of the teeth to the rest position of the mandible (or the interocclusal space), optimal working length of the jaw elevator muscles, swallowing, speaking, or to some other neurobehavior parameter of function, vertical dimension is usually described in terms of the height of the lower third of the face, mandibular overclosure, or a need to "raise the bite" (increase the height of the teeth with restorations) because of worn down or intruded posterior teeth (Fig. 16–61, *A*), or "impinging overbite" (Fig. 16–61, *B*). At the present time, there is no acceptable "test" of "lost" vertical dimension. The neurobehavioral aspects of the inter-occlusal space and occlusal vertical dimension are complex and require much further study.

It is not possible to determine with scientific assurance that aggressive bruxing and clenching in centric occlusion have caused intrusion or wear of the teeth that has not been compensated for by eruption of the posterior teeth. Even short-term intrusion or loss of stops on posterior teeth may result in reflex produced responses from anterior teeth because of premature contacts on anterior teeth, especially where horizontal overlap is minimal and vertical overlap prevents anterior movement. As already indicated, rest position has an anterior as well as a vertical component. With fatigue of the jaw-closing muscles and hyperactivity of the jaw-opening muscles, the mandible tends to move forward in the rest position. Under these conditions, functional disturbances may occur. Again,

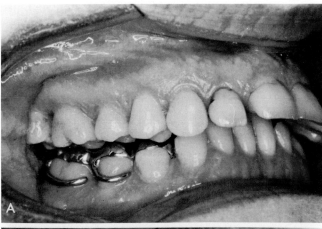
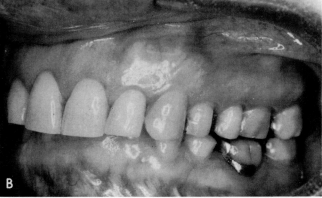

Figure 16–61 Loss of occlusal vertical dimension. *A*, Use of a posterior bilateral onlay splint in an attempt to "raise the bite" and eliminate temporomandibular joint (TMJ) and muscle dysfunction symptoms. *B*, An impinging overbite may require comprehensive orthodontics for correction.

there are no acceptable "tests" to determine with scientific assurance, even in the presence of dysfunction, that an apparent loss of contact vertical dimension and/or deep overbite requires correction. The clinical evaluation of vertical dimension may be found more appropriately in references dealing with the diagnosis and treatment of occlusion.

Oral Motor Behavior

The term "oral motor behavior" is a convenience of speech by which it is possible to refer with a brief phrase to observable actions involving orofacial structures, including "simple" actions like mandibular rest position and much more complex movements such as mastication. Human behavior reflects the translation of past, present, and ongoing ideas and learning (as well as sensations and emotions) into movements and actions. Although many of the responses or actions are common among all persons, the subjective response of a particular individual to a stimulus (including a change in the occlusion) may involve an inner experiential aspect of emotion in which the sensory experience may not fall into the usual acceptable range of pleasant or unpleasant. This aspect of sensation, referred to as "affect," is the basis of much suffering as well as pleasure, including that related to the occlusion and occlusal therapy. In mentalistic terms, feelings of pleasantness and unpleasantness are correlated with "motivation-intention to respond" and with emotion. Even a simple reflex may be considered as a unit of behavior. The advantage of viewing occlusion (in terms of function and parafunction) as human behavior is that the clinician has a better understanding of functional disturbances (i.e., TMJ and muscle disorders) and the recognition that how patients feel and respond to their occlusion is an important aspect of diagnosis and dental treatment.

Emotion is a motivational phenomenon that plays a significant role in the determination of behavior. Motivation or "drive" and "emotional states" may be the basis for oral motor behavior, which is a fundamental component of ingestive responses and for other behaviors essential for adaptation and survival. In effect, oral motor behavior can be initiated not only by situations involving cognitive processes but also by "emotive" processes including homeostatic drives (e.g., hunger) concerned with the internal environment and nonhomeostatic drives (e.g., fear) related to adaptation to the external environment. The external environment may begin at the interface between oral sensory receptors and external stimuli involved in oral function and parafunction. However, ideas suggesting a "hard" interface between the internal and external environment are rapidly being re-evaluated in terms of functional criteria. It is no longer possible to restrict thinking to the external environment as being "out there." From a psychophysiological standpoint, an interface between the external and internal worlds may not exist.

As already indicated, oral motor behavior involves the translation of thought, sensation, and emotion into actions. Implied is the idea that actions or behavior may change because of learning and that there is some drive or motivation to alter existing responses to environmental variables. And although the neural substrate for the translation of "innate drives" appears to exist and such regulatory behavior as eating has clear value to the immediate survival of an individual, other oral motor behavior may not have clear antecedents in individual or species survival. However, during the development of the nervous system and motor functions, oral motor behavior may be highly dependent on homeostatic drives concerned with ingestive processes. Later oral motor behavior is an expression of the plasticity of the organism over a long period of time and consists of a whole complex of emotive as well as cognitive determinants that cannot be related easily to a hypothetical construct of homeostatic needs in the adult organism even in a teleological sense.

Although oral motor behavior is judged on the basis of observable actions, the strategy and tactics of the occlusal aspects of human behavior are based on past dental experiences and the present state of the joints, muscles, periodontium contact relation of the teeth, and central nervous system. The neural mechanisms that underly the initiation, programming and execution of motor behavior can be described only briefly here.

Complex behavior may involve neuronal circuits called *pattern generators,* which when activated elicit stereotyped, rhythmic, and/or coordinated movements. The pattern generators for locomotion appear to be in the spinal cord and to be activated by discrete nuclei or regions in the brain stem, and they can be accessed by higher level structures in the central nervous system. The pattern generators for chewing and swallowing are located in the brainstem medullary-pontine reticular formation. As already mentioned, limbic structures appear to have access to pattern generators.

Chewing is a type of oral motor behavior that demonstrates centrally programmed movement and in part peripherally driven movement. Controlled interaction is more often the case than either pure centrally programmed movement or pure peripheral control. Pattern generators may be part of the particular programs accessed by higher brain centers to generate complex behavior.

Swallowing involves the coordination of nearly 20 different muscles with motor neurons distributed from mesencephalic to posterior medullary levels. The patterning of muscular contractions is independent of the stimulus necessary to evoke swallowing. The neurons responsible for coordination form a ''swallowing center'' in which neuronal groups fire automatically in a particular sequence when stimulated to achieve the necessary pattern of muscle activity to produce swallowing. ''Triggering,'' or initiation of a central program, involves neurons in the motor cortex that act as command elements and control patterns of neuronal activity and also receive feedback from the systems controlled. Thus movement may be centrally programmed (''driven'') and also at the same time modulated by peripheral influences.

The cyclic movements of the jaw in mastication reflect past experiences, adaptive behavior, neuronal activity of the mesencephalic rhythm generator and the trigeminal motor nucleus, and the influence of oral reflexes, either conditioned or unconditioned. The pattern generator may be influenced by sensory input from the orofacial area as well as from influences from higher centers in the central nervous system.

Summary

In order to understand occlusion in its broadest sense, it is necessary to consider, in addition to TMJ articulation, muscles, and teeth, some of the neurobehavioral mechanisms that give meaning to the presence and function of the masticatory system. Although many of the neural interactive mechanisms between occlusion and thoughts, sensations, and emotions are complex and often indeterminate, it is possible to suggest strategies that could account for the variety of responses (physiologic and psychological) that occur in function and parafunction.

The ''obvious'' strategy to compensate for wear of proximal contact areas is mesial migration of the teeth, and the strategy to compensate for wear of the occlusal surfaces is eruption of the teeth. The strategy for regulating the contraction of the jaw elevators to achieve a normal resting position of the mandible with a small interocclusal space is a postural reflex (stretch reflex). The overall strategy for motivation to have access to the muscles of mastication might be to provide ''drive'' for ingestive processes, especially during the early stages of development of the masticatory system and maturation of the nervous system—swallowing in fetal life, suckling in the newborn, and chewing in the young infant.

It appears plausible at least that emotion may be important not only as a motivational phenomenon but also as a reflection of what is agreeable or disagreeable about something that is placed in the mouth, including items not considered to be food and perhaps even restorations that interfere with function or parafunction. Demonstrating evidence for and against strategies to explain completely neurobehavioral mechanisms of "occlusion" requires much more space than provided here.

The extensive "education" of people through the television media, newspapers, and magazines and through professional dental care and instructions to patients not only has produced an awareness of the teeth and mouth but also has coupled these structures to a sense of health and comfort. The "affect" involved in such a sense of "well-being" about oral health involves part of the same neurobehavioral substrate underlying innate "drives," motivation, and "emotional states" necessary for biological adaptation and survival of the species. Ingestive processes, which include oral motor responses involved in mastication, are essential for survival. Functional disturbances of the masticatory system may involve psychophysiological mechanisms that are related to the teeth and their functions. Therefore, occlusal interferences to function or parafunction may then involve more than simply contact relations of the teeth; they may involve psychophysiological mechanisms of human behavior as well. There is no scientific evidence for making a specific structure or psychophysiological mechanism the sole cause of TMJ muscle dysfunction. But any attempt to negate the role of the teeth in human behavior, including dysfunction, perhaps is done by those who have not had the opportunity to observe the effect on "affect," favorable neuromuscular response, and elimination of discomfort when appropriate occlusal therapy is rendered.

Unfortunately, neuroscientific evidence to separate the subjective from objective clinical observations has not lived up to its full potential. "Scientific" clinical studies are difficult to design where true "cause and effect" relationships can be determined, especially where such relationships may be indirect, "on-and-off again," and significantly influenced by the observer and other factors under "natural conditions." Considerably more appropriate research is needed to establish the role of occlusion, as well as other factors, in TMJ muscle dysfunction.

References

Ackerman, R. J. (1976). Tooth migration during the transitional dentition. Dent. Clin. North Amer. 20:661.

Anderson, D. J., and Matthews, B. (eds.) (1976). *Mastication*. Bristol, England: John Wright and Sons.

Andrews, L. F. (1976). The diagnostic system: Occlusal analysis. Dent Clin N. Am. 20:671.

Angle, E. H. (1887). *The Angle System of Regulation and Retention of the Teeth*, 1st ed. Philadelphia: S. S. White Manufacturing.

Arnold, N. R., and Frumker, S. C. (1976). *Occlusal Treatment*. Philadelphia: Lea & Febiger.

Ash, M. M., and Ramfjord, S. P. (1982). *Introduction to Functional Occlusion*. Philadelphia: Saunders.

Bates, J. F., Stafford, G. D., and Harrison, A. (1975). Masticatory function—A review of the literature. 1. The form of the masticatory cycle. J. Oral Rehabil. 2:281.

Baume, L. R. (1950). Physiologic tooth migration and its significance for the development of occlusion. J. Dent. Res. 29:123.

Beyron, H. L. (1954). Characteristics of functionally optimal occlusion and principles of occlusal rehabilitation. J. Am. Dent. Assoc. 48:648.

Beyron, H. L. (1964). Occlusal relations and mastication in Australian aborigines. Acta. Odont. Scand. 22:597.

Beyron, H. L. (1969). Optimal occlusion. Dent. Clin. North Amer. 13:537.

Bonwill, W. G. A. (1899). Scientific articulation of human teeth as founded on geometrical mathematical laws. Dent. Items Interest 21:817.

Brodie, A. G. (1939). Temporomandibular joint. Illinois Dent. J. 8:2.

Burch, J. G. (1972). Patterns of change in human mandibular arch width during jaw excursions. Arch Oral Biol. 17:623.

Butler, P. M. (1974). A zoologist looks at occlusion. Br. J. Orthodont. 1:205.

Celenza, F. B. (1973). The centric position: Replacement and character. J. Prosthet. Dent. 30:591.

Currier, J. H. (1969). A computerized geometric analysis of human dental arch form. Am. J. Orthodont. 56:164.

D'Amico, A. (1958). The canine teeth—Normal functional relation of the natural teeth in man. J. South. Calif. Dent. Assoc. 1:6–23; 2:49–60; 4:127–142; 5:175–182; 6:194–208; 7:239–241.

Dawson, P. (1974). *Evaluation, Diagnosis and Treatment of Occlusal Problems*. St. Louis, Mo.: Mosby.

Dempster, W. T., Adams, W. J., and Duddles, R. A. (1963). Arrangement in the jaws of the roots of the teeth. J. Am. Dent. Assoc. 67:779.

Dewel, B. F. (1949). Clinical observations on the axial inclination of teeth. Am. J. Orthod. 35:98.

Dolwick, M. F., and Sanders, B. (1985). *TMJ Internal Derangement and Arthrosis*. St. Louis, Mo.: C. V. Mosby.

Dubner, R., et al. (1978). *The Neural Basis of Oral and Facial Function*. New York: Plenum Press.

Falkner, F. (1957). Deciduous tooth eruption. Arch. Dis. Child. 32:386.

Finn, S. B. (1973). *Clinical Pedodontics,* 4th ed. Philadelphia: Saunders.

Friel, S. (1927). Occlusion—Observations on its development from infancy to old age. Int. J. Orthod. Surg. 13:322.

Friel, S. (1954). The development of ideal occlusion of the gum pads and teeth. Am. J. Orthodont. 40:196.

Gibbs, C. H., et al. (1971). Functional movements of the mandible. J. Prosthet. Dent. 26:604.

Graf, H. (1975). Occlusal forces during function. In Rowe, N. H. (ed.), *Occlusal Research in Form and Function*. Ann Arbor: University of Michigan Press.

Gysi, A. (1910). The problem of articulation. Dent. Cosmos 52:1.

Hannam, A. G., et al. (1977). The relationship between dental occlusion, muscle activity, and associated jaw movement in man. Arch. Oral Biol. 22:25.

Hatton, M. (1955). Measure of the effects of heredity and environment in eruption of the deciduous teeth. J. Dent. Res. 34:397.

Hellman, M. (1941). Factors influencing occlusion. In Gregory, W. K., Broadbent, B. H., and Hellman, M. (eds.). *Development of Occlusion*. Philadelphia: University of Pennsylvania Press.

Hemley, S. (1944). *Fundamentals of Occlusion*. Philadelphia: Saunders.

Higley, L. B. (1940). Some controversies over the temporomandibular joint. J. Am. Dent. Assoc. 27:594.

Klatsky, M. (1940). A cinefluorographic study of the human masticatory apparatus in function. Am. J. Orthod. 26:664.

Knott, J., and Meredith, H. V. (1966). Statistics on the eruption of the permanent dentition from serial data from North American white children. Angle Orthod. 36:68.

Kornfeld, M. (1967). *Mouth Rehabilitation,* Vols. 1 and 2. St. Louis, Mo.: Mosby.

Kraus, J. A. (1969). *Dental Anatomy and Occlusion*. Baltimore, Md.: Williams & Wilkins.

Kurth, L. E. (1942). Mandibular movements in mastication. J. Am. Dent. Assoc. 29:1769.

Lo, R. T., and Moyers, R. E. (1953). Studies in the etiology and prevention of malocclusion. 1. The sequences of eruption of the permanent dentition. Am. J. Orthod. 39:460.

Logan, W. H. G., and Kronfeld, R. (1933). Development of the human jaws and surrounding structures from birth to age of fifteen years. J. Am. Dent. Assoc. 20:379.

Lord, F. P. (1937). Movements of the jaw and how they are effected. Int. J. Orthod. 23:557.

Lucia, V. O. (1962). The gnathological concept of articulation. Dent. Clin. North Amer. 6:183.

MacLean, P. D. (1952). Some psychiatric implications of physiological studies of frontotemporal portions of the limbic system (visceral brain). Electroencephalogr. Clin. Neurophysiol. 4:407.

MacMillan, H. W. (1934). Foundations of mandibular movement. J. Am. Dent. Assoc. 231:429.

Mann. A. W., and Pankey, L. D. (1960). Oral rehabilitation. J. Prosthet. Dent. 10:135.

Matthews, B. (1975). Mastication. In Lavelle, C. L. B. (ed.), *Applied Physiology of the Mouth*. Bristol, England: John Wright and Sons.

Meredith, H. V. (1946). Order and age of eruption for the deciduous dentition. J. Dent. Res. 25:43.

Mills, J. R. E. (1976). Attrition in animals. In Poole, D. F. G., and Stack, M. V. (eds.), *The Eruption and Occlusion of Teeth*. Colston Symposium No. 27. London: Butterworths.

Mogenson, G. J., et al. (1980). From motivation to action: Functional interface between the limbic system and the motor system. Progr. Neurobiol. 14:69.

Monson, G. S. (1920). Occlusion as applied to crown and bridgework. J. Nat. Dent. Assoc. 7:399.

Moorrees, C. (1959). The dentition of the growing child: A longitudinal study of dental development between 3 and 18 years of age. Cambridge, Mass.: Harvard University Press.

Moorrees, C., and Chadha, J. M. (1965). Available space for the incisors during dental development—A growth study based on physiologic age. Angle Orthod. 35:12.

Moss, J. P., and Picton, D. C. A. (1970). Mesial drift in teeth in adult monkeys (Macaca irus) when forces from the cheeks and tongue have been eliminated. Arch. Oral Biol. 15:979.

Moss, J. P., and Picton, D. C. (1974). The effect on approximal drift of cheek teeth of dividing mandibular molars of adult monkeys (Macaca irus). Arch. Oral Biol. 19:1211.

O'Leary, T. J. (1969). Tooth mobility. Dent. Clin. North Amer. 13:567.

Picton, D. C. A., and Moss, J. P. (1980). The effect of approximal drift of altering the horizontal component of biting force in adult monkeys (Macaca irus). Arch. Oral Biol. 25:45.

Poole, D. F. G. (1976). Evolution of mastication. In Anderson, D. J., and Matthews, B. (eds.), *Mastication*. Bristol, England: John Wright and Sons.

Prentiss, H. L. (1923). Regional anatomy emphasizing mandibular movements with specific reference to full denture construction. J. Am. Dent. Assoc. 15:1085.

Ramfjord, S. P., and Ash, M. M. (1983). *Occlusion,* 3rd ed. Philadelphia: Saunders.

Rees, L. A. (1954). The structure and function of the mandibular joint J. Brit. Dent. A., 96:125.

Richardson, A. S., and Castaldi, C. R. (1967). Dental development during the first two years of life. J. Canad. Dent. Assoc. 33:418.

Robinson, M. (1946). The temporomandibular joint: Theory of reflex controlled nonlever action of the mandible. J. Am. Dent. Assoc. 33:1260.

Savalle, W. P. M. (1988). Some aspects of the morphology of the human temporomandibular joint capsule. Acta Anatomica 131:292.

Sessle, B. J., and Hannam, A. G. (eds.) (1976). *Mastication and Swallowing: Biology and Clinical Correlates.* Toronto: University of Toronto Press.

Stallard, H., and Stuart, C. (1963). Concepts of occlusion. Dent. Clin. North Amer. (November).

Taylor, A. (1981). Proprioception in the strategy of jaw movement control. In Kawamura, Y., and Dubner, R. (eds.), *Oral-Facial Sensory and Motor Functions.* Tokyo: Quintessence.

Van Beek, H., and Fidler, V. J. (1977). An experimental study of the effect of functional occlusion on mesial tooth migration in macaque monkeys. Arch. Oral Biol. 22:269.

Yamada, Y., and Ash, M. M. (1982). An electromyographic study of jaw opening and closing reflexes in man. Arch. Oral Biol. 27:13.

Yilmaz, R. S., et al. (1980). Mesial drift of human teeth assessed from ankylosed deciduous molars. Arch. Oral Biol. 25:127.

Index

Note: Page numbers in *italics* refer to illustrations.
Page numbers followed by (t) refer to tables.

ISBN 0-7216-4374-4

90038